HYPERTENSION

SECOND EDITION

HYPERTENSION

SECRETS

EDGAR V. LERMA, MD
Clinical Professor of Medicine
Section of Nephrology
University of Illinois at
Chicago College of Medicine
Associates in Nephrology, SC
Chicago, IL

JAMES M. LUTHER, MD
Associate Professor of Medicine
Clinical Pharmacology
Vanderbilt University Medical Center
Nashville, TN

SWAPNIL HIREMATH, MD
Associate Professor of Medicine
University of Ottawa;
Associate Scientist
Clinical Epidemiology
Ottawa Hospital Research Institute
Ottawa, ON
Canada

ELSEVIER

Elsevier
1600 John F. Kennedy Blvd.
Ste 1800
Philadelphia, PA 19103-2899

Hypertension Secrets, Second Edition ISBN: 978-0-323-75852-9

ISBN: 978-0-323-75852-9

Content Strategist: Marybeth Thiel
Content Development Manager: Meghan Andress
Content Development Specialist: Nicole Congleton
Publishing Services Manager: Shereen Jameel
Project Manager: Nadhiya Sekar
Design Direction: Bridget Hoette

Printed in India

Last digit is the print number: 9 8 7 6 5 4 3 2

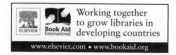

To all my mentors, colleagues, and friends, at the University of Santo Tomas Faculty of Medicine and Surgery in Manila, Philippines, Mercy Hospital and Medical Center and Northwestern University Feinberg School of Medicine in Chicago, IL, who have in one way or another, influenced and guided me to become the physician that I am.

To all the medical students, interns, and residents at Advocate Christ Medical Center whom I have taught or learned from, especially those who eventually decided to pursue nephrology as a career.

To my parents and my brothers, without whose unwavering love and support through the good and bad times, I would not have persevered and reached my goals in life.

Most especially, to my two lovely and precious daughters, Anastasia Zofia and Isabella Ann, whose smiles and laughter constantly provide me unparalleled joy and happiness, and my very loving and understanding wife Michelle, who has always been supportive of my endeavors both personally and professionally, and who sacrificed a lot of time and exhibited unwavering patience as I devoted a significant amount of time and effort to this project. Truly, they provide me with constant motivation and inspiration.

Edgar V. Lerma, MD

To my family, the primary source of joy in life. To my teachers, colleagues and mentors who instilled the appreciation and love of hypertension physiology. And especially to the late Dr. John Oates, who established an academic culture of inquisitiveness in both the research and clinical settings and has trained multiple generations of physicians.

James M. Luther, MD

To my mentors, colleagues, and teachers, in particular Marcel Ruzicka, Peter Magner, George Fodor, and Alan Almeida.

To my long-suffering wife and children who have let me pursue the 5 to 9 passion of FOAMed.

Swapnil Hiremath, MD

CONTRIBUTORS

Blaise W. Abramovitz, DO
Division of Renal-Electrolyte, Department of Medicine, University of Pittsburgh School of Medicine, Pittsburgh, PA

Rajiv Agarwal, MD, MS
Division of Nephrology, Department of Medicine, Indiana University School of Medicine and Richard L. Roudebush Veterans Administration Medical Center, Indianapolis, IN

Sarah Ahmad, MD
Renal-Electrolyte and Hypertension Division, Department of Medicine, Perelman School of Medicine, University of Pennsylvania, Philadelphia, PA

Matthew R. Alexander, MD, PhD
Department of Medicine, Division of Cardiovascular Medicine, Vanderbilt University Medical Center, Nashville, TN

Ibrahim A. AlQassas, MD
Internal Medicne Specialist (Senior Registrar), International Medical Center, Jeddah, Saudi Arabia

Juan P. Arroyo, MD PhD
Nephrology Fellow, Medicine, Vanderbilt University Medical Center, Nashville, TN

Christopher Asuzu, MD
Division of Nephrology, Department of Medicine, Duke University School of Medicine, Durham, NC

Ali Ayesh, MD
Nephrology
Wayne State University
Farmington, MI

George Bakris, MD, MA
Professor and Director, AHA Comprehensive Hypertension Center, Medicine, The University of Chicago Medicine, Chicago, IL

Atul Bali, MD, CHS, FASN, FNKF
Divisions of Nephrology, Department of Medicine, University of Virginia Health System, Charlottesville, VA

Joshua A. Beckman, MD
Director, Section of Vascular Medicine, Cardiovascular Division, Vanderbilt University Medical Center, Nashville, TN

Fabian Bock, MD, PhD
Division of Nephrology and Hypertension, Vanderbilt University Medical Center, Nashville, TN

Ann Bugeja, MD
University of Ottawa, Ottawa, Ontario, Canada; The Ottawa Hospital, Ottawa, Ontario, Canada

Anna Burgner, MD, MEHP
Assistant Professor, Internal Medicine, Vanderbilt University Medical Center, Nashville, TN; Assistant Professor, Division of Nephrology and Hypertension, Vanderbilt University Medical Center, Nashville, TN

Robert M. Carey, MD, MACP
Divisions of Endocrinology and Metabolism, Department of Medicine, University of Virginia Health System, Charlottesville, VA

Jordana B. Cohen, MD, MSCE
Renal-Electrolyte and Hypertension Division, Department of Medicine, Perelman School of Medicine, University of Pennsylvania, Philadelphia, PA; Department of Biostatistics, Epidemiology and Informatics, Perelman School of Medicine, University of Pennsylvania, Philadelphia, PA

Beatrice P. Concepcion, MD
Division of Nephrology and Hypertension, Vanderbilt University Medical Center, Nashville, TN

Christine Dillingham, MD
Eastern Nephrology Associates, North Myrtle Beach, SC

Luciano F. Drager, MD, PhD
Heart Institute (InCor), Hypertension Unit, University of Sao Paulo Medical School, Brazil; Hypertension Unit, Renal Division, University of Sao Paulo Medical School, Brazil

George K. Dresser, MD, PhD, FRCPC, FACP
Associate Professor of Medicine, Schulich School of Medicine and Dentistry, University of Western Ontario, London, Ontario, Canada

Garabed Eknoyan, MD
Selzman Institute of Kidney Health, Section of Nephrology, Department of Medicine, Baylor College of Medicine, Houston, TX

David Ellison, MD
Professor, Internal Medicine, Oregon Health & Science University, Portland, OR; Staff Physician, VA Portland Health Care System, Portland, OR

Uta Erdbrugger, MD
Divisions of Nephrology, Department of Medicine, University of Virginia Health System, Charlottesville, VA

Maureen C. Farrell, MS
Drexel University College of Medicine, Philadelphia, PA

Ryan P. Flood, DO
Division of Nephrology, Department of Medicine, University of Colorado Anschutz Medical Campus, Aurora, CO

Joseph T. Flynn, MD, MS
Professor of Pediatrics, University of Washington School
of Medicine; Division of Nephrology, Seattle Children's
Hospital, Seattle, WA

Panagiotis I. Georgianos, MD, PhD
Section of Nephrology and Hypertension, 1st Department
of Medicine, AHEPA Hospital, Aristotle University of
Thessaloniki, Thessaloniki, Greece

Sarah Gilligan, MD MPH
Division of Nephrology and Hypertension,
University of Utah Health, Salt Lake City, UT

Christin Giordano McAuliffe, MD
Fellow, Medicine, Vanderbilt University Medical Center,
Nasvhille, TN

Swapnil Hiremath, MD
Associate Professor of Medicine
University of Ottawa;
Associate Scientist
Clinical Epidemiology
Ottawa Hospital Research Institute
Ottawa, ON
Canada

Tara A. Holder, MD
Cardiovascular Fellow, Cardiovascular Medicine,
Vanderbilt University Medical Center, Nashville, TN

Jiun-Ruey Hu, MD, MPH
Resident Physician, Department of Medicine, Vanderbilt
University Medical Center, Nashville, TN

Irma Husain, MD
Division of Nephrology, Department of Medicine,
Duke University School of Medicine, Durham, NC

Nashat Imran, MD, FASN, FACP
Associate Professor of Medicine, Division of Nephrology
and Hypertension, Wayne State University School of
Medicine, Detroit, MI

Eric Judd, MD, MS
Associate Professor of Medicine, University of Alabama at
Birmingham, Division of Nephrology, Birmingham, AL

Talar B. Kharadjian, MD
Fellow, Nephrology-Hypertension, University of California,
San Diego, San Diego, CA

Esther S. Kim, MD, MPH
Department of Medicine, Division of Cardiovascular Medicine,
Vanderbilt University Medical Center, Nashville, TN

Cassandra Kovach, MD
Nephrology and Hypertension, Cleveland Clinic,
Cleveland, OH

Arun Kumar, MD
Attending Physician, Nephrology, Emory North Decatur
Hospital, Decatur, GA

Edgar V. Lerma, MD
Clinical Professor of Medicine
Section of Nephrology
University of Illinois at Chicago College of
Medicine
Associates in Nephrology, SC
Chicago, IL

Julia B. Lewis, MD
Division of Nephrology and Hypertension,
Vanderbilt University Medical Center, Nashville, TN

Renata Libiano, MBBS, BMedSci, FRACP
Fellow, Endocrinology, Monash Health, Melbourne,
Australia

Matthew Lloyd, BSc, PhD
Department of Cardiac Sciences, Libin Cardiovascular
Institute of Alberta, University of Calgary, Calgary,
Alberta, Canada

James M. Luther, MD
Associate Professor of Medicine
Clinical Pharmacology
Vanderbilt University Medical Center
Nashville, TN

Rakesh Malhotra, MD, MPH
Division of Nephrology- Hypertension, University of California,
San Diego, San Diego, CA

Hina N. Mehta, MD
Division of Hospital Medicine, Department of Internal
Medicine, UT Southwestern Medical Center,
Dallas, TX

John R. Montford, MD
Division of Nephrology, Department of Medicine,
University of Colorado Anschutz Medical Campus,
Aurora, CO; Division of Nephrology, Eastern Colorado VA
Healthcare System, Rocky Mountain Regional VA Medical
Center, Aurora, CO

Jonathan D. Mosley, MD
Assistant Professor, Internal Medicine,
Vanderbilt University Medical Center, Nashville, TN;
Assistant Professor, Biomedical Informatics,
Vanderbilt University Medical Center, Nashville, TN

Bilal Munir, MD
Department of Internal Medicine, London Health Sciences
Centre, London, ON, Canada

Raj Padwal, MD, MSc
Department of Medicine, University of Alberta, Edmonton,
Alberta, Canada; Women and Children's Health Research
Institute (WICHRI), Edmonton, Alberta, Canada

Trisha Patel, DO
Resident Physician, Department of Internal Medicine,
Advocate Christ Medical Center, Oak Lawn, IL

Aldo J. Peixoto, MD
Department of Internal Medicine and Section of
Nephrology, Yale School of Medicine. New Haven, CT;
Hypertension Program at the Yale New Haven Hospital
Heart and Vascular Center. New Haven, CT

Nishigandha Pradhan, MD
Division of Nephrology and Hypertension,
University Hospitals Cleveland Medical Center,
Case Western Reserve University, Cleveland, OH

J. Howard Pratt, MD
Division of Endocrinology, Department of Medicine,
Indiana University School of Medicine, Indianapolis, IN

Akshan Puar, MD
Division of Endocrinology, Department of Medicine,
Indiana University School of Medicine, Indianapolis, IN

Simon W. Rabkin, MD, BSc(Med)
Division of Cardiology, Department of Medicine,
University of British Columbia, Vancouver, British Columbia,
Canada

Mahboob Rahman, MD
Division of Nephrology and Hypertension,
University Hospitals Cleveland Medical Center,
Case Western Reserve University, Cleveland OH;
Louis Stokes Cleveland VA Medical Center, Cleveland OH

Satish R. Raj, MD, MSCI, FHRS, FRCPC
Department of Cardiac Sciences, Libin Cardiovascular
Institute of Alberta, University of Calgary, Calgary,
Alberta, Canada; Autonomic Dysfunction Center, Division
of Clinical Pharmacology, Department of Medicine,
Vanderbilt University Medical Center, Nashville, TN

Nirupama Ramkumar, MD MPH
Division of Nephrology and Hypertension,
University of Utah Health, Salt Lake City, UT

Fitra Rianto, MD
Division of Nephrology, Department of Medicine,
Duke University School of Medicine, Durham, NC

Jennifer Ringrose, BSc, MSc, MD
Department of Medicine, University of Alberta, Edmonton,
Alberta, Canada; Women and Children's Health Research
Institute (WICHRI), Edmonton, Alberta, Canada

Marcel Ruzicka, MD, PhD, FRCPC
Associate Professor, Division of Nephrology, University of
Ottawa, Ottawa, Ontario, Canada; Medical Director,
Renal Hypertension Program, TOH-Riverside Campus,
Ottawa, Ontario, Canada

Carlos A. Schiavon, MD
Bariatric Surgery Center - BP Hospital – Sao Paulo, Brazil;
Research Institute - Heart Hospital (HCor) - Sao Paulo,
Brazil

Michel Shamy, MD, MA, FRCPC
Department of Medicine, University of Ottawa and The
Ottawa Hospital & Research Institute

Saed Shawar, MD
Division of Nephrology and Hypertension,
Vanderbilt University Medical Center, Nashville, TN

Cyndya A. Shibao, MD, MSCI
Department of Medicine, Division of Clinical Pharmacology,
Vanderbilt Autonomic Dysfunction Center,
Vanderbilt University Medical Center, Nashville, TN

Matthew A. Sparks, MD
Division of Nephrology, Department of Medicine,
Duke University School of Medicine, Durham, NC;
Renal Section, Durham VA Medical Center, Durham, NC

Hillel Sternlicht, MD
Assistant Professor of Medicine
Internal Medicine, Division of Nephrology & Hypertension
Wayne State University School of Medicine
Detroit, MI

Craig Sussman, MD
Associate Professor of Clinical Medicine, Vanderbilt
University Medical Center, Nashville, TN

Andrew Terker, MD PhD
Fellow, Nephrology, Vanderbilt University Medical Center,
Nashville, TN

Yuta Tezuka, MD, PhD
Division of Metabolism, Endocrinology and Diabetes,
University of Michigan, Ann Arbor, MI

Karen C. Tran, MD, MHSc, FRCPC
Division of General Internal Medicine,
Department of Medicine, University of British Columbia,
Vancouver, British Columbia, Canada

Adina F. Turcu, MD, MS
Division of Metabolism, Endocrinology and Diabetes,
University of Michigan, Ann Arbor, MI

Anand Vaidya, MD MMSc
Director, Center for Adrenal Disorders, Brigham and
Women's Hospital, Boston, MA;
Associate Professor of Medicine, Harvard Medical School,
Boston, MA

Jun Yang, MBBS (Hon), PhD, FRACP
Endocrine Hypertension Service, Hudson Institute of
Medical Research, Clayton, Victoria, Australia

PREFACE

In medicine, the time-honored Socratic method has been the predominant influence in the teaching styles used by various institutions of higher learning, both locally and internationally. In keeping with this very effective teaching method, the first edition of Anthony Zollo's *Medical Secrets* was published in 1991. The subtitle was "Questions you will be asked on rounds, in the clinic, and on oral exams." The book was very successful, as it appealed not only to the learners but also to the teachers. Subsequently, various fields of medicine came out with their own editions, with particular focus on individual specialties.

In 2020 we gathered a select group of highly motivated individuals who were well-renowned authoritative figures in the field of hypertension and who had exemplary reputations with regard to the profession of teaching medicine. In keeping with the design of the original Medical Secrets, we have included questions on everyday topics in addition to some "zebras" with particular academic interest.

We hope that this book will be used not only by nephrologists and nephrology fellows, medical residents and interns, and medical students, but also by primary care providers with particular interest in this very exciting field of medicine.

From personal experience, we know that very few people read a textbook from cover to cover. For a variety of reasons, the majority would read only one or a few chapters at any given time. Therefore, we tried to ensure that each chapter would be complete in itself. As a consequence, there is unavoidable overlap among some of the information provided in some chapters; we, however, feel that this was truly necessary, at least from an information-retrieving standpoint, and in this way it will not be necessary for readers to read bits of information between one or more chapters just to get complete information regarding a particular subject.

Certainly this book would not have been possible were it not for so many people. First, we would like to thank the contributing authors, who have spent countless hours in producing high-quality, up-to-the-last-minute information that we would characterize as "edutaining." We spent a significant amount of time communicating via telephone and e-mail as we reviewed the chapters and discussed recommendations, most of which were agreed upon, but, on occasion, disputed. We express our sincere gratitude for their openness to this very collegial collaboration, which has been a truly rewarding learning experience for us.

In particular, we appreciate the help and support of all the staff of Elsevier, most especially Sara Watkins and Nicole Congleton, our Developmental Editors, and Marybeth Thiel, our Production Editor, all of whom have been very patient with our procrastinations and stubbornness at times.

We thank our teachers and mentors, who devoted their own time to educate and train us to become who we are. We thank all the medical students, residents, and fellows who in one way or another have given us inspiration to persevere in the teaching profession. Mostly, we thank all of our patients, who have been truly instrumental in our learning and devotion to medicine. On behalf of all the contributors to this book, we fervently hope that all our efforts will contribute to relieving your suffering and perhaps lead to your recovery.

Edgar V. Lerma, MD
James M. Luther, MD
Swapnil Hiremath, MD

CONTENTS

4   HYPERTENSION IN SPECIFIC POPULATIONS

5   THERAPEUTIC PRINCIPLES

6 MISCELLENIA

TOP 100 SECRETS

1. Use of automated blood pressure (BP) measurement, particularly automated office BP (AOBP), minimizes many common observer-related sources of error in office BP measurement.
2. Office BP measurement should be supplemented with out-of-office measurements to better inform diagnostic and treatment decisions.
3. Out-of-office BP monitoring with ambulatory or home BP monitors (ABPM or HBPM) should be used for the diagnosis and monitoring of hypertension due to the ability to identify abnormal BP patterns that cannot be identified using clinic BP monitoring alone.
4. It is critical to use a validated device to perform home BP monitoring.
5. Pseudohypertension is thought to occur in elderly individuals who have stiff or rigid arteries; it should be suspected in elderly patients who present with relatively elevated BP readings in the absence of target organ damage.
6. A hypertensive urgency might not differ from asymptomatic hypertension and it is important to try to rule out the 'acute recognition' of chronic hypertension.
7. Common etiologies of a hypertensive emergency include: acute aortic dissection, acute coronary syndrome, acute kidney injury, acute left ventricular failure, catecholamine-associated hypertension, hemorrhagic stroke or acute ischemic stroke, hypertensive encephalopathy, preeclampsia/eclampsia.
8. With each decade of life, hypertension (HTN) becomes more common. By 75 years of age, more than 70% of Americans meet criteria for HTN based on the ACC/AHA definitions.
9. Fewer than 50% of people living with HTN are aware of their underlying condition and only 15% have achieved optimal BP control.
10. Minorities including African Americans and Mexican Americans are at higher risk of developing HTN, uncontrolled BP, and its associated complications.
11. Short-term regulation of blood pressure is mediated by the central nervous system through the baroreceptor reflex arc and chemoreceptors.
12. Long term blood pressure control is mediated by the kidney and hormonal systems.
13. Chronically and acutely elevated blood pressures can cause target organ damage to the heart, blood vessels, brain, kidneys, and eyes.
14. Stringent and consistent blood pressure control is the most effective way to reduce the risk of developing primary and secondary target organ damage.
15. Only a minority of patients with primary aldosteronism (30%) present with hypokalemia; routine screening identifies even more patients with normokalemia.
16. Most patients with primary aldosteronism (PA) are indistinguishable from patients with other forms of hypertension.
17. The aldosterone-to-renin ratio (ARR) remains as the recommended screening test for primary aldosteronism on the basis that isolated measurements of either plasma aldosterone concentration (PAC), direct renin concentration (DRC), or plasma renin activity (PRA) show overlap with unaffected patients.
18. Cortisol circulates in higher concentrations than aldosterone; whereas cortisol and aldosterone have similar affinity for the mineralocorticoid receptors, the enzyme 11β-hydroxysteroid dehydrogenase type 2 (HSD11B2) serves as a gatekeeper, by inactivating cortisol to cortisone.
19. Whereas exogenous or iatrogenic Cushing syndrome (CS) is relatively common, endogenous CS is a rare disease, with an incidence of 1 to 2 per million per year. Endogenous CS is most commonly caused by an ACTH-producing pituitary adenoma, and this form of CS is also known as Cushing disease.
20. Testing for CS should take into account the possibility of circadian rhythm disruptions (such as night-shifts or recent travel across time zones).
21. Apparent mineralocorticoid excess (AME) shares several clinical and laboratory features with primary aldosteronism: hypertension, hypokalemia, metabolic alkalosis and low renin.
22. When pheochromocytoma or paraganglioma is suspected, measuring plasma metanephrines or 24-hour urinary metanephrines are both appropriate and have similar diagnostic accuracy, with sensitivity ∼97% and specificity ∼90%.
23. Surgery is the treatment of choice for symptomatic and functional pheochromocytomas and paragangliomas.
24. Use of anabolic androgen steroids (AAS) is associated with increased 24-hour ambulatory blood pressure, prevalent hypertension, reduced ventricular function, vascular calcification, and aortic stiffness.

25. Recombinant erythropoietin increases blood pressure in patients with chronic kidney disease independent of hemoglobin increase, but typically responds to non-specific antihypertensive medications.

26. Polycythemia is associated with severe hypertension (Gaisböck's syndrome) and may be driven by a secondary cause of hypertension.

27. Hypothyroidism is the most common thyroid disorder and is associated with hyperlipidemia and diastolic hypertension.

28. *JAK2* V617F-positive polycythemia vera is associated with increased risk of both cardiovascular events and renal artery stenosis.

29. Renovascular disease is typically assessed by imaging of the renal arteries by renal duplex ultrasound, computed tomographic angiography (CTA), or magnetic resonance angiography (MRA), or digital subtraction angiography.

30. Renal angiography remains the definitive diagnostic study and provides direct access for pressure monitoring and possible intervention, but this test is invasive with attendant increased risks.

31. Angiotensin converting enzyme (ACE) inhibitors or angiotensin II receptor blockers (ARBs) directly target the pathogenesis of renovascular hypertension and should be offered as first-line antihypertensive therapy to every patient in the absence of contraindications.

32. The blood pressure raising effect (stimulation of alpha-1 receptors thereby causing vasoconstriction) of pseudoephedrine (OTC decongestant) is augmented when coadministered with acetaminophen, which increases the bioavailability of pseudoephedrine.

33. Caffeine is a xanthine that antagonizes adenosine receptors in vascular tissue, resulting in vasoconstriction; it also increases sympathetic activity.

34. Naloxone, an opioid antagonist used to treat opioid overdose, can also cause hypertension.

35. The use of a beta-blocker during clonidine withdrawal, pheochromocytoma, or a hyperadrenergic state, can lead to unopposed alpha activation and result in hypertension.

36. Prevalence of obstructive sleep apnea (OSA) is increased in patients with obesity, diabetes mellitus, chronic kidney disease, and in particular resistant hypertension.

37. Treatment with continuous positive airway pressure (CPAP) causes modest decrease in blood pressure in hypertensive patients with impaired nocturnal blood pressure pattern (non-dippers) and symptomatic OSA, and also in patients with HTN resistant to pharmacotherapy.

38. The clinical presentation of a patient with a monogenetic cause of hypertension typically includes a low plasma renin activity, a family history of resistant hypertension or a family member with a stroke before age 50 years old, and abnormal serum electrolyte values.

39. Since cardiovascular events are rare in the pediatric age group, a statistical definition for hypertension has been adopted, based upon the distribution of BPs in healthy children, with BP values at the upper end of the distribution ($\geq$90th percentile) considered abnormal.

40. Over the past decade, the childhood obesity epidemic has resulted in an increased prevalence of hypertension in the young with a prevalence of hypertension as high as 4.5% among obese children as compared with less than 2% in non-obese children.

41. The predominant form of hypertension in children, at least those over 6 years of age, is primary hypertension, with secondary causes accounting for a smaller proportion of all hypertension.

42. The two factors that appear to be most influential in children and adolescents with primary hypertension are family history and obesity.

43. The sensitivity and specificity of renal Doppler to detect renovascular disease in the pediatric age group is poor.

44. Given their effectiveness at preventing and delaying the progression of kidney disease in diabetes, renin-angiotensin-aldosterone system (RAAS) inhibitors are preferred first-line treatment of hypertension in diabetes and may also be considered in the absence of hypertension.

45. In hypertensive patients with type 2 diabetes mellitus (T2DM), SGLT2 inhibitors are effective at reducing the cardiovascular risk and protect the kidney in addition to RAAS inhibition in those with significant kidney disease and may thus be considered second-line after RAAS inhibitors in this setting.

46. ACE inhibitors and ARBs are usually avoided in the first 3 to 6 months after transplant due to concerns for worsening of anemia, hyperkalemia, and a possible decline in kidney function.

47. Bariatric surgery has the potential to reduce BP (with a significant rate of hypertension remission) and other cardiovascular risk factors.

48. Patients with body mass index (BMI) between 35 and 39.9 kg/m^2 should be referred to surgery if significant comorbidities such as hypertension, type 2 diabetes, dyslipidemia, heart failure, atrial fibrillation, sleep apnea, or orthopedic problems are present. Patients with BMI greater than 40 kg/m^2 should be referred for surgical evaluation regardless of the presence of comorbidities.

49. Most Blacks with hypertension have a suppressed renin-angiotensin system due to plasma volume expansion—a result of excessive sodium retention mediated, at least in part, by aldosterone.

50. Treatment of the hypertension with drugs that mitigate the activity of epithelial sodium channel (ENaC) can be highly effective in lowering BP in Blacks.

51. Both systolic (SBP) and diastolic BP (DBP) increase with age up to the sixth decade of life. After that, DBP starts to decline, resulting in increased pulse pressure (PP).
52. Significant inter-arm BP differences (>10 mm Hg) are associated with underlying peripheral arterial disease and are more common among older men than other groups.
53. Orthostatic hypotension (defined as a BP fall >20/10 mm Hg with standing), often asymptomatic, occurs in up to a third of older patients with hypertension.
54. Low DBP (<70 mm Hg, and especially <60 mm Hg) is associated with increased rates of de novo and recurrent cardiovascular events in older hypertensive patients. In isolated systolic hypertension, treatment targeting systolic BP usually also lowers DBP, thus raising concerns about coronary risk.
55. Based on published data, there is a modest effect of BP reduction on the incidence or progression of cognitive impairment and dementia in elderly hypertensive patients.
56. During normal pregnancy both the systolic and diastolic blood pressure are significantly lower than baseline.
57. Low dose aspirin in women at moderate or high risk for preeclampsia has been shown to decrease the frequency of preeclampsia and its gestational complications.
58. The definitive treatment of preeclampsia is delivery.
59. All antihypertensive agents cross the placenta, and there is not adequate data to recommend one antihypertensive over another. The most commonly used antihypertensive agents which are considered to have acceptable safety profile in pregnancy include methyldopa, labetalol, and nifedipine.
60. The principle of utilizing a single drug that would address hypertension and angina pectoris has led to guideline recommendations for the use of beta-blockers or calcium channel blockers in coronary artery disease (CAD).
61. Since the degree of coronary stenosis is unknown in most patients with hypertension and CAD, clinicians should be cautioned about the potential for myocardial ischemia at low diastolic blood pressure.
62. It is not simply BP reduction that is useful in chronic heart failure as there are some antihypertensive agents that do not lower mortality in patients with heart failure so that the general recommendation has been to use agents with demonstrated efficacy to reduce cardiovascular mortality as well as the morbidity of hospital readmissions.
63. In heart failure with reduced ejection fraction (HfrEF), guidelines often encourage titrating heart failure drugs according to tolerance irrespective of achieved BP.
64. Intravenous beta-blockers, including metoprolol, esmolol, labetalol, or propranolol, are first-line therapy for aortic dissection (AoD) due to their ability to decrease heart rate and shear stress on the aorta.
65. Short acting vasodilators should not be used as first-line therapy for acute aortic syndromes (AAS) in the absence of adequate heart rate control, because they routinely cause reflex tachycardia, increased LV contractility, and increased shear stress.
66. Confirmation of resistant hypertension needs to be done by ensuring assessment for medication adherence, accurate BP measurement with automated office BP and out-of-office BP measurements.
67. The majority of randomized controlled trials, physiologic data, and metaanalysis support the use of spironolactone as a fourth-line agent due to it having the greatest BP lowering.
68. ECG alone should not be relied upon to correctly identify which patients with hyperkalemia require immediate attention.
69. Novel potassium exchange resins such as Patiromer and sodium zirconium cyclosilicate (SZC) show great promise in both the acute and chronic treatment of hyperkalemia and might allow for better RAAS inhibitor adherence among individuals with hypertension.
70. The Dietary Approaches to Stop Hypertension (DASH) diet is a widely used intervention for hypertension, which emphasizes fruits, vegetables, and low-fat dairy products with reduced intake in saturated fat and cholesterol. It is most effective when combined with sodium restriction (<1500 mg/d or 65 mmol/d).
71. Population studies and trials show an inverse relationship to potassium intake to blood pressure. The daily recommended potassium intake is 3500 mg/dL (90 mmol) or higher per WHO.
72. BP goals are intended as general guides, and with this knowledge individual BP goals should be set by the clinician in consultation with the patient.
73. Overcoming therapeutic inertia is important because every mm Hg BP reduction towards goal can prevent cardiovascular disease (CVD) events and death.
74. ACE inhibitors and ARBs are highly effective antihypertensive drugs that also have proven benefit in reducing albuminuria, progression to kidney disease, and death.
75. Avoid using combined therapy with ACE inhibitors and ARBs due to increased adverse events.
76. With nifedipine's duration of action being less than 24 hours, it provides inadequate BP control in the ambulatory setting, while lending itself to use in the hospital setting (lowers BP within 6–8 hours) where a prompt antihypertensive effect may be desired.
77. Symptomatic side effects with calcium channel blockers (CCBs), if present, are often dose-dependent and relieved with either dosage de-escalation or if necessary, agent discontinuation.
78. CCBs preferentially dilate the precapillary vessels such that a greater transcapillary pressure gradient is generated, promoting extravasation of fluid into the interstitium and peripheral edema. Concurrent ACEi or ARB therapy decreases the incidence of edema significantly.

79. Hydralazine combined with nitrates conferred a mortality benefit in a selected group of patients with heart failure and reduced EF in the V-HEFT trial.

80. Administration of hydralazine is contraindicated in patients with conditions sensitive to the significant drop in afterload, or the attendant increase in sympathetic activity and cardiac output. Examples include myocardial ischemia, aortic or mitral stenosis, and high output heart failure.

81. Amlodipine is an ideal outpatient medication because of its extended antihypertensive effect (half-life 30–50 hours, duration of action >30 hours). However, it is a poor choice for inpatient BP control because the onset of action is 1 to 2 days.

82. Nondihydropyridine calcium channel blockers have been shown to reduce proteinuria by 25% to 50%, perhaps by decreasing glomerular permeability to filtered serum proteins.

83. Dihydropyridine calcium channel blockers have been shown to modestly (<10%) increase urinary protein excretion.

84. Spironolactone has been shown to reduce cardiovascular mortality in patients with systolic heart failure and eplerenone reduces mortality in patients after acute myocardial infarction.

85. Due to lack of clinical outcome data supporting the use of alpha blockers, they should be considered only as additional therapy in patients with resistant hypertension receiving maximally tolerated doses of diuretics, inhibitors of the renin-angiotensin system, and calcium channel blockers.

86. Beta-blockers are no longer recommended as first-line agents in pharmacotherapy of uncomplicated hypertension but should be considered for the management of hypertension in patients with specific indications for their use, such as among patients with concomitant heart failure, angina, and atrial fibrillation, or after an acute myocardial infarction.

87. Beta-blockers do appear to be more effective in improving BP control, and possibly in reducing the occurrence of serious adverse cardiovascular events among hypertensive dialysis patients.

88. When tapering a clonidine patch, transition to lower dose patch requires a new prescription for the lower dose patch because the patches should not be cut.

89. Clonidine and other α2-agonists may produce an initial paradoxical vasoconstrictor response which increases blood pressure, particularly at a high dose.

90. Clonidine causes initial vasoconstriction when given intravenously and should not be administered via this route.

91. Drug metabolism is mediated, in part, by the cytochrome P450 proteins, which are monooxygenases which participate in activation, inactivation, and clearance of drugs.

92. Chronic triamterene use is associated with a high incidence of eosinophiluria, the significance of which is unclear.

93. Despite initial reports of huge blood pressure decrease from uncontrolled and unblinded studies, properly conducted trials demonstrate a more modest 4 to 7 mm Hg decrease with renal denervation, approximately the effect seen with the addition of one blood pressure lowering drug.

94. Central arteriovenous fistula may lower blood pressure, but with high complication rates, and should not be pursued at this time.

95. Baroreceptor modulation/activation seems to have interesting physiologic effects; however, data from ongoing trials on safety and efficacy are needed before widespread use.

96. Orthostatic hypotension (OH) describes a sustained reduction in systolic blood pressure of at least 20 mm Hg or diastolic blood pressure of 10 mm Hg within 3 minutes of standing or head-up tilt to at least 60 degrees on a tilt table.

97. The Valsalva maneuver is the mainstay of autonomic tests and allows for evaluation of both the cardiac and vascular baroreflex responses to a change in blood pressure.

98. Cardiac baroreflex sensitivity (BRS) decreases with age. Baroreflex-mediated heart rate responses are therefore larger in younger individuals versus older individuals.

99. Afferent baroreflex failure is one of the most challenging hypertensive or autonomic disorders to manage, and treatment should focus on management of patients' expectations, reduction of stimuli (auditory, visual) that induce hypertensive crises, and pharmacological management of hypertension with long-acting sympatholytics.

100. Richard Bright's report in 1836 of the association of ventricular hypertrophy with the fullness of a hard pulse in patients with kidney disease launched the studies that would eventuate in identifying the systemic effects of hypertension as a disease rather than merely a sign of disease.

MEASUREMENT OF BLOOD PRESSURE IN THE OFFICE

Jennifer Ringrose, MD, MSc, and Raj Padwal, MD, MSc

CHAPTER 1

QUESTIONS

1. **What is office blood pressure measurement?**
   Blood pressure (BP) measurement in the office has been standard practice for over 100 years, and most physicians continue to use office BP for diagnosis and to follow patients with known or suspected hypertension.[1]

2. **What are the major types of office BP measurement?**
   Two major types of office BP measurement exist. The auscultatory technique is performed with a mercury or aneroid sphygmomanometer by listening for Korotkoff sounds with a stethoscope. Onset of the sounds (K1) coincides with systolic BP (SBP), and the pressure at which the sounds are no longer heard (K5) is the diastolic BP (DBP).[2] The oscillometric technique utilizes an automated device that, if singly or repeatedly activated, can take one or more readings, or an automated office BP (AOBP) device that is preprogrammed to take multiple sequential readings. In the latter case, a provider can leave the room, which is known as "unattended" BP measurement.[3] It is important that only automated devices that have been validated according to an internationally accepted clinical protocol be used.[2] Oscillometric devices work by recording, filtering, and analyzing arterial pulsations. BP is determined by applying a proprietary algorithm to these recordings.[4]

   BP measurement techniques, advantages, and disadvantages are summarized in Table 1.1.

3. **How should BP measurement be performed in the office?**
   BP measurement has been described as "...likely the clinical procedure of greatest importance that is performed in the sloppiest manner."[5] Because BP is a highly variable physiologic parameter sensitive to numerous endogenous and exogenous stimuli, it must be performed meticulously with strict adherence to standardized technique. This is not often done in conventional clinical practice, and this type of nonstandardized measurement has been termed "casual" BP measurement. A major barrier to adopting proper measurement technique in the office setting is lack of time. Casual measurement technique readings are, on average, 5 to 10 mm Hg higher than standardized technique and have greater variability in BP measurements and lower correlation with target organ damage compared to standardized measurement.[6] This can lead to inaccurate diagnosis and management of hypertension.

   The proper technique for performing BP measurement is summarized in Table 1.2 and in Fig. 1.1.

4. **What are the sources of error with office BP measurement?**
   The many potential sources of error in BP measurement can be divided into patient-related, procedure-related, equipment-related, and observer-related factors (Table 1.3). Use of automated devices standardizes the measurement process and eliminates some of the potential sources of observer-induced inaccuracy (e.g., hearing deficits, terminal digit preference, rapid deflation rate). Consequently, clinical practice guidelines endorse use of automated BP measurement in place of auscultation whenever possible.[3,7,8]

5. **How is AOBP monitoring performed?**
   AOBP monitoring is the preferred method of office BP measurement. Several AOBP devices exist and differ in terms of technique and available options. They are summarized in Table 1.4.

   Even though using an AOBP device is the best way to ensure standardized technique in the office, two aspects of AOBP measurement are variably performed, which can impact the results:
   - **Rest period:** Use of a rest period, which is typically 5 minutes but can be longer, before initiating the AOBP sequence results in a lower mean BP. Published studies vary widely in terms of use of an antecedent rest period. Because the BpTRU is typically set to perform six readings, an additional rest period is not recommended.
   - **Attended versus unattended measurement:** Attended measurement results in higher mean BP.[9]

Table 1.1 Types of Blood Pressure Measurement

DEVICE	BENEFITS	CHALLENGES
Mercury auscultation	• Does not require calibration as long as the mercury column is intact and the meniscus is zeroed. • Accuracy: Two-observer mercury-based auscultation is the gold standard measurement method but is too impractical to be used in clinical settings.	• Human error in technique. • Risk of spills (extremely rare). Nevertheless, mercury has been banned in many jurisdictions because of this theoretical risk. LED devices may be an alternative. • White coat and masked effect. • Does not facilitate unattended measurement.
Aneroid auscultation	• Can be accurate if a calibrated device and proper technique are used.	• Human error in technique. • Requires regular calibration (every 3–6 months) to maintain accuracy. • White coat and masked effect. • Does not facilitate unattended measurement.
Single activation automated device (can include a home BP device)	• Standardizes the measurement process and eliminates some human error. • Less expensive than AOBP device.	• Must be reactivated to take multiple readings. • Unattended readings cannot be performed.
AOBP device	• Enables multiple, sequential measurements. • Auto calculates mean blood pressure. • Measurements can be unattended, potentially reducing white coat effect.	• Due to limited outcome data and high variability relative to out-of-office measurement modalities, AOBP is not a replacement for out-of-office measurement.

AOBP, Automated office blood pressure; *LED,* light-emitting diode.
Data from Padwal R, Campbell NRC, Schutte AE, et al. Optimizing observer performance of clinic blood pressure measurement: a position statement from the Lancet Commission on Hypertension Group. *J Hypertens.* 2019;37:1737-1745.

Table 1.2 Recommended Technique for Performing Blood Pressure Measurement

Device
• Automated devices must be validated. A validation process involves comparing the automated device against two-observer mercury auscultation following a published protocol. There are several registries that list validated devices:
  • Hypertension Canada (https://hypertension.ca/hypertension-and-you/managing-hypertension/measuring-blood-pressure/devices/)
  • British and Irish Society of Hypertension (https://bihsoc.org/bp-monitors/)
  • Validated Device Listing (VDL) for United States Blood Pressure Devices (Validatebp.org)
  • Japanese listing (Japanese only) (http://www.jpnsh.jp/com_ac_wg1.html)
  • dabl Educational Trust (http://www.dableducational.org)
  • MEDAVAL (https://medaval.ie)
  • STRIDE BP (www.stridebp.org/index.php)
• Aneroid devices must be calibrated every 3–6 months to remain accurate.

Cuff
• The cuffs that belong with the device should be used for all measurements.
• The cuff should be appropriately sized for each patient. Ensure the device used has a wide range of cuff options to accommodate various arm sizes.
• The inflatable cuff bladder width should be 40% of the arm circumference.
• The inflatable cuff length should be 80%–100% of the arm circumference.
• For automated measurements, the cuff should be applied per the manufacturer's specifications.
• For auscultatory measurements, the cuff should be placed so that its lower edge is 2–3 cm above the elbow crease and the brachial artery marker in line with the brachial artery.

Preparation
• Patient should have an empty bladder and should not have exercised, eaten, consumed caffeine, or smoked for more than 30 minutes prior.
• Cuff should be applied to the exposed arm with loose clothing above or the cuff applied over very thin clothing.
• Feet should be on the floor, back supported, legs uncrossed, and arm supported with BP cuff at the level of the heart.
• In this position, the patient should be instructed to rest for 5 minutes. During the rest period and measurements, the patient and observer (person taking measurement) should not talk.

Table 1.2 Recommended Technique for Performing Blood Pressure Measurement—cont'd

Measurement
- On initial assessment, BP should be taken in both arms and subsequent BP measurements should be taken in the arm with the higher BP.
- Two or three measurements should be taken, and the mean should be recorded as the office BP measurement.
  - Auscultation:
    - While palpating the radial or brachial pulse, inflate rapidly to 30 mm Hg above where the pulse disappears.
    - Place the stethoscope on the brachial artery and listen while deflating the cuff 2 mm Hg/s.
    - The first Korotkoff sound heard corresponds to the systolic BP and the point the sounds disappear corresponds to the diastolic BP. If the sounds persist toward 0 mm Hg, the point of muffling should be used as the diastolic BP.
    - BP should be recorded to the nearest 2 mm Hg.
  - Automated: initiate measurements per the manufacturer's specifications.

BP, Blood pressure.
Data from Pickering TG, Hall JE, Appel LJ, et al. Recommendations for blood pressure measurement in humans and experimental animals: Part 1: blood pressure measurement in humans: a statement for professionals from the subcommittee of professional and public education of the American Heart Association Council on High Blood Pressure Research. *Circulation.* 2005;111:697-716; Padwal R, Campbell NRC, Weber MA, et al. The Accuracy in Measurement of Blood Pressure (AIM-BP) collaborative: background and rationale. 2019;21:1780-1783; and Ogedegbe G, Pickering T. Principles and techniques of blood pressure measurement. *Cardiol Clin.* 2010;28:571-586.

6. **What is the evidence for office BP as a predictor of cardiovascular outcomes, and how does it compare to out-of-office BP measurement?**
A great deal of evidence exists supporting the concept that standardized, research quality BP measurement predicts cardiovascular events and mortality, including data from high-quality prognostic studies and randomized controlled trials evaluating antihypertensive drugs.[10,11] However, for casual office measurement, the data are much less robust. Indeed, when casual office measurement and out-of-office measurement (e.g., ambulatory BP measurement) are entered into the same model, casual office measurement is a weak, almost nonstatistically significant predictor of outcomes.[12] This is one reason why use of out-of-office measurement instead of office BP is strongly preferred. A second reason why out-of-office measurement is preferred is because it detects white coat hypertension and masked hypertension, thereby enabling more appropriate and personalized management (masked hypertension is treated, but white coat hypertension is not treated).[13,14] The third reason is that out-of-office measurement enables performance of many readings, thereby more closely estimating an individual's "usual" BP, particularly in settings that correspond to her or his usual daily life.
  The evidence base for AOBP as a predictor of outcomes is limited to one study. In this Canadian study of 3627 subjects aged 66 years or older, the AOBP thresholds that predicted increased risk of fatal and nonfatal cardiovascular events were 135 mm Hg or higher (hazard ratio [HR] 1.7; 95% confidence interval [CI] 1.1–2.5) for SBP and 80 mm Hg or higher (HR 1.7; 95% CI 1.2–2.5) for DBP.[15] Therefore the evidence base for AOBP as a hard outcome predictor is very limited compared to the data supporting out-of-office BP. There is some evidence that AOBP can predict target organ damage similar to ambulatory BP measurement.[16] However, to date, these data are cross sectional and need to be confirmed in outcome studies.
  In terms of use in clinical trials, the evidence base for AOBP is limited to Action to Control Cardiovascular Risk in Diabetes (ACCORD) and Systolic Blood Pressure Intervention Trial (SPRINT).[17,18] SPRINT is the more important of these two studies, and the Omron HEM-907XL (Omron Healthcare, Lake Forest, IL) was the specific AOBP device used in this study. SPRINT was a 9361-subject, 5-year randomized control trial demonstrating that intensive BP control (SBP target <120 mm Hg) reduces the risk of cardiovascular disease and death compared to standard BP control (SBP target <140 mm Hg). Some controversy exists with respect to whether AOBP was performed attended or unattended at each SPRINT study center.[19] The results of the SPRINT ambulatory BP substudy (897 SPRINT participants) demonstrated mean AOBP was 7/6 mm Hg (systolic/diastolic) lower than daytime ambulatory BP and highly variable between subjects.[20] This shows that AOBP can be markedly discordant from ambulatory blood pressure monitoring (ABPM) and is not a replacement for out-of-office measurement.

7. **What are the thresholds for normal vs. elevated BP values in the office in order to guide treatment?**
These thresholds vary across guidelines and are summarized in Table 1.5.

8. **What are the treatment threshold and treatment targets for AOBP?**
The Hypertension Canada clinical practice recommendations are the only guidelines that endorse separate thresholds for AOBP relative to non-AOBP in office measurement:
- The threshold for elevated non-AOBP levels is 140/90 mm Hg or greater, whereas the threshold for elevated AOBP levels is 135/85 mm Hg or greater.

BLOOD PRESSURE MEASUREMENT

When you measure your blood pressure:

✓ Sitting position

✓ Back supported

✓ Arm bare and supported

✓ Use a cuff size appropriate for your arm

✓ Middle of the cuff at heart level

✓ Apply cuff according to manufacturer's instructions

✓ Do not talk or move before or during the measurement

✓ Legs uncrossed

✓ Feet flat on the floor

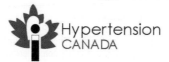

Hypertension
CANADA

Fig. 1.1 Correct blood pressure technique. (With permission from Hypertension Canada.)

- The guidelines are unclear with respect to AOBP thresholds in specific subgroups. For example, the non-AOBP threshold in patients with diabetes is 130/80 mm Hg, but no specific analogous threshold for AOBP (e.g., 125/75 mm Hg could be considered) is given.
- In SPRINT-eligible patients, the Canadian guidelines recommend that, to be consistent with application of the study results in clinical practice, only AOBP measurements be used.

9. **What is the bottom line with respect to office BP measurement?**
   Office BP measurement is commonly performed, and great care should be taken to use standardized technique so that measurements are as accurate as possible. In most cases in contemporary clinical practice, standardized technique is not used ("casual" measurement) to the detriment of patient diagnosis and management. Use of

Table 1.3 Sources of Inaccuracy in Blood Pressure Measurement

POTENTIAL SOURCE OF INACCURACY SBP (mm Hg)	RANGE OF REPORTED MEAN EFFECT ON SBP	RANGE OF REPORTED EFFECT ON DBP
White coat effect	−12.7 to +26.7	−8.2 to +21
Cold exposure	+5 to +32	+4 to +23
Insufficient rest	+4.2 to +11.6	+1.8 to +4.3
Talking during measurement	+4 to +19	+5 to +14.3
Undercuffing (cuff too small)	+2.08 to +11.2	+1.61 to +6.6
Overcuffing (cuff too big)	−3.7 to −1.45	−4.7 to −0.96
Reliance on a single measurement	+3.3 to +10.4	−2.4 to +0.6

DBP, Diastolic blood pressure; *SBP,* systolic blood pressure.
Data from Kallioinen N, Hill A, Horswill MS, Ward HE, Watson MO. Sources of inaccuracy in the measurement of adult patients' resting blood pressure in clinical settings. *J Hypertens.* 2017;35:421-441.

Table 1.4 Automated Office Blood Pressure Devices in Use

DEVICE	NUMBER OF READINGS	CUFF TYPE	CUFF SIZES (NUMBER)	CIRCUM-FERENCE OF LIMB ACCOMMODATED (cm)	INTERVAL BETWEEN READINGS	MISCELLANEOUS
BpTRU	1–6	2-piece, upper arm	5	13–52 cm	1, 2, 3, 4, or 5 mins	First AOBP device invented; no longer available on the market
Omron HEM 907XL	1–3	2-piece, upper arm	4	17–50 cm	5 s, 30 s, 1 min or 2 min	Used in the SPRINT trial[19]
Microlife AG Watch BP Office	1–3	2-piece, upper arm	2	22–42 cm	15, 30, 45 or 60 s	Atrial fibrillation detection Capable of performing simultaneous measurements in both arms and legs, which enables measurement of ankle-brachial index
Welch Allyn ProBP 2400	1–3	2-piece, upper arm	4	14–52 cm	15, 30, 45 or 60 s	Validated in pregnancy and pre-eclampsia

AOBP, Automated office BP; *mins,* minutes; *s,* seconds; *SPRINT,* Systolic Blood Pressure Intervention Trial.

validated automated devices, especially AOBP measurement, facilitates more standardized technique and should be encouraged. Outcome-based data supporting standardized office BP measurement is strong, but the data supporting casual office BP and AOBP is much weaker. For this reason, diagnosis and clinical management should not be guided solely by office BP measurement; out-of-office measurement results should be incorporated into the clinical decision-making process.

Table 1.5 Thresholds to Define Elevated Office Blood Pressure Levels for the Purposes of Initiating and Guiding Drug Treatment

	Guidelines		
	HYPERTENSION CANADA	**ESH**	**ACC/AHA**
Threshold to initiate drug treatment (mm Hg)	≥160/90 (low risk) ≥130/80 (diabetes) ≥140/90 for non-AOBP ≥135/85 and (moderate risk) ≥130 (high-risk SPRINT eligible; AOBP device should be used)	≥140/90 (all patients) ≥130/85 (high CV risk) ≥160/90 (≥80 years)	>130/80 (high CV risk, diabetes, chronic kidney disease) >140/90
Treatment target (mm Hg)	<140/90 (low and moderate risk) <130/80 (diabetes) <120 (high-risk SPRINT eligible)	<140/90 (all patients) <130/80 (<65 years) 130–139/<80 (65–80 years) 130–139/<80 if tolerated (>80 years)	<130/80

ACC/AHA, American College of Cardiology/American Heart Association; AOBP, automated office blood pressure; CV, cardiovascular; ESH, European Society of Hypertension; SPRINT, Systolic Blood Pressure Intervention Trial.
Data from Nerenberg KA, Zarnke KB, Leung AA, et al. Hypertension Canada's 2018 Guidelines for diagnosis, risk assessment, prevention, and treatment of hypertension in adults and children. Can J Cardiol. 2018;34:506-525; Whelton PK, Carey RM, Aronow WS, et al. 2017 ACC/AHA/AAPA/ABC/ACPM/AGS/APhA/ASH/ASPC/NMA/PCNA Guideline for the prevention, detection, evaluation, and management of high blood pressure in adults: a report of the American College of Cardiology/American Heart Association Task Force on Clinical Practice Guidelines. Hypertension. 2018;71:e13-e115; Williams B, Mancia G, Spiering W, et al. 2018 ESC/ESH guidelines for the management of arterial hypertension: the task force for the management of arterial hypertension of the European Society of Cardiology and the European Society of Hypertension. J Hypertens. 2018;36:1953-2041.

KEY POINTS

1. Proper technique is essential.
2. Use of automated BP measurement, particularly automated office BP (AOBP), minimizes many common observer-related sources of error in office BP measurement.
3. Use a validated automated device or a calibrated aneroid device to perform measurements.
4. Office BP measurement should be supplemented with out-of-office measurements to better inform diagnostic and treatment decisions.

REFERENCES

1. Kaczorowski J, Myers MG, Gelfer M, et al. How do family physicians measure blood pressure in routine clinical practice? National survey of Canadian family physicians. Can Fam Physician. 2017;63:e193–e199.
2. Pickering TG, Hall JE, Appel LJ, et al. Recommendations for blood pressure measurement in humans and experimental animals: Part 1: blood pressure measurement in humans: a statement for professionals from the subcommittee of professional and public education of the American Heart Association Council on High Blood Pressure Research. Circulation. 2005;111:697–716.
3. Padwal R, Campbell NRC, Schutte AE, et al. Optimizing observer performance of clinic blood pressure measurement: a position statement from the Lancet Commission on Hypertension Group. J Hypertens. 2019;37:1737–1745.
4. Alpert BS, Quinn D, Gallick D. Oscillometric blood pressure: a review for clinicians. J Am Soc Hypertens. 2014;8:930–938.
5. Commentary on the sixth report of the Joint National Committee (JNC-6) [editorial]. Am J Hypertens. 1998;11(1 Pt 1):134.
6. Rinfret F, Cloutier L, L'Archevêque H, et al. The gap between manual and automated office blood pressure measurements results at a hypertension clinic. Can J Cardiol. 2017;33:653–657.
7. Nerenberg KA, Zarnke KB, Leung AA, et al. Hypertension Canada's 2018 guidelines for diagnosis, risk assessment, prevention, and treatment of hypertension in adults and children. Can J Cardiol. 2018;34:506–525.
8. Whelton PK, Carey RM, Aronow WS, et al. 2017 ACC/AHA/AAPA/ABC/ACPM/AGS/APhA/ASH/ASPC/NMA/PCNA guideline for the prevention, detection, evaluation, and management of high blood pressure in adults: a report of the American College of Cardiology/American Heart Association Task Force on Clinical Practice Guidelines. Hypertension. 2018;71:e13–e115.
9. Andreadis EA, Thomopoulos C, Geladari CV, Papademetriou V. Attended versus unattended automated office blood pressure: a systematic review and meta-analysis. High Blood Press Cardiovasc Prev. 2019;26:293–303.
10. Prospective Studies Collaboration. Age-specific relevance of usual blood pressure to vascular mortality: a meta-analysis of individual data for one million adults in 61 prospective studies. Lancet. 2002;360:1903–1913.
11. Ettehad D, Emdin CA, Kiran A, et al. Blood pressure lowering for prevention of cardiovascular disease and death: a systematic review and meta-analysis. Lancet. 2015;387:957–967.
12. Banegas JR, Ruilope LM, de la Sierra A, et al. Relationship between clinic and ambulatory blood-pressure measurements and mortality. N Engl J Med. 2018;378:1509–1520.

13. Muntner P, Anderson A, Charleston J, et al. Hypertension awareness, treatment, and control in adults with CKD: results from the Chronic Renal Insufficiency Cohort (CRIC) study. *Am J Kidney Dis.* 2010;55:441–451.
14. Rinfret F, Cloutier L, Wistaff R, et al. Comparison of different automated office blood pressure measurement devices: evidence of nonequivalence and clinical implications. *Can J Cardiol.* 2017;33:1639–1644.
15. Myers MG, Kaczorowski J, Paterson JM, Dolovich L. Thresholds for diagnosing hypertension based on automated office blood pressure measurements and cardiovascular risk. *Hypertension.* 2015;66(3):489–495.
16. Andreadis EA, Agaliotis GD, Angelopoulos ET, Tsakanikas AP, Kolyvas GN, Mousoulis GP. Automated office blood pressure is associated with urine albumin excretion in hypertensive subjects. *Am J Hypertens.* 2012;25:969–973.
17. ACCORD SG, Cushman WC, Evans GW, et al. Effects of intensive blood-pressure control in type 2 diabetes mellitus. *N Engl J Med.* 2010;362:1575–1585.
18. The SPRINT Research Group. A randomized trial of intensive versus standard blood pressure control. *N Engl J Med.* 2015;373:2103–2116.
19. SPRINT blood pressure: sprinting back to Smirk's basal blood pressure [editorial]. *Hypertension.* 2017;69(1):15.
20. Drawz PE, Pajewski NM, Bates JT, Bello NA. Effect of intensive versus standard clinic-based hypertension management on ambulatory blood pressure: novelty and significance. *Hypertension.* 2017;69:42–50.

CHAPTER 2

AMBULATORY AND HOME BLOOD PRESSURE MONITORING

Blaise W. Abramovitz, DO, and Jordana B. Cohen, MD, MSCE

QUESTIONS

1. **What is out-of-office blood pressure monitoring?**
   Out-of-office blood pressure (BP) monitoring is the assessment of BP outside of the clinic setting using either ambulatory BP monitoring (ABPM) or self-monitoring of BP at home, also known as home BP monitoring (HBPM).

2. **Why is out-of-office BP monitoring performed?**
   Out-of-office BP monitoring is performed to confirm the diagnosis of hypertension and to assist with titration of antihypertensive medications.[1–3] Out-of-office BP monitoring is particularly useful for identifying discrepancies between BPs measured in versus outside of the clinic, including masked and white coat hypertension (Fig. 2.1).
   Masked hypertension (MH) and masked uncontrolled hypertension (MUCH)[4]:
   - Defined as normal clinic BP with elevated out-of-office BP
     - MH occurs in patients not yet on antihypertensive therapy
     - MUCH occurs in patients on antihypertensive therapy
   - Associated with similarly elevated cardiovascular risk as sustained hypertension
   - Most common in men, individuals of African descent, individuals with chronic kidney disease, and individuals with obstructive sleep apnea
   - Consider screening patients with:
     - Evidence of target organ damage disproportionate to their degree of BP control in the clinic
     - Clinic BPs less than 10 mm Hg below their goal
     - Labile clinic BPs
     White coat hypertension (WCH) and white coat effect (WCE)[5]:
   - Defined as elevated clinic BP with normal out-of-office BP
     - WCH occurs in patients not yet on antihypertensive therapy
     - WCE occurs in patients on antihypertensive therapy
   - WCH is associated with:
     - Elevated cardiovascular risk that is lower in magnitude than sustained hypertension
     - High risk of transitioning to sustained hypertension
   - WCE is not associated with elevated cardiovascular risk
   - Most common in women, children, older adults, and patients with apparent treatment resistant hypertension
   - Consider screening in patients with:
     - Apparent treatment resistant hypertension
     - Treated hypertension and symptoms of low BPs outside of the office
     - Labile clinic BPs
     - Newly elevated clinic BPs

3. **What is ABPM?**
   ABPM is a noninvasive method of out-of-office BP monitoring in which BPs are measured repeatedly over a 24- to 48-hour period, during routine daily activities and sleep, using a fully automated device.[6]

4. **Why is ABPM performed?**
   ABPM is considered to be the reference standard for the diagnosis of hypertension because it is the method of BP measurement that is most strongly associated with adverse cardiovascular outcomes and provides an assessment of overall BP load beyond the office snapshot.[6] ABPM can determine the presence of MH, MUCH, WCH, and WCE. A distinctive part of the prognostic value of ABPM is the ability to identify elevated nocturnal BPs and non-dipping (i.e., the absence of a 10% decline in BP during sleep). Non-dipping and elevated nocturnal BPs are independently associated with an elevated risk of major cardiac events, including myocardial infarction, stroke, and heart failure.[7] ABPM is also helpful for identifying short-term BP variability, which is associated with elevated cardiac risk,[8] as well as for monitoring the effectiveness of antihypertensive therapy over a full day.

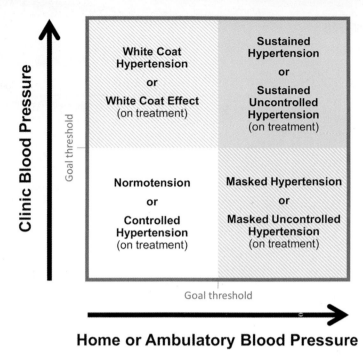

Fig. 2.1 Blood pressure (BP) patterns determined using the combination of clinic and out-of-office BP monitoring.

5. How is ABPM performed?

Key steps for clinicians when performing ABPM[6,9]:

- Program the monitor to perform readings at predetermined intervals, typically every 15 to 30 minutes during the day and every 30 to 60 minutes at night over 24 hours
- Apply the cuff to the patient's nondominant arm unless there is a contraindication, such as an arteriovenous fistula or prior lymph node dissection
- Provide advanced instructions to the patient to prepare according to the following:
  - Wear a loose-fitting or sleeveless shirt so that the cuff can be applied to a bare arm
  - Plan to wear the monitor for a full 24-hour period during a routine day
  - The device may disrupt some activities and sleep
  - Plan to return to the office within a reasonably short time period (e.g., 1–2 days) to return the monitor
- Provide verbal and written instructions to the patient on the day the monitor is applied to do the following:
  - Maintain a diary documenting, at minimum:
    - Time of awakening
    - Time to sleep
    - Time, name, and dose of any prescribed and over-the-counter medications taken
    - Symptoms such as lightheadedness, dizziness, or palpitations
  - Avoid showering or immersion in water while wearing the device
  - Continue with a normal daily routine
  - Keep the arm still when the device is initiating and inflating
  - Avoid rigorous exercise while wearing the device
  - Refit the cuff if it migrates downward, rotates, or needs to be temporarily removed
- Upon return of the monitor to the clinic, the data should be downloaded to a secure device and interpreted by the provider

6. How is ABPM interpreted?

Key components of ABPM interpretation[6,9]:

- Mean 24-hour systolic and diastolic BP
  - Used to determine the diagnosis of the BP patterns outlined in Fig. 2.1

(A) Dipping

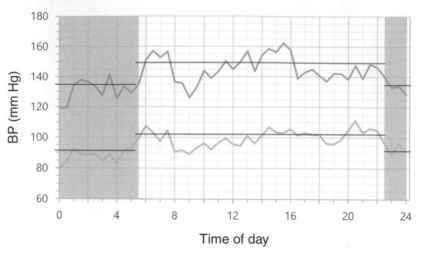

(B) Non-dipping

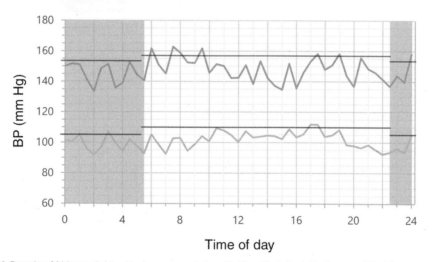

Fig. 2.2 Examples of 24-hour ambulatory blood pressure monitoring, with (A) ≥10% decline in blood pressure (*BP*) while sleeping (i.e., nocturnal "dipping") and (B) <10% decline in BP while sleeping (i.e., nocturnal "non-dipping").

- Mean daytime (i.e., awake) systolic and diastolic BP
  - Used to determine the diagnosis of the BP patterns outlined in Fig. 2.1, typically with a higher threshold than the overall 24-hour mean
- Mean nocturnal (i.e., asleep) systolic and diastolic BP (Fig. 2.2)
  - BP typically declines by 10% to 20% during sleep compared to daytime BP
  - Elevated nocturnal BP and non-dipping (absence of a ≥10% decline in BP during sleep) are associated with elevated risk of adverse outcomes
  - Nocturnal dosing of antihypertensives may improve non-dipping in some patients, although further evidence is needed to determine if this reduces long-term risk
  - Cardiovascular risk attenuation addressing other cardiovascular risk factors (such as hyperlipidemia and obstructive sleep apnea) is recommended

Other components of ABPM interpretation to be aware of:
- Systolic and diastolic BP load
  - Proportion of BPs during the day that are above the patient's goal (>40% is considered "abnormal")
  - Considered to provide additional information about the duration of elevated readings and BP variability
  - Does not seem to provide added prognostic value beyond the mean daytime BP
- Morning surge
  - Difference between early morning BPs and nocturnal BPs
  - No consensus on best approach to calculating
  - May be associated with elevated risk of adverse cardiovascular events
- Short-term BP variability
  - May be due to several factors, such as poor exercise tolerance, stress, anxiety, vascular stiffness, and autonomic dysfunction
  - No consensus on best approach to calculating, but average real variability (the sum of the difference of each successive BP measurement divided by the total number of measurements minus one) is the most strongly linked with adverse outcomes

7. What is HBPM?

HBPM allows patients to monitor their BPs at home over a long period of time using a semiautomated device that is activated by the patient.

8. Why is HBPM performed?

Similar to ABPM, HBPM is performed to detect discrepant BPs outside of the clinic compared to those measured in the clinic and thus to identify MH, MUCH, WCH, and WCE. In contrast to ABPM, HBPM is better suited for long-term monitoring of BP and titration of medications due to greater reproducibility of the readings over time,[10] better tolerability,[11] and easier access to monitors for many patients. However, HBPM is not as strongly linked to adverse cardiovascular outcomes as ABPM,[12] in part, because HBPM does not typically include the measurement of BPs during sleep.

9. How is HBPM performed?

Unlike ABPM, HBPM requires individual patient education on correct BP measurement technique. Patients should be provided with verbal and written instructions on how to perform HBPM appropriately.

Key steps for performing HBPM[6,13,14]:
- Empty the bladder and avoid rigorous exercise, caffeine, alcohol, and cigarette smoking for at least 30 minutes before measurement
- Wear short or loose sleeves or take the arm out of the sleeve so the BP can be performed on a bare arm
- Sit in a comfortable chair with the back supported
- Place the arm through the cuff loop of the nondominant arm
- Slide the cuff up the arm so the bottom edge is about 1 inch (2–3 cm) above the elbow and the tube runs along the inside of the arm; tighten the cuff
- Rest for 3 to 5 minutes before the measurement with no distractions in a quiet room
- Arm supported near the level of the heart
- Feet flat on the floor
- After the first reading is complete, wait approximately 1 minute and then perform a second BP reading
- Record the two readings with the time and date
- Perform measurements in the morning before taking medications and in the evening for a minimum of 3 days, ideally 5 to 7 consecutive days

Patient education should be reiterated over time to ensure ongoing adherence to correct BP measurement technique. Preferably, patients should bring their home device into the clinic to confirm the accuracy of the device against a manual clinic reading and to confirm that they are using appropriate measurement technique.

10. How is HBPM interpreted?

HBPM is interpreted using the mean of the systolic and diastolic BP measurements. Some guidelines recommend discarding BP measurements performed on the first day of HBPM when calculating the mean of the home BPs.[13,14]

Similar to daytime ABPM, the mean HBPM BPs are used to determine the diagnosis of normotension and sustained, white coat, and masked hypertension, typically with a higher threshold than the overall 24-hour mean. Current guidelines recommend antihypertensive treatment targeting home BP thresholds over clinic thresholds due to greater prognostic utility of HBPM and elevated cardiovascular risk associated with MH.

11. Are there important differences in the information obtained using ABPM vs. HBPM?

Both ABPM and HBPM have stronger prognostic value than clinic BPs. However, in contrast to ABPM, HBPM measurements occur exclusively while awake and at rest. Consequently, the readings obtained by ABPM are not always consistent with those obtained by HBPM.[15,16] The prognostic significance of conflicting ABPM and HBPM values is not well understood. Whereas some studies show similar associations of BPs obtained by ABPM and HBPM with cardiac risk, those measured by ABPM are more consistently associated with long-term risk.[5,12]

Table 2.1 International Validated Blood Pressure Monitor Device Listings

SPONSORING MEDICAL SOCIETY	WEBSITE
European Society of Hypertension and International Society of Hypertension	https://www.stridebp.org
Hypertension Canada	https://hypertension.ca/hypertension-and-you/managing-hypertension/measuring-blood-pressure/devices2/
British and Irish Hypertension Society	https://bihsoc.org/bp-monitors/
American Medical Association	https://www.validatebp.org

12. **Does it matter what device is used to perform ABPM and HBPM?**
Accurate BP measurement depends on using a cuff that is the appropriate size for the patient's arm circumference and selecting a monitor that has undergone validation using a widely accepted protocol.[17] Automated BP monitors use proprietary algorithms to estimate the systolic and diastolic BPs. These devices require population-wide and individual-level validation to ensure accuracy. Most countries do not require that devices be validated in order to be marketed to the public, and less than 15% of commercially available BP measurement devices have undergone validation.[18] Hypertension Canada, the British and Irish Hypertension Society, the International Society of Hypertension, the American Medical Association, and other international medical societies maintain online listings of validated devices available in their region (Table 2.1). Wrist and finger BP devices are generally not recommended, as they often perform poorly in validation studies.

KEY POINTS

1. Out-of-office BP monitoring with ABPM or HBPM should be used for the diagnosis and monitoring of hypertension due to the ability to identify abnormal BP patterns that cannot be identified using clinic BP monitoring alone
2. ABPM uses fully automated devices to measure BPs repeatedly over a 24-hour period, whereas HBPM relies upon patients to activate a semiautomated device to measure BP longitudinally
3. HBPM has greater reproducibility, tolerability, and accessibility to most patients compared to ABPM
4. ABPM is more strongly associated with adverse cardiac outcomes than HBPM, in large part, due to the distinct ability to identify nocturnal BPs
5. It is critical to use a validated device

REFERENCES

1. Whelton PK, Carey RM, Aronow WS, et al. 2017 ACC/AHA/AAPA/ABC/ACPM/AGS/APhA/ASH/ASPC/NMA/PCNA guideline for the prevention, detection, evaluation, and management of high blood pressure in adults: a report of the American College of Cardiology/American Heart Association Task Force on Clinical Practice Guidelines. *Hypertension.* 2018;71:e13–e115.
2. Nerenberg KA, Zarnke KB, Leung AA, et al. Hypertension Canada's 2018 guidelines for diagnosis, risk assessment, prevention, and treatment of hypertension in adults and children. *Can J Cardiol.* 2018;34:506–525.
3. Williams B, Mancia G, Spiering W, et al. 2018 ESC/ESH guidelines for the management of arterial hypertension. *Eur Heart J.* 2018;39:3021–3104.
4. Pierdomenico SD, Pierdomenico AM, Coccina F, et al. Prognostic value of masked uncontrolled hypertension. *Hypertension.* 2018;72:862–869.
5. Cohen JB, Lotito MJ, Trivedi UK, Denker MG, Cohen DL, Townsend RR. Cardiovascular events and mortality in white coat hypertension: a systematic review and meta-analysis. *Ann Intern Med.* 2019;170(12):853–862.
6. Muntner P, Shimbo D, Carey RM, et al. Measurement of blood pressure in humans: a scientific statement from the American Heart Association. *Hypertension.* 2019;73(5):e35–e66.
7. Hansen TW, Li Y, Boggia J, Thijs L, Richart T, Staessen JA. Predictive role of the nighttime blood pressure. *Hypertension.* 2011;57:3–10.
8. Parati G, Stergiou GS, Dolan E, Bilo G. Blood pressure variability: clinical relevance and application. *J Clin Hypertens (Greenwich).* 2018;20:1133–1137.
9. Parati G, Stergiou G, O'Brien E, et al. European Society of Hypertension practice guidelines for ambulatory blood pressure monitoring. *J Hypertens.* 2014;32:1359–1366.
10. Guo QH, Cheng YB, Zhang DY, et al. Comparison between home and ambulatory morning blood pressure and morning hypertension in their reproducibility and associations with vascular injury. *Hypertension.* 2019;74:137–144.
11. Kronish IM, Kent S, Moise N, et al. Barriers to conducting ambulatory and home blood pressure monitoring during hypertension screening in the United States. *J Am Soc Hypertens.* 2017;11:573–580.
12. Shimbo D, Abdalla M, Falzon L, Townsend RR, Muntner P. Studies comparing ambulatory blood pressure and home blood pressure on cardiovascular disease and mortality outcomes: a systematic review. *J Am Soc Hypertens.* 2016;10:224–234e17.

13. Parati G, Stergiou GS, Asmar R, et al. European Society of Hypertension practice guidelines for home blood pressure monitoring. *J Hum Hypertens*. 2010;24:779–785.
14. Stergiou GS, Nasothimiou EG, Kalogeropoulos PG, Pantazis N, Baibas NM. The optimal home blood pressure monitoring schedule based on the Didima outcome study. *J Hum Hypertens*. 2010;24:158–164.
15. Kang YY, Li Y, Huang QF, et al. Accuracy of home versus ambulatory blood pressure monitoring in the diagnosis of white-coat and masked hypertension. *J Hypertens*. 2015;33:1580–1587.
16. Anstey DE, Muntner P, Bello NA, et al. Diagnosing masked hypertension using ambulatory blood pressure monitoring, home blood pressure monitoring, or both? *Hypertension*. 2018;72:1200–1207.
17. Cohen JB, Padwal RS, Gutkin M, et al. History and justification of a national blood pressure measurement validated device listing. *Hypertension*. 2019;73:258–264.
18. Sharman JE, O'Brien E, Alpert B, et al. Lancet Commission on Hypertension group position statement on the global improvement of accuracy standards for devices that measure blood pressure. *J Hypertens*. 2020;38:21–29.

CHAPTER 3

CLINICAL EVALUATION OF THE PATIENT WITH HYPERTENSION

Trisha Patel, DO, Arun Kumar, MD, ABIM, Edgar V. Lerma, MD, and George L. Bakris, MD, MA

QUESTIONS

1. **What are the objectives of clinical evaluation of a patient with hypertension?**
   - To identify potentially correctable causes of hypertension
   - To identify other cardiovascular risk factors or concomitant disorders that may influence prognosis and guide treatment
   - To assess end-organ damage (which may affect therapy) and identify baseline abnormalities
   - To assess previous treatment experiences and obstacles to therapy

2. **What is the appropriate method to check blood pressure?**
   See Chapter 1: Measurement of Blood Pressure in the Office

3. **What are the appropriate requisites when taking blood pressure readings?**
   Below are the recommendations for blood pressure (BP) monitoring:
   - Condition
     - Quiet room where there is comfortable seating without distraction
     - Avoid caffeine, cigarettes, and other stimulants 30 minutes before taking the BP
     - Wait at least 30 minutes after a meal
     - If on BP medication, take the BP reading before taking the medication
     - Empty the bladder beforehand
   - Position
     - Keep the back supported
     - Keep feet flat on the floor
     - Sit with legs uncrossed
     - Keep arm supported, palm up, and muscles relaxed
     - Position arm so BP cuff is at the heart level
     - Put the BP cuff on the bare arm, above the elbow at mid-arm
   - Device
     - Validated electronic (oscillometric) upper-arm cuff device
     - Alternatively use a calibrated auscultatory device (aneroid, or hybrid as mercury sphygmomanometers are banned in most countries) with first Korotkoff sound for systolic BP and fifth for diastolic BP with a low deflation rate
   - Cuff
     - Size according to arm circumference (i.e., smaller cuff overestimates BP, and larger cuff underestimates BP [Table 3.1])
   - Protocol
     - Rest for 5 minutes while in position before starting
     - Take two or three measurements, 1 minute apart
     - Keep relaxed and in position during measurements
     - Sit quietly without distractions during measurements (i.e., avoid conversations, television, telephones, and other devices)
     - Record measurements when finished
       See Chapter 1: Measurement of Blood Pressure in the Office, and Chapter 2: Ambulatory and Home Blood Pressure Monitoring

4. **What pertinent information should be obtained during history taking in the patient who initially presents with hypertension?**
   Patients with hypertension are typically asymptomatic; it is important to pay particular attention to historical clues that can point to underlying secondary hypertension as well as hypertensive complications that warrant further investigation.

Table 3.1 Recommended Cuff Sizes for Accurate Measurement of Blood Pressure

ARM CIRCUMFERENCE	BP CUFF SIZE
22–26 cm	12 × 22 cm (Small adult)
27–34 cm	16 × 30 cm (Adult)
35–44 cm	16 × 36 cm (Large adult)

BP, Blood pressure.
(From https://targetbp.org/wp-content/uploads/2016/10/How-to-Measure-Blood-Pressure-at-Home.pdf.)

- **Blood pressure**
  This should be obtained in all patients at all appropriate visits to assess cardiovascular risk and monitor effects of antihypertensive treatment.
  - New onset hypertension, duration, previous BP readings, antihypertensive agents (current and previous), other medications (including herbal medications, nutritional supplements) that may potentially affect BP, history of adverse events related to medications (angiotensin-converting enzyme inhibitor induced angioedema, erectile dysfunction due to beta-blockers), hypertension diagnosed with pregnancy or while taking oral contraceptives)
- **Risk factors**
  - Personal history of cardiovascular disease (myocardial infarction, heart failure, stroke, transient ischemic attack, peripheral vascular disease), diabetes, dyslipidemia, chronic kidney disease (nephrolithiasis); tobacco use; alcohol intake; illicit drug use; analgesic use; soda consumption; physical activity; psychosocial aspects (employment, level of education) that may affect access to care/medications or influence adherence to treatment
  - Family history of hypertension, premature cardiovascular disease (early-onset stroke), diabetes, hypercholesterolemia, chronic kidney disease (polycystic kidney disease, nephrolithiasis)
- **Signs and symptoms**
  - Hypertension/comorbid illnesses
    - Headaches, visual disturbances, chest pain, shortness of breath, palpitations, claudication, peripheral edema, nocturia, hematuria
  - Secondary hypertension (commonly associated with resistant hypertension)
    - Hypokalemia (spontaneous or diuretic induced); muscle cramps or weakness *(primary aldosteronism)*
      See Chapter 8: Primary Aldosteronism and Mineralocorticoid Excess
    - Central obesity; "moon" facies; dorsal and supraclavicular fat pads (buffalo hump); wide 1-cm violaceous striae, easy bruisability; hirsutism; proximal muscle weakness *(Cushing syndrome)*
      See Chapter 9: Glucocorticoid Excess
    - Paroxysmal hypertension or crisis superimposed on sustained hypertension; "spells" of BP lability, headache, sweating, palpitations, pallor *(pheochromocytoma)*
      See Chapter 10: Pheochromocytoma and Paraganglioma
    - Skin stigmata of neurofibromatosis (i.e., café-au-lait spots); neurofibromas *(paraganglioma)*
      See Chapter 10: Pheochromocytoma and Paraganglioma
    - Dry skin, cold intolerance, constipation, weight gain, delayed ankle reflex, periorbital puffiness, slow movement *(hypothyroidism)*
      See Chapter 11: Other Endocrine Causes of Hypertension
    - Warm, moist skin; heat intolerance; diarrhea; weight loss; proximal muscle weakness; lid lag; fine tremors of outstretched hands *(hyperthyroidism)*
      See Chapter 11: Other Endocrine Causes of Hypertension
    - New onset of worsening or difficult to control BP, flash pulmonary edema, holosystolic epigastric bruit with diastolic component, bruits over other arteries (i.e., carotid, femoral *[renovascular disease])*
      See Chapter 12: Renovascular Hypertension
    - Poor sleep quality, snoring, breathing pauses during sleep, daytime sleepiness or tiredness *(obstructive sleep apnea)*
    - Young patient (∼ <30 years) with hypertension; higher BP in upper vs. lower extremities; absent femoral pulses; continuous murmur heard over patient's back, chest, or abdominal bruit *(coarctation of the aorta)*
      See Chapter 14: Obstructive Sleep Apnea

- Recurrent urinary tract infections; obstructive uropathy gross hematuria; urinary urgency, frequency, or dysuria; peripheral edema; elevated serum creatinine; abnormal urinalysis (i.e., microscopic hematuria, proteinuria *[chronic kidney disease])*

5. **What pertinent findings on physical examination should one look for during evaluation of a patient with hypertension?**
   A thorough and detailed physical examination should be performed in the initial evaluation of the patient with hypertension. This helps not only in establishing the diagnosis of hypertension but also in identifying features that point to underlying secondary hypertension. This should include:
   - General
     - Height, weight (body mass index, BMI), waist circumference
   - Heart and circulation
     - Heart rate/rhythm, jugular venous pulse/pressure, apical impulse, extra heart sounds (murmurs, gallops), adventitious sounds (rales), peripheral edema, bruits, radiofemoral delay
   - Other organ systems
     - Skin: striae and fatty deposits
     - Funduscopy
       The Keith, Wagener, and Barker hypertensive retinopathy classification is based on the level of severity of the retinal findings:

GRADE	CLASSIFICATION
Grade I (mild hypertension)	Mild, generalized, retinal, arteriolar narrowing or sclerosis
Grade II (more marked hypertensive retinopathy)	Definite focal narrowing and arteriovenous crossings, moderate to marked sclerosis of the retinal arterioles, exaggerated arterial light reflex
Grade III (mild angiospastic retinopathy)	Retinal hemorrhages, exudates, and cotton wool spots; sclerosis and spastic lesions of retinal arterioles
Grade IV	Severe grade III and papilledema

   - Neck circumference (>40 cm may point to obstructive sleep apnea)
   - Palpably enlarged thyroid gland (goiter)
   - Palpably enlarged kidneys (polycystic kidney disease)

6. **What laboratory and diagnostic tests should be performed as part of hypertension evaluation?**
   Although there appears to be some general consensus between various guidelines as far as routine laboratory and ancillary tests in the evaluation of a patient with hypertension, there are also some minor differences.

	ACC/AHA 2017	ESC/ESH 2018	Hypertension Canada 2020	ISH 2020
ROUTINE Blood tests	• Complete blood count • Chemistries (sodium, potassium, calcium, creatinine with eGFR, TSH)	Serum creatinine and eGFR	Chemistries (sodium, potassium, creatinine: **Grade D;** fasting blood glucose and/or HgbA1C: **Grade D;** Lipid profile: **Grade D)**	Chemistries (sodium, potassium, serum creatinine, eGFR) If available, lipid profile and fasting blood glucose
Urine tests	Urinalysis	Urine albumin to creatinine ratio	Urinalysis **(Grade D)**	Dipstick urine test
Others	12-Lead EKG	• 12-Lead EKG • Funduscopy	12-Lead EKG **(Grade C)**	12-Lead EKG

	ACC/AHA 2017	ESC/ESH 2018	Hypertension Canada 2020	ISH 2020

NON ROUTINE	• 2D ECHO
	• Serum uric acid
	• Urine albumin to creatinine ratio
		• 2D ECHO, carotid ultrasound, abdominal ultrasound, and doppler studies
		• Pulse wave velocity (PWV)
		• Ankle brachial index
		• Cognitive function testing
		• Brain imaging
			• Urine albumin excretion in diabetics *(Grade C)*
			• Pregnancy test prior to initiation of health behavior management changes or drug therapy *(Grade D; NEW 2020 recommendation)*
			• 2D ECHO for all hypertensive patients is not recommended *(Grade D)*
			• 2D ECHO (for assessment of LVM, systolic and diastolic LV function) for hypertensive patients suspected of having LV dysfunction or CAD *(Grade D)*
			• 2D ECHO or Nuclear imaging (for assessment of LVEF) for patients with evidence of heart failure *(Grade D)*
				• 2D ECHO, carotid ultrasound, kidneys/kidney artery and adrenal imaging, fundoscopy, brain CT/MRI
				• Functional tests, additional laboratory investigations
				  • Ankle-brachial index
				  • Further testing for secondary hypertension if suspected (aldosterone-renin ratio, plasma free metanephrines, late-night salivary cortisol, or other screening tests for cortisol excess)
				• Urine albumin/creatinine ratio
				• Serum uric acid
				• Liver function tests

Grade C (Hypertension Canada 2020): Recommendations are on the basis of trials that have lower levels of internal validity and/or precision, or trials for which unvalidated surrogate outcomes were reported, or results from nonrandomized observational studies.
Grade D (Hypertension Canada 2020): Recommendations are on the basis of expert opinion alone.
CAD, Coronary artery disease; *CT*, computed tomography; *2D ECHO*, Two-dimensional echocardiogram; *eGFR*, estimated glomerular filtration rate; *EKG*, electrocardiogram; *ESC*, European Society of Cardiology; *ESH*, European Society of Hypertension; *ISH*, International Society of Hypertension; *JNC*, Joint National Committee; *LV*, left ventricular; *LVEF*, left ventricular ejection fraction; *LVM*, left ventricular myocardium; *MRI*, magnetic resonance imaging; *TSH*, thyroid stimulating hormone.

7. **Which patients require additional diagnostic testing?**
   • Those with historical and clinical features that suggest secondary causes of hypertension
   • Those with resistant hypertension defined by BP >140/90 mm Hg (160/90 mm Hg for patients >60 years old) on maximal doses of at least three appropriate antihypertensives agent
   • Those with previous good BP control with acute unexplained exacerbation
   • Those with hypertension associated with grade 3 or grade 4 retinopathy
   • Those with new onset hypertension after the age of 60 years
   • Those with new or worsening target end-organ damage

8. **What is pseudohypertension?**
   Pseudohypertension is thought to occur in elderly individuals who have stiff or rigid arteries. In particular, measuring the BP with a calibrated auscultatory device can lead to an overestimation of the true intraarterial pressure because of the increased pressure required for the cuff to compress the stiff artery.
   With several proposed definitions, there has been no general consensus. A cutoff of 10 to 15 mm Hg has been arbitrarily used as the cutoff difference between cuff pressures and intraarterial pressures in most published studies.

It should be suspected in elderly patients who present with relatively elevated BP readings in the absence of target organ damage. It is important to be aware of this condition because most elderly or chronically ill individuals who are already at risk for orthostatic or postural hypotension may have acute declines in BP when their antihypertensive regimen is increased on the basis of a cuff pressure that is actually much higher than the real BP and this can prove detrimental.

9. **What is Osler maneuver?**
Osler maneuver can be used to discern pseudohypertension in suspected cases. A positive Osler maneuver test describes the presence of a palpable pulseless brachial or radial artery distal to a point of occlusion of the artery either manually or by cuff inflation. Although this physical finding is compatible with pseudohypertension, some clinicians argue that this maneuver is neither sensitive nor specific enough to rule out true hypertension.

KEY POINTS

1. Patients with hypertension are typically asymptomatic; it is important to pay particular attention to historical clues that can point to underlying secondary hypertension as well as hypertensive complications that warrant further investigation.
2. Pseudohypertension is thought to occur in elderly individuals who have stiff or rigid arteries.

BIBLIOGRAPHY

Ali W, Gao G, Bakris GL. Improved Sleep Quality Improves Blood Pressure Control among Patients with Chronic Kidney Disease: A Pilot Study. *American Journal of Nephrology.* 2020;51(3):249–254.

Bakris GL, Ali W, Parati G. ACC/AHA Versus ESC/ESH on Hypertension Guidelines. *Journal of the American College of Cardiology.* 2019;73(23):3018–3026.

Chobanian AV, Bakris GL, Black HR, et al. Seventh Report of the Joint National Committee on Prevention, Detection, Evaluation, and Treatment of High Blood Pressure. *Hypertension.* 2003;42(6):1206–1252.

Rabi DM, McBrien KA, Sapir-Pichadze R, et al. Hypertension Canada's 2020 Comprehensive Guidelines for the Prevention, Diagnosis, Risk Assessment, and Treatment of Hypertension in Adults and Children. *The Canadian Journal of Cardiolog.* 2020;36(5):596–624.

Unger T, Borghi C, Charchar F, et al. *Hypertension.* 2020 International Society of Hypertension Global Hypertension Practice Guidelines. 2020;75(6):1334-1357.

Weber MA, Schiffrin EL, White WB, et al. Clinical Practice Guidelines for the Management of Hypertension in the Community. *J Clin Hypertens.* 2014;16:14–26.

Whelton PK, Carey RM, Aronow WS, et al. 2017 ACC/ AHA/ AAPA/ ABC/ ACPM/ AGS/ APhA/ ASH/ ASPC/ NMA/ PCNA Guideline for the Prevention, Detection, Evaluation, and Management of High Blood Pressure in Adults: Executive Summary: A Report of the American College of Cardiology/American Heart Association Task Force on Clinical Practice Guidelines. *Circulation.* 2018;138(17):e426–e483.

Williams B, Mancia G, Spiering W, et al. 2018 ESC/ESH Guidelines for the Management of Arterial Hypertension: The Task Force for the Management of Arterial Hypertension of the European Society of Cardiology and the European Society of Hypertension: The Task Force for the Management of Arterial Hypertension of the European Society of Cardiology and the European Society of Hypertension. *J Hypertens.* 2018;36(10):1953–2041.

CHAPTER 4

HYPERTENSIVE EMERGENCIES AND URGENCIES

Ann Bugeja, MD

QUESTIONS

1. **What is a hypertensive emergency?**
   A hypertensive emergency refers to large elevations in systolic and/or diastolic blood pressure with impending or progressive, acute, end-organ damage. The systolic blood pressure is usually 180 mm Hg or higher and/or diastolic blood pressure 120 mm Hg or higher.
   This definition implies that hospitalization for intravenous medication is required and that altering the blood pressure will improve end-organ damage. In-hospital mortality is estimated at 0.2% to 11%.

2. **Why do hypertensive emergencies happen?**
   The most common reason is nonadherence to blood pressure–lowering medication. Greater than 70% of patients diagnosed with a hypertensive emergency in the emergency room have previously diagnosed hypertension and have been prescribed medications. Common associations include a previous history of hypertension; being an elderly, non-White man; a lack of a primary care practitioner, and cocaine use.

3. **What is a hypertensive urgency and how does this differ from a hypertensive emergency?**
   The definition is the same as that for an emergency but there is NO acute end-organ involvement. The absolute level of blood pressure does not distinguish an emergency from an urgency as blood pressure thresholds are different in children and pregnant women, among whom sudden, modest increases in blood pressure can cause severe vascular injury.
   There is a poor correlation between symptoms and the presence of a hypertensive emergency. Patients with chronic hypertension may be asymptomatic with a blood pressure of 220/140 mm Hg. So a hypertensive urgency might not differ from asymptomatic hypertension, and it is important to try to rule out the "acute recognition" of chronic hypertension.

4. **What is the pathophysiology of a hypertensive emergency?**
   With normotension or chronic hypertension, the endothelium modulates vascular resistance through release of vasodilators. An acute and sustained rise in blood pressure leads to endothelial damage, low production of vasodilators, and a significant increase in vasoconstrictors, such as angiotensin II (i.e., loss of endothelial vascular tone). The coagulation system and platelets are activated, leading to fibrinoid necrosis.

5. **What is the role for the terms "accelerated hypertension", "malignant hypertension", and "hypertensive crisis"?**
   Hypertensive crisis has largely been replaced by hypertensive emergency or hypertensive urgency. Malignant, or accelerated, hypertension is not a meaningful term and refers historically to a poor prognosis when blood pressure–lowering medications were not available.

6. **What are the common etiologies of hypertensive emergencies?**
   - Acute aortic dissection
   - Acute coronary syndrome
   - Acute kidney injury
   - Acute left ventricular failure
   - Catecholamine-associated hypertension
   - Hemorrhagic stroke or acute ischemic stroke
   - Hypertensive encephalopathy
   - Preeclampsia, eclampsia

7. **How do you assess for end-organ damage?**
   - Starting with the brain, consider posterior reversible encephalopathy syndrome. Look for symptoms and signs of increased intracranial pressure caused by a severe rise in blood pressure including headache, vomiting, and confusion. This is a diagnosis of exclusion. Focal neurologic signs may suggest a hemorrhagic or ischemic stroke. Hypertensive retinopathy does not correlate well with hypertensive encephalopathy.
   - Retinal changes of hypertensive retinopathy (exudates, hemorrhages, papilledema) should be sought.
   - Chest pain or discomfort may be due to myocardial ischemia or aortic dissection. Acute aortic dissection may be associated with acute, severe back pain. Dyspnea may be due to pulmonary edema.
   - Investigations, depending on the clinical context, include:
     - Complete blood count to look for microangiopathy (microangiopathic hemolytic anemia and thrombocytopenia)
     - Cardiac biomarkers if an acute coronary syndrome is suspected
     - Electrocardiography
     - Chest radiography
     - Urinalysis, serum electrolytes, and creatinine to look for renal dysfunction
     - Computed tomography or magnetic resonance imaging of the brain with neurological signs
     - Computed tomography of the chest if aortic dissection is suspected (do not delay rapid blood pressure lowering)

8. **How do you lower blood pressure safely in a hypertensive emergency?**
   An intravenous medication with short time-to-effect with short off-time is desirable in case blood pressure drops more than desired. Ordering "as needed" intravenous medication can lead to overtreatment. Although choice of therapy may vary according to the specific hypertensive emergency (Table 4.1), prescriber comfort level with medication may also play a role in selecting an intravenous medication in a hypertensive emergency.

   Largely based on consensus, the diastolic blood pressure should be reduced by 10% to 15% or to 110 mm Hg over 30 to 60 minutes. Vascular beds need to adjust to a new, lower blood pressure without causing ischemia as vessels have constricted over time to deliver proper blood flow in chronic hypertension. Excessive blood pressure lowering is associated with an increased risk of death.

   Blood pressure is usually not lowered in the setting of an acute ischemic stroke unless required for acute reperfusion therapy. Because of high mortality, blood pressure lowering is faster for patients with an acute aortic dissection. Blood pressure should be lowered to less than 120/80 mm Hg. Intravenous beta blockade is required to decrease the shear stress on the ruptured intimal flap and minimize propagation of the dissection.

   Intensive care unit admission is often required for minute-to-minute blood pressure monitoring to avoid precipitous drops in blood pressure. Once end-organ damage has "ceased," oral medications must be started before tapering off intravenous medication to avoid rebound hypertension, usually 6 to 12 hours after starting intravenous therapy. Blood pressure–lowering medication that causes precipitous hypertension should be avoided, including nifedipine capsules.

9. **How do you lower blood pressure safely in a hypertensive urgency?**
   Blood pressure in a hypertensive urgency can be safely lowered using oral medications to achieve a gradual blood pressure reduction over 24 to 48 hours, preferably with long-acting agents. Although it takes time to see oral medications achieve a full blood pressure–lowering effect, blood pressure should be lowered with appropriate medication dosing over 24 to 48 hours. Adherence does require subsequent close follow-up. If a patient in the emergency room has a hypertensive urgency and nonadherence is a concern, consider giving oral medications and observe for 4 to 6 hours. Follow-up for hypertension management within 1 to 5 days is vital with a primary care practitioner, internal medicine, or hypertension clinic.

10. **Is it safe to treat a patient with a hypertensive urgency as an outpatient?**
    A recent study examined approximately 2 million outpatient visits between 2008 and 2013, among whom 60,000 had a hypertensive urgency. The study found that patients sent to the emergency room were more likely to get admitted and readmitted without any difference in cardiovascular events or in blood pressure control at 6 months. Once acute end-organ damage is ruled out, patients can be effectively managed with timely outpatient care for management and follow-up. Long-term fatal and nonfatal cardiovascular risk is 50% higher than controls, despite similar blood pressure levels during follow-up. Among those with treatment-resistant hypertension during follow-up, secondary causes of hypertension, such as obstructive sleep apnea, renal artery stenosis, hyperaldosteronism, coarctation of the aorta, pheochromocytoma, and glucocorticoid excess, should be considered.

11. **When do I send my patient to the emergency room for high blood pressure?**
    In an outpatient setting, it can be challenging to distinguish a hypertensive emergency from a hypertensive urgency. Ensure accurate, resting blood pressure measurements. It has been demonstrated that 30 minutes in a quiet room can decrease blood pressure by 20/10 or greater in 32% of patients. Ensure that no drugs are being taken that can raise blood pressure such as nonsteroidal antiinflammatory medications, cocaine, monoamine oxidase inhibitors, and amphetamines. Recent discontinuation of clonidine may cause rebound hypertension.

Table 4.1 Routine Drugs for Hypertensive Emergencies with Dosing

DRUG	CLASS	CONDITIONS	ONSET OF ACTION (min)	DURATION OF ACTION (min)	USUAL DOSING (IV)	RISKS
Labetalol	Combined nonselective beta-blocker and alpha-1 blocker; ratio of IV alpha- to beta-blockade 1:7	Most hypertensive emergencies, including acute kidney injury Not to be used in acute pulmonary edema, asthma, heart block or bradycardia	5–10	2–4 h	10–20 mg bolus or 0.5–2.0 mg/min infusion	Asthma, LV dysfunction
Nicardipine	Dihydropyridine calcium-channel blocker. vasodilator	Most hypertensive emergencies, excluding acute coronary syndromes and acute pulmonary edema due to reflex tachycardia	2–5	1–4 h	5–15 mg/h infusion	
Nitroglycerin	Venous > arteriolar dilation	Acute coronary ischemia or acute pulmonary edema	2–5	5–10	5–100 µg/min infusion	
Nitroprusside	Vasodilator, predominantly arteriolar	Acute pulmonary edema but generally avoided	<1 min	1–10	0.25–10 µg/kg/min infusion	
Phentolamine	Nonselective alpha-adrenergic blocker, vasodilator; positive inotropic and chronotropic effect due to alpha-2 receptor blockade	Catecholamine excess (adrenergic crisis due to pheochromocytoma cr cocaine overdose)	1–2	10–30	5–15 mg bolus every 5–15 minutes	Tachycardia, flushing, headache, vomiting
Enalaprilat	ACE inhibitor, vasodilator	Acute pulmonary edema (in combination with loop diuretic)	15–30	6– ≥12 h	1.25–5 mg every 6 h	Avoid in ACS, pregnancy, acute kidney injury
Hydralazine	Arterial vasodilator	**Avoided** due to unpredictable blooc pressure lowering Generally prefer labetalol as an IV agent for preeclampsia	10–20	1– ≥4 h	10–20 mg	Precipitous hypotension, tachycardia, vomiting, headache

ACE, Angiotensin-converting enzyme; *ACS,* acute coronary syndrome; *h,* hour; *IV,* intravenous, *LV,* left ventricular; *min,* minute(s).

Access to laboratory investigations and the practitioner's knowledge of the patient and their history are important to ruling out a hypertensive emergency. When treating as an outpatient, clonidine can be used to lower blood pressure over hours, whereas most other medications will lower blood pressure over days. Consider combination therapy in patients with previously untreated hypertension.

Rebound hypertension may occur if reinstituting several blood pressure–lowering medications at one time, such as in the setting of nonadherence. It is also important to consider issues that could contribute to nonadherence: (1) medication cost; (2) forgetfulness or cognition issues where a blister pack may help patients recall medications versus pill bottles; (3) beliefs around taking more or less medication; and/or (4) unwanted effects about which practitioners need to inquire such as gynecomastia with spironolactone.

KEY POINTS

1. Distinguishing hypertensive emergency from a hypertensive urgency is important because an emergency can be life-threatening and requires immediate treatment in an intensive care unit.
2. Common etiologies of a hypertensive emergency include acute aortic dissection, acute coronary syndrome, acute kidney injury, acute left ventricular failure, catecholamine-associated hypertension, hemorrhagic stroke or acute ischemic stroke, hypertensive encephalopathy, and preeclampsia/eclampsia.
3. Hypertensive emergencies are managed with intravenous medications according to the type of emergency, but labetalol can be used in most emergencies.
4. A hypertensive urgency can be managed in the outpatient setting with prompt follow-up and without adverse short-term outcomes. Rule out acute recognition of chronic hypertension.
5. Adherence is often an issue with severe, chronic hypertension. Close follow-up is required to work through reasons for adherence, including medication cost, cognition/forgetfulness, beliefs around taking medication, and unwanted medication effects.

BIBLIOGRAPHY

Feldman RD, Zou GY, Vandervoort MK, et al. A simplified approach to the treatment of uncomplicated hypertension: a cluster randomized, controlled trial. *Hypertension*. 2009;53(4):646–653.

Grassi D, O'Flaherty M, Pellizzari M, et al. Hypertensive urgencies in the emergency department: evaluating blood pressure response to rest and to antihypertensive drugs with different profiles. *J Clin Hypertens*. 2008;10(9):662–667.

Marik PE, Rivera R. Hypertensive emergencies: an update. *Curr Opin Crit Care*. 2011;17(6):569–580.

Park SK, Lee DY, Kim W, et al. Comparing the clinical efficacy of resting and antihypertensive medication in patients of hypertensive urgency: a randomized control trial. *J Hypertens*. 2017;35(7):1474.

Patel KK, Young L, Howell EH, et al. Characteristics and outcomes of patients presenting with hypertensive urgency in the office setting. *JAMA Int Med*. 2016;176(7):981–988.

Peixoto AJ. Acute severe hypertension. *N Engl J Med*. 2019;381:1843–1852.

Varon J. Treatment of acute severe hypertension. *Drugs*. 2008;68(3):283–297.

Vaughan CJ, Delanty N. Hypertensive emergencies. *Lancet*. 2000;356(9227):411–417.

Vlcek M, Bur A, Woisetschlager C, et al. Association between hypertensive urgencies and subsequent cardiovascular events in patients with hypertension. *J Hypertens*. 2008;26:657–662.

THE EPIDEMIOLOGY OF HYPERTENSION

Talar B. Kharadjian, MD, and Rakesh Malhotra, MD, MPH

CHAPTER 5

QUESTIONS

1. **What is the prevalence of hypertension?**
   Hypertension is a major global public health problem and is estimated to impact nearly a third of the world's population (1.13 billion people). In the 1970s, higher-income Western countries were known to have the highest prevalence of hypertension when compared to low-income countries, as evidenced by a pooled analysis of 1479 population studies from 200 countries. However, between 1975 and 2015, this trend effectively reversed. Among those who had hypertension, the proportion of people living in low-income countries was 66% in 2000 and more recently has grown to 75%. The average systolic blood pressures (SBPs) have dropped by 2 to 3 mm Hg in Western and high-income Asian-Pacific countries, whereas the highest average SBPs in 2015 were found in Southeast Asia and sub-Saharan Africa.

   According to a 2017 report by the National Center for Health Statistics (NCHS), the prevalence of hypertension in American adults from 2015 to 2016 was estimated to be around 29%. Although the percentage of hypertensive adults in the United States has not significantly changed between 1999 and 2016, the proportion of controlled blood pressure (BP) has improved from 32% to 48% during this period.

   With the recent changes in hypertension definitions introduced by the American College of Cardiology/ American Heart Association (ACC/AHA) 2017, the prevalence of hypertension in the United States expanded from 31% to 45%, thus identifying a growing need for more widespread awareness as well as need for preventive and treatment strategies to reduce the burden of hypertension and downstream health outcomes.

2. **Which groups have a higher risk of developing hypertension and its complications?**
   With each decade of life, hypertension becomes more common. By 75 years of age, more than 70% of Americans meet the criteria for hypertension based on the ACC/AHA definitions. Male gender is associated with higher rates of hypertension before the age of 65 as compared to women (age 20–44 years: 30% vs. 19%; age 45–54 years: 50% vs. 44%; and age 55–64 years: 70% vs. 63%, respectively). However, women older than the age of 75 have a higher prevalence of hypertension (85%) and higher average BPs compared to older men in the same age group (79%). Overall, men are less likely to be aware that they have hypertension and have higher rates of uncontrolled BP.

   African Americans (AAs) are known to have higher risk of developing hypertension and related end-organ complications. The National Health and Nutrition Examination Survey (NHANES) of American adults between 2013 and 2016 found that the prevalence of hypertension was highest in Blacks (31%) compared to Whites (22%) and Mexican Americans (22%). This racial disparity persisted in spite of adjustments for demographics, socioeconomic status, and comorbidities. Similarly, in the Multiethnic Study of Atherosclerosis (MESA) study, investigators have shown an increased incidence rate ratio (IRR) for hypertension among Blacks (IRR = 2.1, 95% confidence interval [CI] = 1.5 to 2.9) as compared to Whites.

   Mexican Americans have lower rates of awareness of the diagnosis of hypertension (28%) as compared to Whites (35%) and Blacks (43%). A larger proportion of hypertensive Blacks and Mexican Americans in NHANES have uncontrolled BP (37% and 38%, respectively) as compared to Whites (28%). These ethnic disparities in hypertension are important to recognize because of disproportionate clinical outcomes in minority populations. AAs experience greater rates of end-stage kidney disease (ESKD), cardiovascular disease (CVD), and all-cause mortality when compared to Whites. Recent studies in different settings demonstrate the incidence of CVD outcomes in AAs is 50% to 100% higher than in Whites. Similarly, the incidence of ESKD in Hispanics is 50% higher than in Whites, although studies have not consistently found an associated increase in mortality risk or CVD events. These findings are largely due to the fact that epidemiological studies to date have not adequately represented the Hispanic population; data from NHANES has largely been limited to Mexican Americans, and further epidemiological studies are needed to examine the disaggregated profiles of specific ethnicities within this culturally, socioeconomically, and genetically heterogeneous group. For instance, cross-sectional analysis of participants in the Hispanic Community Health Study/Study of Latinos (HCHS/SOL) showed that Dominicans, Cubans, and Puerto Ricans have higher rates of hypertension than those of Mexican background.

3. **What are the risk factors for hypertension?**

The risk factors for developing hypertension include diabetes mellitus, hyperlipidemia, chronic kidney disease (CKD), obesity, obstructive sleep apnea, tobacco use, and alcohol use. Physical inactivity is another important contributor for the development of hypertension. In NHANES, a large percentage of Blacks and Mexican Americans reported having no weekly physical activity (27% and 33%, respectively) compared to Whites (15%). Dietary risk factors for high BP include high sodium, low potassium, and low fiber intake.

Environmental and behavioral factors, such as education, occupation, and psychologic stress, are thought to be drivers of disparities in hypertension. Neighborhood disparities may be related to access to healthy food, social cohesion, childhood adversity, and regional safety. Analysis of the MESA study showed that acculturation is associated with a higher risk of hypertension, whereas speaking a non-English language at home and place of birth outside of the United States are inversely correlated with hypertension. For those born outside of the United States, each 10-year increment lived in the United States confers higher odds of hypertension.

Access to health care significantly impacts hypertension outcomes. Fewer than half of individuals with hypertension are aware of their condition, one third are receiving treatment, and fewer than 15% have achieved BP control. Effective interventions have mitigated barriers to care, including programs that connect trained community members to reach individuals with hypertension outside of a traditional health care setting, such as in barber shops within AA communities and patient homes in Argentina.

4. **How does hypertension impact health outcomes?**

Hypertension is the most important contributor to CVD morbidity and mortality. The Framingham study found that all-cause mortality of individuals with hypertension was double that of the general population and threefold higher for CVD-related mortality specifically. In 2015 the estimated all-cause mortality associated with SBP of 140 mm Hg or higher was 8 million (14% of deaths), with deaths related to ischemic heart disease at 40% (3.6 million), ischemic stroke at 38% (1.1 million), and hemorrhagic stroke at 43% (1.4 million).

Epidemiological studies have shown a log-linear relationship between BP and CVD. Individuals with hypertension are three times more likely to have coronary artery disease or peripheral arterial disease and four times more likely to have congestive heart failure (CHF). Cardiovascular mortality risk doubles for every 20 mm Hg of SBP and 10 mm Hg of diastolic BP above 115/75 mm Hg. The Systolic Blood PRessure Intervention Trial (SPRINT) trial showed that the incidence of CHF improves with intensive control of SBP (SBP <120 mm Hg) compared to a SBP target of less than 140 mm Hg (1.3% and 2.1%, respectively).

Similarly, hypertension is responsible for 50% of deaths attributed to stroke. In the Framingham study, individuals with hypertension between the ages of 55 and 64 were seven times as likely to develop stroke. In the Multiple Risk Factor Intervention Trial (MRFIT), hypertension was associated with higher incidence of stroke for every decile of BP, with SBP associated with an eightfold relative risk of stroke.

CKD progression has been shown to be more rapid in people with hypertension. In the Chronic Renal Insufficiency Cohort (CRIC) study, the hazard ratio (HR) for developing ESKD in individuals with SBP of 130 to 139 mm Hg and those of 140 mm Hg or higher was 2.4 and 3.4, respectively, compared to individuals with SBP less than 120 mm Hg.

Relative risk reductions in ischemic heart disease and ESKD have been shown to be proportional to the magnitude of SBP reduction. Every 10 mm Hg reduction in SBP is associated with a 20% risk reduction in CVD events, 27% in stroke, 28% in CHF, and 13% in all-cause mortality.

5. **What percentage of pregnant women are affected by hypertension?**

Hypertension is associated with worse maternal and fetal mortality. It is the leading cause of premature birth and accounts for 16% of maternal death. hypertension during pregnancy is a significant risk factor for developing future hypertension and CVD. Preeclampsia is present in 12% of pregnancies worldwide and disproportionately affects AAs and Hispanic women (11% and 9%, respectively) as compared to Whites (5%). Women with preeclampsia are at higher risk of developing type 2 diabetes mellitus and stroke and three times more likely to develop chronic hypertension. Eclampsia is present in 1 in 2000 deliveries in high-resource countries.

6. **What is the clinical significance of white coat hypertension?**

White coat hypertension is defined as elevated BP measurements at repeated clinic visits in patients untreated for hypertension who have reliable out-of-clinic BP measurements that are at goal. The prevalence of white coat hypertension is 10% to 15% of the general population. Systematic review has demonstrated elevated all-cause mortality and CVD in patients with white coat hypertension compared to normotensive individuals.

7. **How prevalent is masked hypertension?**

Masked hypertension is defined as a normal BP in the clinic or office (<140/90 mm Hg) but an elevated BP out of the clinic (ambulatory daytime BP or home BP >135/85 mm Hg). Of patients with BP readings within normal range when measured in the clinic, 15% to 30% have masked hypertension based on ambulatory or home BP monitoring.

The prevalence of masked hypertension varies by geography. According to the International Ambulatory blood pressure Registry: TEleMonitoring of hypertension and cardiovascular rISk project (ARTEMIS) international registry of ambulatory daytime BP monitoring, the prevalence of masked hypertension varied from 9% in Europe to 16% in Asia and 17% in Africa. A pooled analysis of US population studies in combination with NHANES data estimated a prevalence of 19% for masked hypertension in American adults. Prevalence was higher among individuals who were 65 years of age or older, male, AA, and taking antihypertensive therapy and those with underlying diabetes, obesity, and/or CKD.

Studies have consistently demonstrated that ambulatory BP monitoring correlates better with clinical outcomes than office measurements. Masked hypertension has been associated with end-organ damage, including CKD and CVD. The HR for CVD events in individuals with masked hypertension compared to normotension is 2.1 as compared to 2.6 for sustained hypertension. Masked hypertension based on nighttime BP readings in AAs has been shown to have a twofold increase in CVD events. In a Japanese cohort study, masked hypertension was found to have an HR of 2.1 for stroke compared to normotension.

8. What is the impact of resistant hypertension?

Resistant hypertension is defined as BP remaining above goal despite the use of three full-dose antihypertensives including a diuretic or the use of at least four antihypertensives to achieve control. Resistant hypertension is present in 15% of individuals receiving hypertension treatment. These patients carry the highest risk of CVD and mortality among those with hypertension. Data from the Antihypertensive and Lipid-Lowering Treatment to Prevent Heart Attack Trial (ALLHAT) study showed that individuals with resistant hypertension had higher risk of coronary artery disease, stroke, heart failure, and ESKD (HR 1.5, 1.6, 1.8, and 2.0, respectively). The HR for all-cause mortality was also elevated at 1.3.

9. How often do patients have a secondary cause of hypertension?

In the past, more than 90% of hypertension was attributed to essential hypertension; however, emerging data has revealed that concurrent conditions are most often implicated in hypertension. Identifying secondary causes of hypertension remains clinically impactful in individuals who have resistant hypertension; in this select group of patients, a secondary cause of hypertension is identified in 10% of cases.

Obstructive sleep apnea is concurrently present in 50% of patients with hypertension; the prevalence is higher in those with resistant hypertension (64%–83%). Renovascular disease accounts for up to 34% of patients with a secondary cause of hypertension, whereas pheochromocytoma, Cushing syndrome, and aortic coarctation are seen in less than 1% of cases. Primary aldosteronism accounts for up to 20% of resistant hypertension cases and should be ruled out in the presence of hypokalemia, incidentally discovered adrenal mass in the setting of resistant hypertension, and family history of early-onset hypertension or early-onset stroke (<40 years). Of those with primary aldosteronism, aldosterone-producing adenoma is identified in 40% of patients and bilateral hyperplasia in 60%. Coarctation of the aorta is mostly seen in children and young adults and is considered the most common congenital heart disease (present in 4 in every 1000 live births with male predominance).

KEY POINTS

1. The updated AHA/ACC definitions in 2017 significantly expanded the number of individuals who stand to benefit from BP management.
2. The proportion of American individuals with controlled BP has been increasing for several decades, and the prevalence of hypertension continues to rise in low-income countries.
3. Minorities including AAs and Mexican Americans are at higher risk of developing hypertension and uncontrolled BP and its associated complications.
4. Fewer than 50% of people living with hypertension are aware of their underlying condition, and only 15% have achieved optimal BP control.
5. A secondary cause of hypertension is found in 10% of patients evaluated for resistant hypertension.

BIBLIOGRAPHY

ACC/AHA/AAPA/ABC/ACPM/AGS/APhA/ASH/ASPC/NMA/PCNA. Guideline for the prevention, detection, evaluation, and management of high blood pressure in adults: a report of the American College of Cardiology/American Heart Association Task Force on Clinical Practice Guidelines. *Hypertension.* 2018;71(19):2199–2269.

American Heart Association Council on Epidemiology and Prevention, American Heart Association Council on Clinical Cardiology, & American Heart Association Council on Cardiovascular and Stroke Nursing. Status of cardiovascular disease and stroke in Hispanics/Latinos in the United States: a science advisory from the American Heart Association. *Circulation.* 2014;130(7):593–625.

Huang Y, Huang W, Mai W, et al. White-coat hypertension is a risk factor for cardiovascular diseases and total mortality. *J Hypertens.* 2017;35:677–688.

Judd E, Calhoun D. Apparent and true resistant hypertension: definition, prevalence and outcomes. *J Hum Hypertens.* 2014;28(8): 463–468.

Lackland D. Racial differences in hypertension: implications for high blood pressure management. *Am J Med Sci.* 2014;348(2):135–138.

Mills K, Stefanescu A, He J. The global epidemiology of hypertension. *Nat Rev Nephrol.* 2020;16(4):223–237.

NCD Risk Factor Collaboration (NCD-RisC). Worldwide trends in blood pressure from 1975 to 2015: a pooled analysis of 1479 population-based measurement studies with 19.1 million participants. *Lancet.* 2017;389(10064):37–55.

Parcha V, Patel N, Kalra R, et al. Prevalence, awareness, treatment, and poor control of hypertension among young American adults: race stratified analysis of the National Health and Nutrition Examination Survey. *Mayo Clin Proceed.* 2020;95(7):1390–1403.

Peacock J, Diaz K, Viera A, et al. Unmasking masked hypertension: prevalence, clinical implications, diagnosis, correlates and future directions. *J Hum Hypertens.* 2014;28(9):521–528.

Redmond N, Baer H, Hicks L. Health behaviors and racial disparity in blood pressure control in the national health and nutrition examination survey. *Hypertension.* 2011;57(3):383–389.

CHAPTER 6

PHYSIOLOGY OF BLOOD PRESSURE REGULATION

Irma Husain, MD, Fitra Rianto, MD, Christopher Asuzu, MD, and Matthew A. Sparks, MD

QUESTIONS

SHORT-TERM REGULATION OF BLOOD PRESSURE

1. **What are the two components of measured blood pressure and what do they represent?**
   An individual's blood pressure, or systemic arterial pressure, refers to the pressure measured within large arteries in the systemic circulation. This number splits into systolic blood pressure (SBP) and diastolic blood pressure (DBP). SBP refers to the maximum pressure within the large arteries when the heart contracts to propel blood through the body. DBP describes the lowest pressure within the large arteries during heart relaxation between beatings.

2. **What is mean arterial pressure and its hemodynamic determinants?**

$$MAP = (CO \times SVR) + CVP$$

   Mean arterial pressure (MAP) is the average blood pressure during a single cardiac cycle. As mentioned in the formula above, MAP is the product of cardiac output (CO) and systemic vascular resistance (SVR) plus the central venous pressure (CVP). CVP can typically be neglected due to the small value. Interestingly, the fraction of time spent in a cardiac cycle between systole and diastole is two thirds and one third, respectively; therefore when noninvasive blood pressure (NIBP) is measured via a cuff, MAP can be estimated as $\frac{2}{3}$ SBP + $\frac{1}{3}$ DBP, and its normal value falls within the range of 65 to 100 mm Hg.

3. **What factors determine CO?**
   The volume of blood being pumped per minute through the circulatory system is defined as CO and is directly proportional to both the heart rate (HR), that is the number of beats per minute, and stroke volume (SV), which is the amount of blood pumped from the ventricles per beat. Therefore it is represented by the formula:

$$CO = HR \times SV$$

   External influences, specifically, the autonomic nervous system, determines the HR through altering the spontaneous depolarization of the cardiac pacemaker cells in the sinoatrial (SA) node. On the other hand, SV is the difference between left ventricular end diastolic volume (EDV) and end systolic volume (ESV), of which the former is determined by venous return and the latter inversely by cardiac contractility.

4. **Define the Frank-Starling law of the heart?**
   This law defines an integral intrinsic mechanical property of the myocardium. The Frank-Starling law states that, for a fixed total load, SV increases as cardiac filling increases. Therefore an increase in preload will increase EDV and SV due to the increase in extent of cardiac sarcomere shortening during contraction.

5. **What are the determinants of SVR?**
   Poiseuille law states that the velocity of the steady flow of a fluid through a narrow tube (as a blood vessel or a catheter) is directly proportional to the pressure and the fourth power of the radius of the tube and inversely to the length of the tube and the coefficient of viscosity. Thus a small change in arterial diameter will result in a significant increase in SVR, making this mechanism the predominant factor responsible for sizeable changes in MAP. The vasoconstriction and vasodilation mechanisms are mediated through the autonomic nervous system and through the effect of various hormones discussed in this chapter.

6. **What are the primary mechanisms involved in the short-term regulation of blood pressure?**
   The predominant mechanism for the short-term regulation of blood pressure occurs via the autonomic nervous system, which subsequently moderates changes to CO and SVR. The autonomic nervous system can be divided into two pathways—the parasympathetic and sympathetic nervous systems.

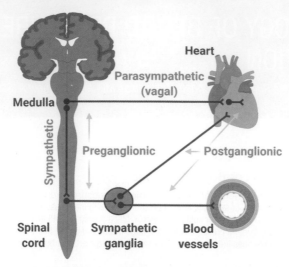

Fig. 6.1 **Autonomic innervation of the heart and vasculature.** (Created with BioRender.com.)

Parasympathetic Nervous System: The cardiovascular effects of the parasympathetic nervous system are primarily mediated by the efferent fibers of the vagus nerve (cranial nerve [CN] X). Although the cardiac pacemaker cells of the SA node exhibit automaticity, they can be influenced by agents that augment their rate of firing. The pacemaker cells of the SA node are innervated by the vagus nerve, which mainly acts to decrease chronotropy via the release of acetylcholine and activation of muscarinic receptors located on cardiac pace-maker cells. As previously noted, this can decrease CO and thus decrease blood pressure.

Sympathetic Nervous System: The cardiovascular effects of the sympathetic nervous system are mediated via the release of catecholamines—epinephrine and norepinephrine. The effects of these catecholamines causes direct and indirect stimulation of their target organs via the release of norepinephrine at peripheral synapses located within the vascular smooth muscle cells and cardiac myocytes and the release of epinephrine and norepinephrine from chromaffin cells located within the adrenal medulla. Their effect is moderated via the activation of α and β adrenergic receptors located at the membranes of their target tissues. Their overall effect is to increase vascular resistance via activation of α_1 receptors located within the vascular smooth muscle and to increase chronotropy and contractility via activation of β_1 receptors located on the cardiac pacemaker cells and cardiac myocytes, respectively. Activation of these receptors leads to an increase in CO and SVR, resulting in an overall increase in blood pressure (Fig. 6.1).

7. **What is the role of the baroreceptor reflex in regulation of MAP?**
   The baroreceptor reflex describes an important way by which the body attempts to maintain a constant blood pressure in the face of acute changes. This homeostatic mechanism relies on the actions of specialized neurons known as baroreceptors, which are stretch-sensitive mechanoreceptors primarily located at the bifurcation of the internal and external carotid arteries and aortic arch. These baroreceptors respond mainly to passive stretching of the arterial wall. The baroreceptors in the carotid sinuses are innervated by the sinus nerve of Haring, a branch of the glossopharyngeal nerve (CN IX), which synapses in the nucleus tractus solitarius (NTS) located in the dorsal medulla. The baroreceptors in the aortic arch are alternatively innervated by the aortic nerve, a branch of the vagus nerve (CN X), which also synapses in the NTS. Together, these comprise the afferent limb of a negative feedback system known as the baroreceptor reflex loop. The efferent limb of the baroreceptor reflex loop starts at the level of the NTS, which modifies the activity of the sympathetic and parasympathetic in the medulla to exhibit autonomic control of the cardiovascular system to maintain a constant blood pressure (Fig. 6.2).

8. **What is the role of chemoreceptors in the regulation of blood pressure?**
   Carotid body chemoreceptors have been implicated in the mechanism of hypertension correlated with sleep apnea syndrome in which a reversible diurnal elevation of blood pressure occurs as a result of periods of brief hypoxic episodes. Additionally, an accumulation of partial pressure of carbon dioxide (pCO_2) within the cerebral vasculature in the case of cerebral ischemia leads to the activation of the sympathetic system, thereby increasing blood pressure to facilitate cerebral perfusion. The primary role of chemoreceptors is to maintain arterial pH, pCO_2, and partial pressure of oxygen (pO_2) by regulating respiratory activity. Chemoreceptors are primarily located in the periphery at the carotid and aortic bodies and centrally in the cardiovascular regulatory center within the medulla. Like baroreceptors, chemoreceptors in the carotid and aortic bodies are innervated by branches of the

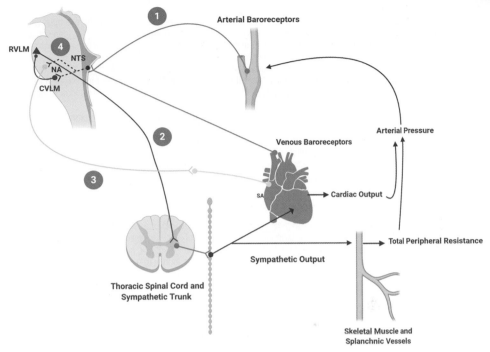

Fig. 6.2 Baroreflex pathways for postural blood pressure control. *(1)* Baroreceptor afferents synapse at the nucleus of the nucleus tractus solitarius *(NTS)*. *(2)* The vagal baroreflex pathway runs from the NTS to the nucleus ambiguus *(NA)*, which sends efferents *(3)* to the sinoatrial node (SA). *(4)* The adrenergic baroreflex pathway runs from the NTS to the caudal ventrolateral medulla *(CVLM)* and from there to the rostral ventrolateral medulla *(RVLM)*. The adrenergic pathway continues with sympathetic efferents from the RVLM to the intermediolateral thoracic spinal cord and from there to autonomic ganglia and to the heart, arterioles, and venules. (Created with BioRender.com.)

glossopharyngeal nerve (CN IX) and vagus nerve (CN X), respectively. Their action is mediated via the chemoreceptor reflex such that decreased arterial pO_2 (hypoxemia), increased arterial pCO_2 (hypercapnia), and decreased arterial blood pH (acidemia) results in decreased parasympathetic outflow to the heart and increased sympathetic tone, resulting in an increased CO via increased HR and SV, systemic vasoconstriction, and an increased respiratory rate to facilitate gas exchange. Additionally, an accumulation of pCO_2 within the cerebral vasculature in case of cerebral ischemia leads to the activation of the sympathetic system, thereby increasing blood pressure to facilitate cerebral perfusion.

9. **Describe and indicate the mechanisms involved in the Bezold–Jarisch reflex.**
   This is a reflex originating from cardiac chemoreceptors concentrated in the posterior wall of the left ventricle of the heart. This reflex can be elicited in pathological conditions such as a myocardial infarction involving that region resulting in bradycardia and hypotension. This is in contrast to the more common reaction to myocardial infarction, which leads to hypotension and tachycardia from an arterial baroreceptor response.

10. **What are the cardiovascular responses associated with emotion?**
    The origin of these responses is in the cerebral cortex, which, through the cortico hypothalamic pathways, reaches the medullary cardiovascular centers. Most importantly, these responses include the flight and fight response and vasovagal syncope. The flight and fight response includes a myriad of effects, but the cardiovascular effect is a general increase in sympathetic nervous activity as well as a decrease in parasympathetic activity. Conversely, an extremely stressful stimuli can result in vasovagal syncope, and this loss of consciousness is due to a precipitous loss of arterial blood pressure from sudden loss of sympathetic tone combined with an increase in parasympathetic tone and decrease in HR.

11. **What is the effect of pain on blood pressure?**
    Depending on the origin of it, pain can have either a positive or negative influence on blood pressure. Typically, pain that is superficial or cutaneous in origin can cause a rise in blood pressure through sympathetic stimulation and blunting of parasympathetic responses. However, severe pain that is of visceral origin, such as from crush injuries, can result in a cardiovascular response similar to vasovagal syncope resulting in low blood pressure.

12. Describe the effect of exercise on cardiovascular response?

The cardiovascular response varies with the type of skeletal muscle activity during exercise; for example, with dynamic exercise, which is any exercise that involves muscle and joint movement, HR, CO, and oxygen consumption all increase linearly with exercise intensity up to maximal levels. Skeletal muscle contraction and relaxation increase the pressure gradient across the muscle vascular bed, which leads to more displacement of blood volume in the muscle vasculature, therefore enhancing the cardiac venous return and hence the CO. This effect has been described as the "muscle pump effect." Despite the increase in CO, only a modest increase in blood pressure occurs. This is due to a decrease in total SVR as a result of vascular dilation in skeletal muscle vascular beds.

On the other hand, the effect of sustained isometric skeletal muscle contraction seen in exercise such as holding a posture, the blood pressure, CO, and HR all increase, but the rise in blood pressure is far greater in proportion to the metabolic energy expenditure of the isometric exercise. Secondly, the cardiovascular adjustments to isometric contraction do not reach a steady state, unlike dynamic exercise. A significant consequence of this is seen in cardiovascular disease in which an isometric muscle activity like shoveling snow can precipitate symptoms of angina. This is secondary to the enhanced metabolic demand placed on ischemic coronary vessels because of atherosclerosis.

LONG-TERM REGULATION OF BLOOD PRESSURE (Fig. 6.3)

13. What are the key factors in the long-term regulation of blood pressure?

A central mechanism to maintaining long-term blood pressure control is the regulation of fluid and salt balance by the kidney, mainly through the following mechanisms: tubuloglomerular feedback, glomerulotubular balance, and pressure natriuresis. Many hormonal systems conspire to act upon the kidney to regulate sodium and volume homeostasis. Most notable is the renin-angiotensin-aldosterone system. Other hormonal systems include natriuretic peptides, vasopressin, prostaglandins, endothelins, and kallikreins.

14. What is pressure natriuresis?

The kidney has a remarkable capacity to resist fluctuations in blood pressure. Pressure natriuresis is a phenomenon whereby increases in blood pressure results in enhanced sodium and water excretion by the kidney. This mechanism was described by Dr. Arthur Guyton. Guyton described how the kidney is an infinite gain system. In this system, urinary salt and water excretion is fine-tuned to respond to stimuli causing high blood

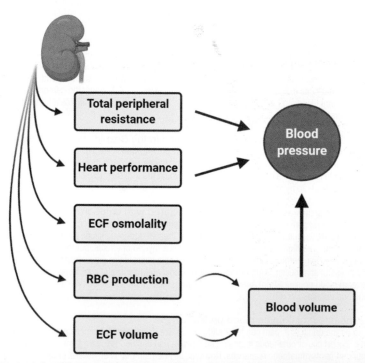

Fig. 6.3 The kidney's role in maintenance of blood pressure. *ECF,* Extracellular fluid, *RBC,* red blood cell. (Created with BioRender.com.)

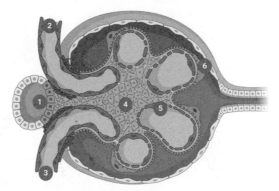

Fig. 6.4 Anatomy of the glomerulus and juxtaglomerular apparatus. Schematic diagram of a section of a glomerulus and its juxtaglomerular apparatus. *(1)* Macula densa; *(2)* efferent arteriole; *(3)* afferent arteriole; *(4)* mesangial cell; *(5)* endothelial cell; *(6)* podocyte. (Created with BioRender.com.)

pressure in an attempt to lower blood pressure to normal values. However, all of the factors that contribute to the mechanism of pressure natriuresis are still being elucidated. Some evidence points toward a direct increase in urinary output secondary to hydraulic pressure from high blood pressure itself, whereas other studies have suggested a decrease in sympathetic tone, diminishing sodium transporter expression and activity.

15. **What is juxtaglomerular apparatus and tubuloglomerular feedback? (Fig. 6.4)**
The juxtaglomerular apparatus (JGA) is anatomical juxtaposition of several cellular constituents aimed to control blood pressure by augmenting renin release and modulating afferent and efferent vascular tone, all located at the glomerular hilum: the afferent and efferent arterioles, granular cells (cells that secrete renin), extraglomerular mesangium, and macula densa (a specialized group of distal convoluted tubule cell). Tubuloglomerular feedback is a mechanism by which the vascular input and output of each individual glomeruli senses the intratubular electrolyte makeup of its own nephron. This is an important way by which the kidney is able to maintain homeostasis. The feedback mechanism relies on intratubular filtrate passing by the macula densa. Specialized cells within the macula densa sense the abundance of sodium chloride in the filtrate through a variety of mechanisms.

16. **How does tubuloglomerular feedback increase glomerular filtration rate? (Fig. 6.5)**
Decreased sodium chloride concentration is perceived as low glomerular filtration rate (GFR) leading the macula densa to produce prostaglandin E_2 (PGE_2) and nitric oxide (NO). Both PGE_2 and NO release lead to relaxation of the afferent arteriole and increased renin secretion from juxtaglomerular cells (further activating the renin-angiotensin system [RAS]), resulting in vasoconstriction of the efferent arteriole, thus increasing intraglomerular pressure and increasing the GFR.

17. **How does tubuloglomerular feedback decrease GFR? (Fig. 6.6)**
Increases in tubular flow and sodium chloride concentration in the intratubular filtrate that reach the macula densa results in the release of adenosine triphosphate (ATP) or its metabolite, adenosine, which constricts the

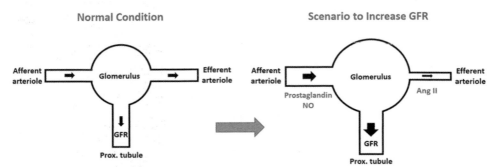

Fig. 6.5 The effects of tubuloglomerular feedback in increasing glomerular filtration rate *(GFR)*. *Ang II,* Angiotensin II; *NO,* nitric oxide; *Prox.,* proximal.

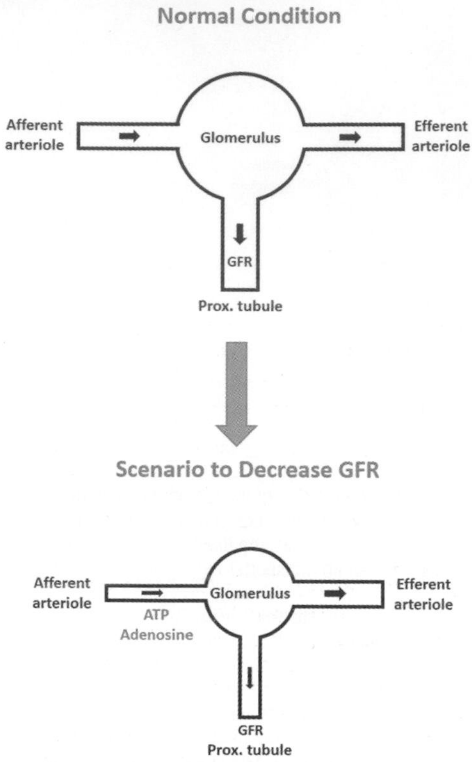

Normal Condition

Afferent arteriole → Glomerulus → Efferent arteriole

↓ GFR

Prox. tubule

Scenario to Decrease GFR

Afferent arteriole → Glomerulus → Efferent arteriole

ATP
Adenosine

↓

GFR
Prox. tubule

Fig. 6.6 The effects of tubuloglomerular feedback in decreasing glomerular filtration rate *(GFR). ATP,* Adenosine triphosphate; *Prox.,* proximal.

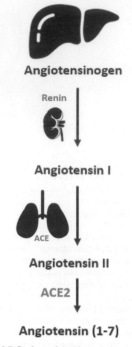

Angiotensinogen

Renin

Angiotensin I

ACE

Angiotensin II

ACE2

Angiotensin (1-7)

Fig. 6.7 Renin-angiotensin system cascade. *ACE,* Angiotensin-converting enzyme; *ACE2,* angiotensin-converting enzyme-2.

afferent arteriole. This results in reducing intraglomerular pressure and diminished flow through the glomerular capillaries, decreasing GFR.

18. **What is the concept of glomerulotubular balance?**
Glomerulotubular balance is the tubule responding to alterations in glomerular filtrate. This concept describes how each proximal tubule segment attempts to respond to changes in glomerular filtrate and solutes parallel to filtered load. The proximal tubule segments are capable of increasing the reabsorption of sodium and other solutes in response to an increase of filtered load and vice versa. Tubuloglomerular feedback and glomerulotubular balance work in concert to ensure the amount of sodium delivered to the distal tubule is relatively constant and thus homeostasis is achieved.

19. **What are the components of the RAS? (Fig. 6.7)**
The RAS plays a central role in the regulation of blood pressure. It is a multienzymatic cascade wherein the major substrate, angiotensinogen, a large 485 amino acid protein produced by the liver, is converted into the 10 amino acid peptide fragment angiotensin (Ang) I by the enzyme renin. Ang I has no known biological activity and is cleaved by angiotensin-converting enzyme (ACE) to produce the major biologically active 8 amino acid peptide Ang II. Most classically identified RAS functions of maintenance of arterial pressure are mediated through angiotensin receptors, the major subclass being angiotensin 1 (AT_1) receptors. These functions include increased sympathetic activity, tubular Na^+ reabsorption and water retention, aldosterone secretion, arteriolar vasoconstriction, and antidiuretic hormone (ADH) secretion. Angiotensinogen is primarily synthesized in the liver. However, more recently it has been demonstrated that several other organ systems are capable of producing all of the components of the RAS including angiotensinogen. This is termed the so-called *intraorgan RAS* and includes the brain, immune system, kidney, and adipose, among others. In the kidney, angiotensinogen is synthesized in the proximal tubules and regulated through negative feedback from Ang II. Typically, the concentration of angiotensinogen in plasma is near half maximal activity (Michaelis Constant, Km); thereby, at any given renin level, the generation rate of Ang I is very

sensitive to small changes in angiotensinogen level. Therefore pathological but only modest elevations in angiotensinogen as a result of angiotensinogen gene mutations can lead to elevated blood pressure.

ACE is the cleaving enzyme that converts the inactive precursor Ang I to active Ang II and is also responsible for metabolism and degradation of bradykinin. ACE is ubiquitously expressed on cell surfaces of endothelial cells, with particular abundance in the lung, intestine, choroid plexus, placenta, and brush border in the tubules of the kidney and also exists in a soluble form circulating in plasma. Furthermore, a homolog of ACE, called ACE2, is expressed on endothelial cells. ACE2 hydrolyzes Ang II and thus leads to generation of Ang -(1-7). Ang -(1-7) acts upon the Mas receptor and has been implicated in promoting vasodilation and natriuresis. However, the physiological role remains unclear. Therefore the ACE-Ang II-AT1 receptor pathway is identified as "classic" RAS, whereas the ACE2-Ang-(1-7)-Mas axis (and the Ang II/Ang III-AT2 receptor pathway) has been recognized as the "non-classic" RAS pathway.

20. How are the plasma levels of renin regulated?

Renin is found in the granular cells within the JGA. The amount of renin in the circulation is regulated by the JGA through kidney baroreceptors that respond to kidney perfusion pressure and sodium chloride delivery to the macula densa. 1. Renin secretion is inversely proportional to perfusion pressure, which explains how, in the case of renal artery stenosis, a drop in perfusion pressure sensed by baroreceptors stimulates renin release resulting in hypertension. 2. The second major pathway of renin release is through sensing of chloride in the macula densa, wherein a reduction in the delivery of chloride, through various signaling pathways, promotes renin release and vice versa. 3. Ang II regulates renin release through a negative feedback by activating AT_1 receptors expressed in the JGA. 4. β-Adrenergic receptors are expressed in the JGA; therefore sympathetic activation is also a stimulus for renin release.

21. What are the hemodynamic effects of Ang II and its receptors?

Ang II is a potent vasoconstrictor and plays a central role in regulating blood pressure within various tissues, including the kidney where it affects glomerular hemodynamics and disproportionately leads to more constriction of efferent arterioles comparative to the afferent arterioles, thereby causing an increased glomerular hydrostatic pressure, which, in turn, preserves the GFR in a state of volume depletion or diminished blood pressure. Furthermore, afferent arteriolar constriction leads to reduced renal blood flow, a consequential increase in filtration fraction, and reduced peritubular capillary pressure, all of which together increases proximal tubular sodium reabsorption. This mechanism delineates the GFR-preserving effect of RAS activation in bilateral renal artery stenosis. On the other hand, RAS blockade in diabetic nephropathy reduces glomerular hemodynamic pressure, which is thought to be a key renoprotective mechanism.

Aside from the glomerular hemodynamic effects, the modulation of kidney medullary circulation by Ang II can control both pressure natriuresis as well as production of vasodilators like NO, therefore suggesting that alterations in the balance between the two can alter systemic blood pressure. In the proximal tubule, Ang II modulates the fluid and solute excretion through its effect on the Na^+/H^+ exchanger. Lastly, Ang II acts on the posterior pituitary to release ADH and, through its effect on the hypothalamus, stimulates thirst and water intake.

Kidney Hemodynamic Consequences of Commonly Used Medications

Pharmacologic Effect	Afferent Arteriole	Efferent Arteriole	Renal Blood Flow	eGFR (short-term)	MAP
ACE inhibitor	Dilation +	Dilation ++	Increase	Reduction	Reduction
ARB	Dilation +	Dilation ++	Increase	Reduction	Reduction
Renin inhibition	Dilation +	Dilation ++	Increase	Reduction	Reduction
Mineralocorticoid receptor antagonism	Unchanged	Unchanged	Unchanged	Minimal reduction	Reduction
SGLT-2 inhibition	Constriction +	Unchanged	Unchanged	Reduction	Reduction (minimal)

ACE, Angiotensin-converting enzyme; *ARB,* angiotensin receptor blocker; *eGFR,* estimated glomerular filtration rate; *MAP,* mean arterial pressure; *SGLT-2,* sodium-glucose cotransporter-2.

22. What are the various stimuli for aldosterone release?

Aldosterone is a steroid hormone synthesized in the zona glomerulosa (ZG) of the adrenal gland that is regulated through three distinct mechanisms:

1. Its synthesis and release is regulated by Ang II acting through AT1Rs in the ZG.
2. The other stimulus for aldosterone release is hyperkalemia, which is independent of Ang II and occurs through membrane depolarization of ZG cells.
3. Elevations in adrenocorticotropic hormone (ACTH) can upregulate aldosterone production in the short term.

23. **What are the effects of aldosterone and how are they mediated?**

   In the distal nephron, aldosterone binds to the mineralocorticoid receptor (MR) located in the principal cells of the collecting tubular epithelium, which, in turn, causes translocation of the epithelial sodium channel (ENaC) to the luminal surface, resulting in uptake of sodium into the circulation. These ENaCs are composed of three structural subunits: α-, β-, and γ-ENaC, each of which are regulated both quantitatively and qualitatively by aldosterone, which results in proteolytic cleavage of the apical loops of the subunits, as well as translocation to the apical membrane of the collecting duct tubular cell. Subsequently, the generation of an electronegative potential in the initial collecting duct and the cortical collecting duct favors secretion of potassium via the renal outer medullary potassium (ROMK) channels of the principal cells into the urine. MRs are also expressed in the vascular endothelial and smooth muscle cells where they contributed to blood pressure control through inhibition of NO-mediated vascular relaxation and reactive oxygen species (ROS) production.

24. **What is the role of the kinin-kallikrein system (KKS) in blood pressure regulation?**

   The kinin polypeptides, bradykinin and kallidin among others, perform a myriad of functions that include the regulation of blood pressure and play a role in inflammation. Their precursor kininogens are synthesized in the liver and subsequently cleaved by plasma and tissue kallikreins. There are two kinin G protein-coupled receptors, B1 and B2 receptors, the latter of which, through calcium stimulation of cyclic guanosine monophosphate, generates NO that mediates renal medullary vasodilation. Bradykinin activates prostaglandin synthesis and excretion as well, which plays a major role in mediating kinin actions like lowering glomerular filtration through preferentially decreasing the efferent arteriolar tone. Kinins have a major role in pressure natriuresis, which contributes to the antihypertensive effect of ACE inhibition by reduced degradation of bradykinin by ACE.

25. **What are endothelins and what role do they play in blood pressure regulation?**

   Endothelins (ETs) are 21 amino acid peptides. Three isoforms exist and are coded on three different chromosomes (ET-1, ET-2, ET-3). Each has a strong vasoactive feature that contributes to blood pressure control and is involved in fluid electrolyte homeostasis and nervous system function. They are primarily produced by vascular endothelial cells, although kidney, lung, colon epithelial cells, and immune cells, as well as certain neurons, can produce ETs. ETs act via activation of G protein-coupled ET_A and ET_B receptors. ET_A and ET_B receptors are ubiquitously expressed in the body. Activation of ET_A receptor in the smooth muscle leads to vasoconstriction, and activation of ET_B leads to vasodilation. In the kidney, ET-1 and ET_B receptors are expressed abundantly in the collecting duct and play a role in kidney sodium excretion. Mouse models have shown that salt sensitive hypertension develops when ET-1 is removed from collecting tubules. Deletion of ET_B receptors from the collecting duct leads to an increased blood pressure that is exacerbated with a high-salt diet. Endothelin has also shown to be elevated in the plasma of patients with hypertension and kidney diseases, although the relationship is not well understood.

26. **What is the role of prostaglandins in blood pressure regulation? (Fig. 6.8)**

   Prostaglandins (PGs) are a group of eicosanoids that synthesized from the oxygenation of the polyunsaturated, essential fatty acid called *arachidonic acid*. This oxygenation is mediated by cyclooxygenase (COX) enzymes. These enzymes are present in a variety of cells throughout the body and have two isoforms, COX-1 and COX-2. There are numerous products derived from arachidonic acid metabolism. Chief among them are PGs, including PGD_2, E_2, F_2, thromboxane A_2, and prostacyclin. PGs play a role in several physiological mechanisms such as inflammation, the gastrointestinal tract, the genitourinary system, the neuronal system, and the cardiovascular system. Their actions are mediated by G protein–coupled receptors. Each prostaglandin binds to their specific receptor. For instance, prostaglandin D_2 binds to DP receptors that are expressed in the ileum, lung, stomach, and uterus. PGE_2 binds to its receptors (EP1-EP4), which are expressed ubiquitously throughout the body, although EP1 is only expressed in the kidney, lung, and stomach. PG F_2 binds to FP receptors that are expressed in the corpus luteum of the ovary. Prostacyclin binds to IP receptors that are mainly expressed on neuron cells. IP receptors are also expressed in the kidney, specifically along the afferent arterioles of glomerulus. Thromboxane binds to TP receptors that are expressed in tissues rich in vasculature including the heart, lung, and kidney and also in the thymus and spleen. The activations of these receptors initiate different actions. The IP, DP, EP2, and EP4 receptors are known as relaxant receptors that induce smooth muscle relaxation, whereas the TP, FP, and EP1 receptors known as contractile receptors that induce smooth muscle contraction. The EP3 receptor has been shown to have inhibitory features. PGs have been shown to regulate blood flow and ion transport in the kidney. PGs, as well as their receptors, are produced along the nephron and kidney vasculature. For example, PGs are produced in macula densa when tubular flow and sodium chloride concentration is reduced and stimulate the dilation of the afferent arteriole. PGs also increase renin secretion, which subsequently activates the RAS. In the distal nephron, PGE_2 reduces sodium reabsorption, which results in salt and water excretion.

27. **What are the roles of the skin and immune system in blood pressure regulation?**

   The classic Guytonian model presumes that the two major components of extracellular volume, intravascular and interstitial spaces, are in equilibrium. The skin can act as a sodium reservoir in hypertonic concentrations that exists complexed with proteoglycans in the subdermal area. Lymphangiogenesis through macrophage activation also acts as a salt-buffering mechanism to maintain blood pressure in the state of high salt load by increasing the lymph capillary transport capacity of sodium. Secondly, the inflammatory

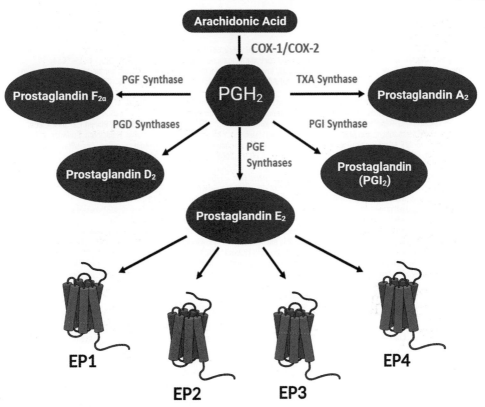

Fig. 6.8 Pathways of eicosanoids synthesis from arachidonic acid. *COX-1,2,* Cyclooxygenase 1,2; *EP1-4,* prostaglandin E receptors 1-4; *PGD,* prostaglandin D; *PGE,* prostaglandin F; *PGF,* prostaglandin F; *PGH₂,* prostaglandin H₂; *PGI,* prostaglandin I; *TXA,* thromboxane A. (Created with BioRender.com.)

mediators and cellular constituents of the immune system, including the nuclear factor κ-light chain enhancer of activated B-cells (NF-κB) signaling cascade, tumor necrosis factor-α (TNF-α), interleukins, cytokines, and triggering of ROS generation, have been implicated in modulating sodium handling by the kidney.

KEY POINTS

1. The two components of arterial pressure are SBP and DBP.
2. MAP is calculated as ⅔ SBP + ⅓ DBP and MAP = CO × SVR.
3. CO = HR × SV, where SV is determined by preload and contractility.
4. Starling's law states that, for a fixed total load, SV increases as cardiac filling increases.
5. The parasympathetic nervous system decreases cardiac output through decreasing HR and SVR and thus decreases blood pressure, whereas the sympathetic system increases cardiac output through increased HR and SVR.
6. Short-term regulation of blood pressure is mediated by the central nervous system through the baroreceptor reflex arc and chemoreceptors.
7. Long-term blood pressure control is mediated by the kidney and hormonal systems.
8. The JGA through tubuloglomerular feedback regulates GFR by primary controlling afferent and efferent arteriole diameters.
9. RAS is a multienzymatic cascade that is central to the regulation of blood pressure and blood volume, with its main active product being Ang II acting through AT1R.
10. Aldosterone regulates salt and water excretion primarily in the distal tubule through the MR in principal cells of the collecting tubular epithelium.
11. The rather Kinin Kallikrein System (KKS) primary affects kidney hemodynamics through modulation of NO and prostaglandins.
12. Outside of the vascular space, the skin and immune system can act as reservoirs of salt to regulate salt and water homeostasis.

BIBLIOGRAPHY

Aperia AC, Broberger CG, Soderlund S. Relationship between renal artery perfusion pressure and tubular sodium reabsorption. *Am J Physiol.* 1971;220(5):1205–1212.

Barajas L. Anatomy of the juxtaglomerular apparatus. *Am J Physiol.* 1979;237(5):F333–F343.

Bhalla V, Hallows KR. Mechanisms of ENaC regulation and clinical implications. *J Am Soc Nephrol.* 2008;19(10):1845–1854.

Brenner BM, Cooper ME, de Zeeuw D, et al. RENAAL Study Investigators. Effects of losartan on renal and cardiovascular outcomes in patients with type 2 diabetes and nephropathy. *N Engl J Med.* 2001;Sep 20;345(12):861–869. doi: 10.1056/NEJMoa011161. PMID: 11565518.

Briet M, Schiffrin E. Aldosterone: effects on the kidney and cardiovascular system. *Nat Rev Nephrol.* 2010;6:261–273.

Carlström M, Wilcox CS, Arendshorst WJ. Renal autoregulation in health and disease. *Physiol Rev.* 2015;95(2):405–511.

Carretero OA, Scicli AG. Renal vasodepressor hormones: the kallikrein-kinin and prostaglandin systems. In: Philipp T, Distler A, eds. *Hypertension: Mechanisms and Management. International Boehringer Mannheim Symposia.* Berlin, Heidelberg: Springer; 1980.

Castrop H, Schweda F, Mizel D, et al. Permissive role of nitric oxide in macula densa control of renin secretion. *Am J Physiol Renal Physioll.* 2004;May;286(5):F848–857. doi: 10.1152/ajprenal.00272.2003. Epub 2004 Jan 13. PMID: 15075180.

Cowley AW, Roman RJ. The role of the kidney in hypertension. *JAMA.* 1996;275(20):1581–1589.

Davenport AP, Hyndman KA, Dhaun N, et al. Endothelin. *Pharmacol Rev.* 2016;68(2):357–418.

Dilauro M, Burns KD. Angiotensin-(1-7) and its effects in the kidney. *Scientific World J.* 2009;9:522–535.

Eaton DC, Pooler JP. *Vander's Renal Physiology.* 9th ed. New York: McGraw-Hill Education; 2018.

Gad SE, Prostaglandins. https://www.sciencedirect.com/topics/veterinary-science-and-veterinary-medicine/prostaglandins.

Granger JP, Alexander BT, Llinas M. Mechanisms of pressure natriuresis. *Current Science Inc.* 2002;4:152.

Guyton AC, Coleman TG, Cowley AW, et al. Arterial pressure regulation. *Am J Med.* 1972; May 01; 52(5):584–594.

Harris RC, McKanna JA, Akai Y, et al. Cyclooxygenase-2 is associated with the macula densa of rat kidney and increases with salt restriction. *J Clin Invest.* 1994;Dec;94(6):2504–2510. doi: 10.1172/JCI117620. PMID: 7989609; PMCID: PMC330084.

Low PA, Tomalia VA. Orthostatic hypotension: mechanisms, causes, management. *J Clin Neurol.* 2015;11(3):220–226.

Miller AJ, Arnold AC. The renin–angiotensin system in cardiovascular autonomic control: recent developments and clinical implications. *Clin Auton Res.* 2019;29:231–243.

Narumiya S, Sugimoto Y, Ushikubi F. Prostanoid Receptors: Structures, Properties, And Functions. *Physiol Rev.* 1999;79(4):1193–1226.

Rautureau Y, Schiffrin EL. Endothelin in hypertension: an update. *Curr Opin. Nephrol. Hypertens.* 2012;21:128–136.

Sparks MA, Crowley SD, Gurley SB, Mirotsou M, Coffman TM, Classical renin-angiotensin system in kidney physiology. *Compr Physiol.* 2014; Jul;4(3):1201–1228. doi: doi: 10.1002/cphy.c130040. PMID: 24944035; PMCID: PMC4137912.

Taylor KA, Wiles JD, Coleman DD, Sharma R, O Driscoll JM. Continuous cardiac autonomic and hemodynamic responses to isometric exercise. *Med Sci Sports Exerc.* 2017;49(8):1511–1519.

Wadei H, Textor S. The role of the kidney in regulating arterial blood pressure. *Nat Rev Nephrol.* 2012;8:602–609.

CHAPTER 7

TARGET ORGAN DAMAGE OR WHY SHOULD WE TREAT HYPERTENSION?

Sarah Ahmad, MD, and Jordana B. Cohen, MD, MSCE

QUESTIONS

1. **Which organs are most affected by elevated blood pressure?**
   - Heart
   - Brain
   - Kidneys
   - Eyes

2. **How does hypertension effect target organs?**
   Elevated blood pressure over many years can cause damage to several organs due to the direct effects of blood pressure on the vasculature of those organs as well as the effects of neurohormonal dysregulation.[1] Sudden severe elevations in blood pressure can cause acute effects on these organs, including microangiopathy and organ failure.[2]

3. **What are the effects of hypertension on the heart and vasculature?**
   Chronically elevated blood pressure results in a number of pathophysiological changes to cardiac structure and function that ultimately result in cardiovascular disease (Table 7.1). Elevated blood pressure leads to increased peak and end-systolic stress in the walls of the left ventricle, ultimately resulting in concentric left ventricular hypertrophy (LVH).[3] Additionally, the renin-angiotensin aldosterone system and sympathetic nervous system are concurrently activated and further contribute to ventricular remodeling. Over several decades, changes in the structure and function of the heart due to elevated blood pressure can result in chronic heart failure[4] and increased risk of nonvalvular arrhythmias.[5] Additionally, elevated blood pressure accelerates the development of vascular diseases (in the coronary vessels and throughout the body) due to medial hypertrophy and intimal thickening from repetitive barotrauma and increased rate of development of atherogenic plaques.

   Sudden elevations in blood pressure, particularly among individuals who do not have chronically elevated blood pressure, can acutely result in target organ effects including myocardial infarction, cardiogenic pulmonary edema, and aortic dissection.[2]

4. **What are the effects of hypertension on the brain?**
   The vascular beds of the brain and kidneys are vulnerable to an elevated systemic blood pressure load, resulting in shear stress and vascular barotrauma. In the brain, the effect of chronically elevated blood pressure on the vasculature results in elevated risk of ischemic and hemorrhagic strokes as well as chronic microvascular disease, which can result in dementia.[6] The mechanisms of ischemic stroke and chronic microvascular disease are similar to the vascular effects of hypertension in the heart due to accelerated vascular stiffness and atherosclerotic disease. Hemorrhagic stroke occurs due to micro- and macrovascular damage caused by elevated intraluminal pressure and hyaline degeneration.[7]

   Acute, severe hypertension, particularly among individuals without chronically elevated blood pressure, can result in acute hemorrhagic stroke and encephalopathy. Hypertensive encephalopathy occurs due to a rise in intracranial pressure that yields cerebral edema, microscopic hemorrhages, and infarctions.[2]

5. **What are the effects of hypertension on the kidneys?**
   Similar to other vascular beds throughout the body, the kidney vasculature experiences medial hypertrophy and intimal thickening due to repetitive barotrauma of elevated blood pressure. However, the kidney is unique in that autoregulation provides a protective mechanism from shear stress and vascular barotrauma via vasoconstriction of the afferent arteriole, which decreases preglomerular hydrostatic pressures (Table 7.2).[8] The decline in renal plasma flow and glomerular pressure activates the renin-angiotensin aldosterone system, resulting in intrarenal vasoconstriction and ultimately leading to focal segmental glomerulosclerosis. Hypertrophy and hyperfiltration of the remaining glomeruli can result in (typically mild but occasionally severe) proteinuria.[9]

   If blood pressure rises acutely and severely, the autoregulation threshold in the kidney is surpassed, which can result in severe vascular hyalinosis due to malignant hypertension.[2,3] Thrombotic microangiopathy also can occur, resulting in intravascular hemolysis and destruction of the microcirculation by thrombi in the glomeruli.[2]

Table 7.1 Preclinical and Clinical Manifestations of Target Organ Damage to the Heart and Large Blood Vessels Due to Hypertension

Cardiac disease	Preclinical • Left ventricular concentric hypertrophy • Left ventricular eccentric hypertrophy • Impaired left ventricular diastolic function • Impaired left ventricular systolic function • Left atrial enlargement Clinical • Chronic heart failure with preserved ejection fraction • Chronic heart failure with reduced ejection fraction

Vascular disease	Preclinical
	• Arterial stiffness
	• Atherosclerotic disease
	  • Coronary artery disease
	  • Peripheral artery disease
	• Aortic aneurysm
	• Aortic dissection
	Clinical
	• Angina
	• Claudication
	• Myocardial infarction

Arrhythmias	Clinical • Atrial fibrillation • Ventricular tachyarrhythmias • Sudden cardiac death

Table 7.2 Preclinical and Clinical Manifestations of Target Organ Damage in the Kidney Due to Hypertension

Kidney parenchymal disease	Preclinical • Focal global glomerulosclerosis • Focal segmental glomerulosclerosis • Interstitial fibrosis • Tubular atrophy Clinical • Albuminuria • Chronic kidney disease • End-stage kidney disease
Vascular disease	Preclinical • Atherosclerotic renal artery disease • Microangiopathy • Hyalinosis • Thrombotic microangiopathy Clinical • Albuminuria • Hematuria • Acute kidney injury • Chronic kidney disease • End-stage kidney disease

6. **What are the effects of hypertension on the eyes?**
   The eyes can experience structural and functional changes to the retinal microvasculature due to chronic exposure to hypertension, including micro- and macroaneurysms, arteriolar narrowing, and arteriovenous nicking, resulting in blurred vision.[10] Retinal micro- and macroaneurysms are caused by elevated intraluminal pressure in the retinal vessels. Fibrinoid necrosis and endothelial dysfunction can result in arteriolar infarctions and arteriovenous nicking. In patients with acute, severe elevations in blood pressure, acute fundoscopic changes can occur due to hypertensive retinopathy and elevated intracranial pressure, including flame hemorrhages, cotton

wool spots, exudates, and papilledema.[2] Similar to the kidney, retinal vessels are also vulnerable to the effects of thrombotic microangiopathy in acute, severe hypertension.[2]

7. How should patients be evaluated for target organ damage due to hypertension?

In all patients with a new diagnosis of hypertension or with chronically uncontrolled hypertension, the following testing is recommended to evaluate for target organ damage due to hypertension[1,10,11]:

- Heart:
  - Volume status history and examination
  - Electrocardiogram
- Brain:
  - Neurological physical examination
- Kidneys:
  - Serum creatinine and estimated glomerular filtration rate
  - Urinalysis, urine albumin/creatinine ratio
- Eyes:
  - Fundoscopic examination

Additional testing should be performed in those patients in whom there is a high level of suspicion for target organ damage (e.g., new symptoms concerning for target organ damage) or with elevated risk for target organ damage:

- Heart:
  - Echocardiogram
- Brain:
  - Cognitive function testing
  - Magnetic resonance imaging or computed tomography
  - Angiography

In patients presenting with acute, severe elevation in blood pressure (i.e., malignant hypertension), additional testing may be appropriate as guided by the presenting symptoms. For example:

- Dyspnea:
  - Chest x-ray to evaluate for pulmonary edema
- Dark or red urine:
  - Creatinine, hemoglobin, platelets, urine sediment, and peripheral smear to evaluate for acute kidney injury and thrombotic microangiopathy
- Chest pain:
  - Electrocardiogram and troponin to evaluate for acute myocardial infarction
  - Chest computed tomography to assess for aortic dissection if chest pain is present

8. What factors increase the risk of target organ damage due to hypertension?

Several factors and comorbid conditions are associated with an elevated risk of target organ damage due to hypertension.[1,11–14] Patients with these risk factors should be closely monitored for the development of target organ damage and should be counseled on particularly stringent blood pressure control. Many of the factors associated with elevated risk of target organ damage due to hypertension are also associated with an increased risk of developing hypertension.

- Severe hypertension
- Prolonged uncontrolled hypertension
- Masked hypertension
- Black race
- Male sex
- Low socioeconomic status
- Smoking
- Obesity
- Hyperlipidemia
- Obstructive sleep apnea
- Diabetes mellitus
- Chronic kidney disease
- Primary hyperaldosteronism

9. What can be done to reduce the risk of target organ damage due to hypertension?

Stringent and consistent blood pressure control is the most effective means of reducing the risk of target organ damage from hypertension.[1,15–18]

Most patients with a diagnosis of hypertension or with blood pressure within 10 mm Hg of their goal blood pressure in the office should undergo out-of-office blood pressure monitoring to evaluate for masked hypertension (i.e., normal blood pressure in the office with elevated blood pressure outside of the office). Those individuals who are found to have masked hypertension may benefit from management of their hypertension based on out-of-office, rather than in-office, blood pressure measurements to ensure adequate longitudinal blood pressure control and reduce the risk of target organ damage.

Optimization of other cardiovascular risk factors, including lipid management, smoking cessation, weight loss, and adequate glycemic control, can help reduce target organ damage due to hypertension.[1,19–21]

Selection of targeted antihypertensive agents can also help reduce organ damage due to hypertension. For example, renin-angiotensin system blockade reduces the risk of progression of chronic kidney disease in patients with proteinuria[22,23] and of adverse cardiac events and mortality in patients with heart failure with reduced ejection fraction.[24]

10. How should hypertension be managed when target organ damage is already present?
Stringent blood pressure control is highly beneficial when treating hypertension for secondary prevention (i.e., when a patient has already experienced target organ damage).[25–27] Similar to primary prevention, optimization of other cardiovascular risk factors, such as lipid management, smoking cessation, weight loss, and glycemic control, can also help reduce the risk of further target organ damage.[27]

KEY POINTS

1. Chronically and acutely elevated blood pressure can cause target organ damage to the heart, blood vessels, brain, kidneys, and eyes.
2. Target organ damage occurs due to several mechanisms, including micro- and macrovascular injury from barotrauma and neurohormonal dysregulation.
3. It is important to perform a careful history and physical examination and appropriate testing in patients with hypertension to evaluate for target organ damage.
4. Stringent and consistent blood pressure control is the most effective way to reduce the risk of developing primary and secondary target organ damage.

REFERENCES

1. Whelton PK, Carey RM, Aronow WS, et al. 2017 ACC/AHA/AAPA/ABC/ACPM/AGS/APhA/ASH/ASPC/NMA/PCNA Guideline for the prevention, detection, evaluation, and management of high blood pressure in adults: a report of the American College of Cardiology/American Heart Association Task Force on Clinical Practice Guidelines. *Hypertension.* 2018;71:e13–e115.
2. van den Born BH, Lip GYH, Brguljan-Hitij J, et al. ESC Council on hypertension position document on the management of hypertensive emergencies. *Eur Heart J Cardiovasc Pharmacother.* 2019;5:37–46.
3. Vasan RS, Levy D. The role of hypertension in the pathogenesis of heart failure. A clinical mechanistic overview. *Arch Intern Med.* 1996;156:1789–1796.
4. Rosendorff C. The renin-angiotensin system and vascular hypertrophy. *J Am Coll Cardiol.* 1996;28:803–812.
5. Benjamin EJ, Levy D, Vaziri SM, D'Agostino RB, Belanger AJ, Wolf PA. Independent risk factors for atrial fibrillation in a population-based cohort. The Framingham Heart Study. *JAMA.* 1994;271:840–844.
6. Iadecola C, Gottesman RF. Neurovascular and cognitive dysfunction in hypertension. *Circ Res.* 2019;124:1025–1044.
7. Johansson BB. Hypertension mechanisms causing stroke. *Clin Exp Pharmacol Physiol.* 1999;26:563–565.
8. Bidani AK, Griffin KA, Picken M, Lansky DM. Continuous telemetric blood pressure monitoring and glomerular injury in the rat remnant kidney model. *Am J Physiol.* 1993;265:F391–398.
9. Mujais SK, Emmanouel DS, Kasinath BS, Spargo BH. Marked proteinuria in hypertensive nephrosclerosis. *Am J Nephrol.* 1985;5:190–195.
10. Wong TY, Mitchell P. Hypertensive retinopathy. *N Engl J Med.* 2004;351:2310–2317.
11. Lawler PR, Hiremath P, Cheng S. Cardiac target organ damage in hypertension: insights from epidemiology. *Curr Hypertens Rep.* 2014;16:446.
12. Monticone S, D'Ascenzo F, Moretti C, et al. Cardiovascular events and target organ damage in primary aldosteronism compared with essential hypertension: a systematic review and meta-analysis. *Lancet Diabetes Endocrinol.* 2018;6:41–50.
13. Echouffo-Tcheugui JB, Greene SJ, Papadimitriou L, et al. Population risk prediction models for incident heart failure: a systematic review. *Circ Heart Fail.* 2015;8:438–447.
14. Fogo A, Breyer JA, Smith MC, et al. Accuracy of the diagnosis of hypertensive nephrosclerosis in African Americans: a report from the African American Study of Kidney Disease (AASK) Trial. AASK Pilot Study Investigators. *Kidney Int.* 1997;51:244–252.
15. Wright Jr JT, Williamson JD, Whelton PK, et al. SPRINT Research Group. A randomized trial of intensive versus standard blood-pressure control. *N Engl J Med.* 2015;373:2103–2116.
16. Cushman WC, Evans GW, Byington RP, et al. ACCORD Study Group. Effects of intensive blood-pressure control in type 2 diabetes mellitus. *N Engl J Med.* 2010;362:1575–1585.
17. Nerenberg KA, Zarnke KB, Leung AA, et al. Hypertension Canada's 2018 guidelines for diagnosis, risk assessment, prevention, and treatment of hypertension in adults and children. *Can J Cardiol.* 2018;34:506–525.
18. Williams B, Mancia G, Spiering W, et al. 2018 ESC/ESH guidelines for the management of arterial hypertension. *Eur Heart J.* 2018;39:3021–3104.
19. Cohen JB. Hypertension in obesity and the impact of weight loss. *Curr Cardiol Rep.* 2017;19:98.
20. Chirinos JA, Gurubhagavatula I, Teff K, et al. CPAP, weight loss, or both for obstructive sleep apnea. *N Engl J Med.* 2014;370:2265–2275.
21. Danaei G, Ding EL, Mozaffarian D, et al. The preventable causes of death in the United States: comparative risk assessment of dietary, lifestyle, and metabolic risk factors. *PLoS Med.* 2009;6:e1000058.

22. Jafar TH, Stark PC, Schmid CH, et al. Progression of chronic kidney disease: the role of blood pressure control, proteinuria, and angiotensin-converting enzyme inhibition: a patient-level meta-analysis. *Ann Intern Med.* 2003;139:244–252.
23. Wright Jr JT, Bakris G, Greene T, et al. Effect of blood pressure lowering and antihypertensive drug class on progression of hypertensive kidney disease: results from the AASK trial. *JAMA.* 2002;288:2421–2431.
24. Garg R, Yusuf S. Overview of randomized trials of angiotensin-converting enzyme inhibitors on mortality and morbidity in patients with heart failure. Collaborative Group on ACE Inhibitor Trials. *JAMA.* 1995;273:1450–1456.
25. Ogden LG, He J, Lydick E, Whelton PK. Long-term absolute benefit of lowering blood pressure in hypertensive patients according to the JNC VI risk stratification. *Hypertension.* 2000;35:539–543.
26. Hypertension, Detection Follow-up Program Cooperative GroupThe effect of treatment on mortality in "mild" hypertension: results of the hypertension detection and follow-up program. *N Engl J Med.* 1982;307:976–980.
27. Smith Jr SC, Benjamin EJ, Bonow RO, et al. AHA/ACCF secondary prevention and risk reduction therapy for patients with coronary and other atherosclerotic vascular disease: 2011 update: a guideline from the American Heart Association and American College of Cardiology Foundation endorsed by the World Heart Federation and the Preventive Cardiovascular Nurses Association. *J Am Coll Cardiol.* 2011;58:2432–2446.

CHAPTER 8

PRIMARY ALDOSTERONISM AND MINERALOCORTICOID HYPERTENSION

Renata Libianto, MBBS, James M. Luther, MD, and Jun Yang, MBBS (Hon), PhD

QUESTIONS

1. **What is the most common identifiable cause of resistant hypertension?**
   Resistant hypertension, defined as elevated blood pressure (BP) despite the concurrent use of three antihypertensive drug classes at maximum tolerated dose or controlled BP on four or more antihypertensive medications, affects approximately 15% of the hypertensive population. Primary aldosteronism (PA) is the most common secondary cause, accounting for up to 15% to 30% of the cases in a hypertension referral clinic setting.[1] Even amongst the general hypertensive population, PA has a reported prevalence of 5% to 10%.[1] PA is substantially under diagnosed due to lack of screening. One Italian study reported 992 diagnoses of PA during a 16-year period, corresponding to only 2% of the overall expected cases.[2] Secondary analysis of the PATHWAY-2 study of resistant hypertension suggested that 25% of participants have previously undiagnosed aldosterone excess.[3] The low detection rate is likely due to the lack of screening; only 7% of European primary care practitioners ever screened for PA using serum renin and aldosterone measurements[4] and the rate of screening in the resistant hypertensive population was only 2% despite guidelines.[5]

2. **What patients should I evaluate for PA?**
   The Endocrine Society recommends screening for PA in patients with[6]:
   - Hypertension with BP greater than 150/100, resistant hypertension despite three agents, or controlled hypertension on four or more agents;
   - Hypertension and spontaneous or diuretic-induced hypokalemia;
   - Hypertension and adrenal incidentaloma;
   - Hypertension and sleep apnea;
   - Hypertension and a family history of early onset hypertension or cerebrovascular accident at a young age (younger than 40 years); or
   - Hypertensive first-degree relatives of patients with PA.
        Given the high prevalence of PA in both primary care and in referral centers, clinicians should have a low threshold to screen for PA. Several studies even found that PA was present in 3% to 6% of patients with newly diagnosed hypertension, suggesting that screening should be initiated before drug treatment or the development of resistant hypertension.[7] A common misconception is that patients with PA present with hypertension at an early age. However, the average age of PA diagnosis is 50 to 60 years, so age alone should not be used to guide screening.

3. **How often do patients with PA present without hypokalemia?**
   Only a minority of patients with PA (30%) present *with* hypokalemia; routine screening identifies even more patients with normokalemia.[8] Thus most patients with PA are indistinguishable from patients with other forms of hypertension. Hypokalemia is more common in patients with aldosterone-producing adenoma than those with bilateral adrenal hyperplasia (affecting 50% and 20%, respectively).

4. **What are the most common causes of PA?**
   The most common causes of PA are bilateral adrenal hyperplasia and unilateral aldosterone-producing adenoma, which account for 70% and 30% of cases, respectively. The most common form of familial hyperaldosteronism is glucocorticoid-remediable aldosteronism, although it accounts for only 1% of the overall PA cases. Sporadic mutations in the adenoma within a limited number of genes (*KCNJ5, CACNA1D, CACNA1H, ATP1A1, ATP1A3,* and *CTNNB1*) are associated with the majority of aldosterone-producing adenomas, although genetic testing is not yet routinely performed.

5. **Why is it important to diagnose PA rather than just treat the hypertension?**
   Patients with PA have higher cardiovascular morbidity and mortality than patients with essential hypertension matched for their age, sex, and degree of elevation in BP.[9,10] Targeted treatment of PA with either adrenalectomy

or mineralocorticoid receptor (MR) antagonists are highly effective at lowering BP and mitigating the adverse cardiovascular consequences of untreated PA. Ineffective antihypertensive medications can be avoided, especially if PA is treated early in the disease process. Patients with aldosterone-producing adenomas who undergo adrenalectomy may even be cured of their hypertension altogether and avoid the need for lifelong antihypertensive medications. An appropriate diagnosis will also allow clinicians to monitor the appropriate outcome parameters, including not just BP but also plasma potassium and renin concentration.

6. **What is the best initial screening test for PA?**
   The aldosterone-to-renin ratio (ARR) was introduced in 1981 and remains the recommended screening test for PA on the basis that isolated measurements of either plasma aldosterone concentration (PAC), direct renin concentration (DRC), or plasma renin activity (PRA) show overlap with unaffected patients. It is a simple blood test best done in the morning about 2 hours after getting up. An abnormal screening test is defined as an elevated ARR above a set threshold, which differs between different centers depending on the assays used to measure aldosterone and renin and the units of measurement. Commonly, an ARR is considered abnormal if it is >70 pmol/L:mU/L, >30 ng/dL:ng/mL/h, >1.6 ng/dL:pmol/L/min, or >60 pmol/L:pmol/L/min.[6] A simplified approach to PA diagnosis is outlined in Fig. 8.1.

7. **How do antihypertensive medications and other conditions affect the ARR?**
   The most commonly used antihypertensive medications can affect the ARR (Table 8.1).[11] Other medications such as nonsteroidal antiinflammatory drugs can inhibit renin secretion. Severe hypokalemia impairs aldosterone secretion and can result in a false negative test; therefore potassium should be normalized and assessed at the same time as the ARR. Plasma renin activity and renin concentration measurements correlate well, but special attention should be given to plasma renin activity measurements, which are inhibited in vitro by the direct renin inhibitor aliskiren.

8. **Do I need to withhold interfering medications before checking the ARR?**
   If safe to do so, it is ideal to stop all interfering medications and switch to noninterfering antihypertensive medications for BP control during the investigative period. They include nondihydropyridine calcium channel blockers (e.g., sustained-release verapamil), alpha-blockers (e.g., prazosin), moxonidine (outside the United States), and/or hydralazine. The new medication regime should ideally be continued for 6 weeks before screening and for all subsequent investigations if the initial screening test is abnormal. However, in patients who cannot safely stop their interfering medications, the ARR should be interpreted accordingly. For example, a low or low-normal renin in the setting of angiotensin-converting enzyme (ACE) inhibitor or angiotensin II (Ang II) receptor blocker use (which should stimulate renin production) increases the likelihood of PA.

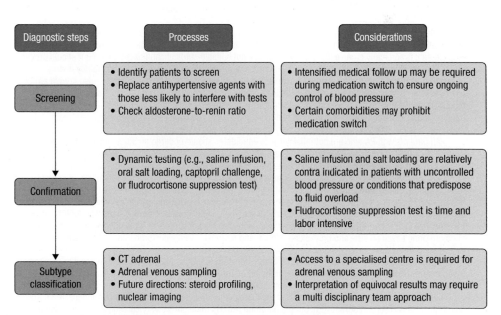

Fig. 8.1 **Simplified pathway for diagnosing primary aldosteronism.** *CT,* Computed tomography.

Table 8.1 Antihypertensive Medications that Can Alter Aldosterone, Renin Activity, and the Aldosterone-to-Renin Ratio (ARR)

	ALDOSTERONE	RENIN	ARR
Medications that may cause a false positive result			
β-Blockers	↓	↓↓	↑
α-Methyldopa	↓	↓↓	↑
Clonidine	↓	↓↓	↑
Medications that may cause a false negative result			
Loop and thiazide diuretics	↑	↑↑	↓
MR antagonists (spironolactone)	↑	↑↑	↓
ACE inhibitors	↓	↑↑	↓
Angiotensin receptor blockers	↓	↑↑	↓
Direct renin inhibitors[a]	↓	↓Activity ↑Renin concentration	↑(Activity) ↓(Concentration)
Dihydropyridine calcium channel blockers	↓	↑	↓

[a]Renin inhibitors decrease activity but increase renin concentration.
ACE, Angiotensin-converting enzyme; *MR,* mineralocorticoid receptor.

9. **What additional testing should be done in a patient with an abnormal ARR?**
   An elevated ARR is not diagnostic of PA. Confirmation of the disease requires the demonstration of at least partly autonomous aldosterone production during interventions to suppress aldosterone, including saline infusion, oral salt loading, fludrocortisone administration, or captopril challenge. Confirmatory test protocols as well as diagnostic thresholds vary across centers. Examples of positive confirmatory tests include:
   - Urinary aldosterone excretion >13 μg (33 nmol)/24 h during high sodium intake documented by urinary sodium excretion >200 mmol/24 h;
   - Plasma aldosterone ≥5 to 10 ng/dL (140–280 pmol/L) after the recumbent saline infusion test or >6 ng/dL (170 pmol/L) after the seated saline suppression test;
   - Plasma aldosterone >6 ng/dL (170 pmol/L) after 3 days of fludrocortisone administration; or
   - Plasma aldosterone >11 ng/dL (300 pmol/L) 1 hour after taking 50 mg captopril.

   Confirmatory testing may be bypassed in hypertensive patients with spontaneous hypokalemia in the setting of elevated PAC greater than 550 pmol/L (20 ng/dL) and suppressed renin[6]—these patients almost certainly have PA.

10. **How can you accurately differentiate between unilateral and bilateral causes of PA?**
    Unilateral disease caused by an aldosterone-producing adrenal adenoma is important to distinguish from bilateral disease as it is surgically curable. For patients who are not suitable surgical candidates, treatment should proceed as for bilateral disease without further testing. Young patients with PA or those with a strong family history of hypertension and early stroke should also be tested for familial hyperaldosteronism type 1, also known as glucocorticoid remediable aldosteronism (GRA), or a familial hyperaldosteronism (FHA) syndrome (Table 8.2). The diagnosis of GRA can be reliably made by testing for the hybrid gene mutation composed of 11β-hydroxylase gene regulatory sequences and aldosterone synthase gene coding sequences. This approach is preferable to dexamethasone suppression testing, which may produce false positive results.

    All patients with PA who are potential surgical candidates should undergo an adrenal computed tomography scan to exclude large masses, which may indicate adrenal carcinoma. However, small adrenal adenomas less than 1 cm may go undetected, and nonfunctioning adrenal incidentalomas are not uncommon.

    Currently the most reliable method to differentiate unilateral from bilateral PA preoperatively is adrenal vein sampling. During adrenal vein sampling, adrenal and peripheral veins are sequentially or simultaneously catheterized through a percutaneous femoral vein approach under fluoroscopic guidance where blood is taken and assayed for aldosterone and cortisol concentrations. The cortisol measurements are used to confirm successful cannulation of the adrenal vein and to correct the aldosterone measurements for dilutional effects. Calculations are done based on left- and right-sided adrenal and peripheral vein aldosterone/cortisol measurements to determine if there is unilateral dominance of aldosterone production.

    Autonomous cortisol secretion, concurrent with aldosterone production, has received increasing recognition. Given the important role of cortisol in the interpretation of adrenal vein sampling results, a 1-mg dexamethasone suppression test is recommended before sampling. In the setting of an abnormal response (e.g., cortisol >50 nmol/L or 1.8 μg/dL), further evaluation of the cortisol burden is required (e.g., 24-hour urinary free cortisol, paired plasma cortisol and adrenocorticotropic hormone [ACTH], midnight salivary cortisol) and an additional adrenal hormone such as androstenedione should be measured during adrenal vein sampling for the purpose of assessing lateralization.

Table 8.2 Familial Hyperaldosteronism (FH) and Genetic Syndromes Associated with Primary Aldosteronism (PA)

SYNDROME	INHERITANCE	GENE/MUTATION	CLINICAL CHARACTERISTICS
FH-I	AD	*CYP11B1-B2* hybrid	Glucocorticoid-remediable aldosteronism ACTH-driven CYP11B2 Hybrid 18-OH-steroids (18-oxy-Cortisol)
FH-II	AD	*CLCN2*	Presents as APA or BAH Likely a genetically heterogeneous group
FH-III	AD	*KCNJ5*	Early-onset (early childhood) refractory PA Severe hypokalemia and polyuria (DI-like) Adrenal hyperplasia treated with ADx
FH-IV	AD-incomplete	*CACNA1H*	Early onset, typical PA
PASNA	*de novo*	*CACNA1D de novo* mutations	PA with seizures and neurologic abnormalities Early onset PA in childhood

ACTH, Adrenocorticotropic hormone; *AD,* autosomal dominant; *ADx,* adrenalectomy; *APA,* aldosterone-producing adenoma; *BAH,* bilateral adrenal hyperplasia; *DI,* diabetes insipidus.

11. **What is the treatment for aldosterone-producing adenoma?**
Unilateral laparoscopic adrenalectomy is the treatment of choice for patients with unilateral disease who are suitable surgical candidates.
Before surgery an MR antagonist should be taken to normalize plasma renin and potassium levels. BP should also be stabilized.
After surgery the MR antagonist can be stopped but other antihypertensive medications may need to be continued. PAC and renin concentration should be measured approximately 3 months postoperatively to confirm a biochemical cure. Hypokalemia usually resolves rapidly, and therefore MR antagonist and potassium supplementation should be stopped immediately after surgery and serum potassium should be monitored. Hypertension due to PA typically resolves in 1 to 6 months, but concurrent essential hypertension often requires continued treatment. The long-term cure rates of hypertension after surgery in well-selected patients ranges from 33% to 85%.

12. **How is bilateral adrenal aldosterone excess treated?**
Bilateral hyperaldosteronism is treated with MR antagonists such as spironolactone (12.5–100 mg daily) as the first choice, as they target the pathophysiology and protect the cardiovascular and renal systems from aldosterone-mediated injury. Spironolactone also acts on the androgen and progesterone receptors and is associated with dose-dependent adverse effects such as gynecomastia and impotence in men and menstrual disturbance in women. A more selective antagonist, eplerenone (25–100 mg twice a day [BD]), has fewer side effects but is less potent and requires twice-daily dosing because it has a short half-life. The dose of spironolactone or eplerenone should be increased until the plasma renin concentration is normal ("unsuppressed") to achieve cardiovascular benefits.[12] Once renin is normalized, other antihypertensives may be required to optimally control BP. If spironolactone is not tolerated and eplerenone is not available, then amiloride, an epithelial sodium channel antagonist, may be considered. It targets the distal tubular sodium channels, which are upregulated by aldosterone, but it does not antagonize the MR receptor elsewhere in the body.
An example of a medical treatment regimen may be:
- Commence spironolactone at 12.5 to 25 mg daily OR eplerenone at 25 mg BD initially
- Increase spironolactone to 50 to 150 mg daily OR eplerenone to 50 to 100 mg BD until normokalemia is achieved without potassium supplementation and *renin is fully unsuppressed* (plasma renin activity >1.5 ng/mL/h or plasma renin concentration >12 mU/L);
- Use amiloride (2.5–10 mg BD) if spironolactone or eplerenone is not tolerated or available;
- Add ACE inhibitors, Ang II receptor blockers, other diuretics (e.g., hydrochlorothiazide), or calcium channel blockers to optimize BP control.[1–9]

13. **What mineralocorticoids other than aldosterone can cause hypertension, and when should this be considered?**
Other steroids can act on the MR as mineralocorticoids, including 11-deocycorticosterone (DOC) and corticosterone. Suppressed or low plasma renin and aldosterone concentrations can indicate an excess mineralocorticoid, MR activation, or ENaC activation (Fig. 8.2). Drugs that interfere with cortisol production often result in compensatory ACTH excess, which, in turn, increases mineralocorticoids (see Chapter 13). Emphasis should be placed on determining the underlying cause of mineralocorticoid excess, which should be specifically treated if possible. MR antagonism or amiloride can be used for treatment of mineralocorticoid excess when a more specific intervention is not possible. Glucocorticoid excess or inhibition of 11-beta hydroxysteroid dehydrogenase 2 also can produce hypokalemic hypertension and is covered in Chapter 9.

High Aldosterone Low Renin	High Aldosterone Low Renin	
ALDOSTERONE EXCESS	**MINERALOCORTICOID EXCESS**	**APPARENT MINERALOCORTICOID EXCESS AND MR ACTIVATION**
Primary Aldosteronism: *Aldosterone-Producing Adenoma* *Idiopathic Hyperaldosteronism* *Adrenal Hyperplasia* **Familial Hyperaldosteronism (FHA):** *FHAI: CYP11B1/B2 Fusion (GRA)* *FHAII: CLCN2 Mutation* *FHAIII: KCNJ5 Mutation* *FHAIV: CACNA1H Mutation*	*ACTH-Cortisol Excess* *(Cushing Syndrome)* *Adrenal Adenoma* *(Cortisol, DOC, Corticosterone)* *GR Resistance/Inhibition* *(Mifepristone)* *Congenital Adrenal Hyperplasia* *CYP17A1 Inhibition (Abiraterone)* *CYP11B1 Inhibition (Fluconazole, Posaconazole, Ketoconazole)* *Adrenocortical Carcinoma*	ENaC Activating Mutation (Liddle Syndrome) MR Activating Mutation (Geller Syndrome) ***HSD11B2 Inhibition or Deficiency:*** *Inhibition (Licorice, Carbenoxolone, Itraconazole, Posaconazole)* *Genetic HSD11B2 Deficiency*

Fig. 8.2 Causes of mineralocorticoid hypertension. *ACTH,* Adrenocorticotropic hormone; *DOC,* deoxycorticosterone; *GR,* glucocorticoid receptor; *ENaC,* epithelial sodium channel; *MR,* mineralocorticoid receptor.

KEY POINTS

1. Only a minority of patients with primary aldosteronism (30%) present with hypokalemia; routine screening identifies even more patients with normokalemia.
2. Most patients with PA are indistinguishable from patients with other forms of hypertension.
3. The aldosterone to renin ratio (ARR) remains as the recommended screening test for primary aldosteronism on the basis that isolated measurements of either plasma aldosterone concentration (PAC), direct renin concentration (DRC) or plasma renin activity (PRA) show overlap with unaffected patients.

REFERENCES

1. Kayser SC, Dekkers T, Groenewoud HJ, et al. Study heterogeneity and estimation of prevalence of primary aldosteronism: a systematic review and meta-regression analysis. *J Clin Endocrinol Metabol.* 2016;101(7):2826–2835.
2. Rossi E, Perazzoli F, Negro A, Magnani A. Diagnostic rate of primary aldosteronism in Emilia-Romagna, Northern Italy, during 16 years (2000-2015). *J Hypertens.* 2017;35(8):1691–1697.
3. Williams B, MacDonald TM, Morant SV, et al. Endocrine and haemodynamic changes in resistant hypertension, and blood pressure responses to spironolactone or amiloride: the PATHWAY-2 mechanisms substudies. *Lancet Diabetes Endocrinol.* 2018;6(6):464–475.
4. Mulatero P, Monticone S, Burrello J, Veglio F, Williams TA, Funder J. Guidelines for primary aldosteronism: uptake by primary care physicians in Europe. *J Hypertens.* 2016;34(11):2253–2257.
5. Jaffe G, Gray Z, Krishnan G, et al. Screening rates for primary aldosteronism in resistant hypertension. Hypertension (Dallas, Tex: 1979).0(0):HYPERTENSIONAHA.119.14359.
6. Funder JW, Carey RM, Mantero F, et al. The management of primary aldosteronism: case detection, diagnosis, and treatment: an Endocrine Society clinical practice guideline. *J Clin Endocrinol Metabol.* 2016;101(5):1889–1916.
7. Käyser SC, Deinum J, de Grauw WJC, et al. Prevalence of primary aldosteronism in primary care: a cross-sectional study. *Br J Gen Pract.* 2018;68(667):e114.
8. Yang J, Fuller PJ, Stowasser M. Is it time to screen all patients with hypertension for primary aldosteronism? *Med J Aust.* 2018;209(2):57–59.
9. Milliez P, Girerd X, Plouin PF, Blacher J, Safar ME, Mourad JJ. Evidence for an increased rate of cardiovascular events in patients with primary aldosteronism. *J Am Coll Cardiol.* 2005;45(8):1243–1248.
10. Monticone S, D'Ascenzo F, Moretti C, et al. Cardiovascular events and target organ damage in primary aldosteronism compared with essential hypertension: a systematic review and meta-analysis. *Lancet Diabetes Endocrinol.* 2018;6(1):41–50.
11. Stowasser M, Gordon RD. Primary aldosteronism: changing definitions and new concepts of physiology and pathophysiology both inside and outside the kidney. *Physiol Rev.* 2016;96(4):1327–1384.
12. Hundemer GL, Curhan GC, Yozamp N, Wang M, Vaidya A. Cardiometabolic outcomes and mortality in medically treated primary aldosteronism: a retrospective cohort study. *Lancet Diabetes Endocrino.* 2018;6(1):51–59.

CHAPTER 9

GLUCOCORTICOID HYPERTENSION

Yuta Tezuka, MD, and Adina F. Turcu, MD MS

QUESTIONS

1. **What are glucocorticoids?**
   The adrenal cortex secretes three major types of steroid hormones, each produced in one of three concentric cortical layers, also known as zones. Glucocorticoids are steroid hormones produced by the zona fasciculata of the adrenal cortex (Fig. 9.1). Cortisol is the major glucocorticoid in humans, and it is a pivotal regulator for a wide variety of functions, such as metabolic homeostasis, immune responses, and hemodynamic stability. The physiological synthesis of cortisol is regulated by the pituitary adrenocorticotropic hormone (ACTH), and it follows a typical circadian pattern with the largest peak in early morning and nadir around midnight.

2. **What are mineralocorticoids?**
   The outermost zone of the adrenal cortex, zona glomerulosa, produces mineralocorticoids (see Fig. 9.1). Aldosterone is the prototype human mineralocorticoid and its main function is salt and water regulation. These effects are mediated primarily via mineralocorticoid receptors (MRs) located in the distal convoluted tubule and cortical collecting duct of the kidneys. MRs are also found in the colon, eccrine glands, and other tissues. In the kidneys, activating MR ligands promote the expression of epithelial sodium channels (ENaCs), which, in turn, facilitate sodium and water reabsorption with compensatory potassium and H^+ urinary excretion. Physiological aldosterone synthesis is regulated via the renin-angiotensin-aldosterone system, which is triggered by low renal perfusion and hyperkalemia. Excessive activation of the MRs leads to intravascular volume expansion and, subsequently, to hypertension with or without hypokalemia and metabolic alkalosis.

3. **How do glucocorticoids influence blood pressure?**
   The affinity of MRs for cortisol is similar to that for aldosterone. Although circulating concentrations of cortisol normally exceed those of aldosterone by roughly 1000 times, peripheral tissues inactivate cortisol to cortisone via the enzyme 11β-hydroxysteroid dehydrogenase type 2 (HSD11B2; see Fig. 9.1).
   Activation of MRs by glucocorticoids occurs when these hormones circulate in excessive amounts due to either endogenous overproduction or pharmacologic administration. Such supraphysiological concentrations of glucocorticoids result in saturation of HSD11B2 and subsequent activation of MR by active glucocorticoids. Other mechanisms by which glucocorticoids contribute to hypertension include suppression of vasodilators, such as nitric oxide and prostaglandins; enhancing the effects of vasoconstrictors, including angiotensin II receptor; and alterations of the sensitivity of the sympathetic nervous system. In addition, patients with chronic glucocorticoid excess often develop central obesity and sleep apnea, which further contributes to hypertension. Indirectly, numerous endogenous and exogenous inhibitors of HSD11B2 facilitate MR activation by physiological cortisol levels, leading to hypertension. Causes of glucocorticoid-induced hypertension are listed in Box 9.1.

CUSHING SYNDROME

4. **What is Cushing syndrome?**
   Cushing syndrome refers to a clinical phenotype associated with chronic glucocorticoid excess. This syndrome can be caused by either excessive cortisol synthesis or by exogenous glucocorticoids administered at supraphysiological doses. Endogenous Cushing Syndrome can be ACTH-dependent (either from a pituitary adenoma producing ACTH, or, rarely, from an ectopic ACTH or corticotropin-releasing hormone [CRH] source), or ACTH-independent (autonomous adrenal cortisol excess from a benign adenoma or a cortical carcinoma).

5. **Is Cushing syndrome common?**
   Although exogenous or iatrogenic Cushing Syndrome is relatively common, endogenous Cushing Syndrome is a rare disease with an incidence of 1 to 2 per million per year. Endogenous Cushing Syndrome is most commonly caused by an ACTH-producing pituitary adenoma, and this form is also known as Cushing disease.

6. **List the etiologies of Cushing syndrome.**
   ACTH-dependent: 80%
   - Pituitary adenoma (Cushing disease): 64%
   - Ectopic ACTH-producing tumors: 16%
     - Small-cell lung carcinomas; bronchial, pancreatic, thymic neuroendocrine tumors; etc.

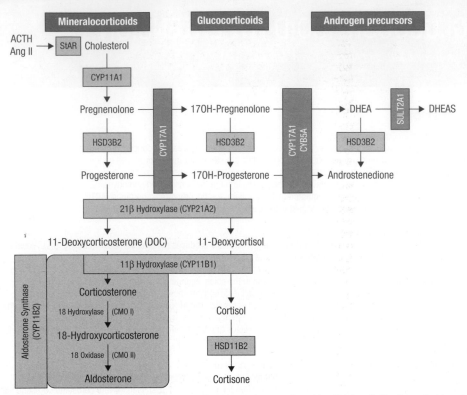

Fig. 9.1 Adrenal steroid pathway. The adrenal cortex produces three major types of steroids: mineralocorticoids, glucocorticoids, and androgen precursors. Each group is produced in distinct layers of the adrenal cortex, which are organized concentrically. Adrenocorticotropic hormone *(ACTH)* and angiotensin II *(Ang II)* prompt steroidogenesis by increasing the expression and activating the steroidogenic acute regulatory *(StAR)*. StAR mobilizes cholesterol to the inner mitochondrial membrane where it is then converted to pregnenolone by the cholesterol side-chain cleavage enzyme *(CYP11A1)*. The enzyme 11β-hydroxysteroid dehydrogenase type 2 *(HSD11B2)* inactivates cortisol to cortisone in peripheral tissues, including the kidney. *HSD3B2,* 3β-Hydroxysteroid dehydrogenase type 2; *CYP17A1,* 17α-hydroxylase or 17,20-lyase; *CYB5A,* cytochrome b_5 type A; *SULT2A1,* sulfotransferase type 2A1.

Box 9.1 Causes of Glucocorticoid Hypertension

Glucocorticoid Excess (Cushing Syndrome)	**Impairment of HSD11B2**
• Pituitary adenoma	• Apparent mineralocorticoid excess syndrome
• Ectopic ACTH syndrome	• Licorice and other HSD11B2 inhibitors
• Ectopic CRH-producing tumors	
• Adrenal cortical adenomas/carcinomas	
• Bilateral macronodular adrenal hyperplasia	
• Primary pigmented nodular adrenal hyperplasia	
• Iatrogenic	

ACTH, Adrenocorticotropic hormone; *CRH,* corticotropin-releasing hormones ; *HSD11B2,* 11β-hydroxysteroid dehydrogenase type 2.

- Ectopic CRH-producing tumors: <1%
    - ACTH-independent: 20%
- Adrenal cortical adenoma: 14%
- Adrenal cortical carcinoma: 4%
- Bilateral macronodular adrenal hyperplasia: <2%
- Primary pigmented nodular adrenal hyperplasia: <1%

7. **Describe the clinical manifestations in Cushing syndrome.**

The clinical manifestations depend on the severity and the duration of hypercortisolism but most commonly occur gradually. The manifestations are most severe in patients with ectopic ACTH production, typically from a neuroendocrine tumor located in the lungs. Conversely, patients with adrenal adenomas often have mild hypercortisolism with subtle clinical manifestations. Staple physical signs found in Cushing Syndrome include central obesity; moon face; dorsocervical adiposity (also known as "buffalo hump"); wide, purple striae, commonly on the abdomen, thighs and/or axillary areas; ecchymoses; and proximal muscle atrophy.

Common cushingoid features:
- Central obesity: 70% to 85%
- Muscle weakness/atrophy: 45% to 82%
- Moon face: 81% to 89%
- Violaceous striae: 44% to 72%
- "Buffalo hump": 51% to 53%

Other manifestations
- Acne: 19% to 27%
- Hirsutism: 75%
- Bruising: 21% to 52%
- Menstrual irregularities: 78%
- Decreased libido: 24%
- Bone loss/fractures: 40% to 70%
- Hyperglycemia: 45% to 70%
- Hypertension: 70% to 85%
- Insomnia: 29%
- Impaired cognition: 22%
- Hypokalemia: 22% to 33%
- Venous thromboembolism: 20%
- Immunosuppression/opportunistic infections: 21% to 51%

8. **Who should be tested for Cushing syndrome?**

The diagnosis is typically pursued when some of the manifestations listed earlier come to the attention of medical providers, patients, or family members. In addition, patients with incidentally found adrenal nodules are commonly screened for mild adrenal cortisol excess. Family members of those affected by genetic conditions known to predispose to Cushing Syndrome have a higher medical scrutiny for this disease.

9. **How do we test for Cushing syndrome?**

When a clinical suspicion exists, the initial step is to exclude exposure to exogenous glucocorticoids. Next, the diagnosis is established by hormonal tests. Because normal hormonal fluctuations can be caused by many different conditions, at least two of three abnormal tests are required to establish the diagnosis. The following tests are conducted when Cushing Syndrome is suspected:
- 1-mg dexamethasone suppression test. Administer 1 mg between 11:00 p.m. and midnight, then draw 8:00 a.m. serum cortisol. This test is commonly used as an initial screening test, particularly in patients with incidentally found adrenal nodules.
- 24-hour urinary free cortisol excretion (this test is often normal in patients with mild hypercortisolism).
- Late-night salivary cortisol.
- Late-night serum cortisol.

10. **What is pseudo-Cushing syndrome?**

Cortisol is a stress hormone, and several conditions can lead to hypercortisolism due to overactivation of the hypothalamus-pituitary-adrenal axis: chronic exercise, severe physical illness, morbid obesity, malnutrition, alcoholism, and poorly controlled diabetes mellitus. When such conditions are associated with clinical features common to Cushing Syndrome, they are referred to as "pseudo-Cushing Syndrome."

11. **What are some other caveats of hypercortisolism testing?**

Testing should take into account the possibility of circadian rhythm disruptions (such as night-shifts or recent travel across time zones).

Many medications can influence testing for Cushing Syndrome:
- Estrogens and mitotane increase cortisol-binding globulin levels and cause an elevated total serum cortisol. Free cortisol, as measured in saliva or urine, is not impacted.
- CYP3A4 inducers (e.g., phenobarbital, carbamazepine, rifampin, etc.) accelerate the metabolism of dexamethasone and lead to false positive results with dexamethasone suppression tests. Measurement of serum dexamethasone level is useful to ascertain if an incompletely suppressed cortisol might be a true or false positive result.

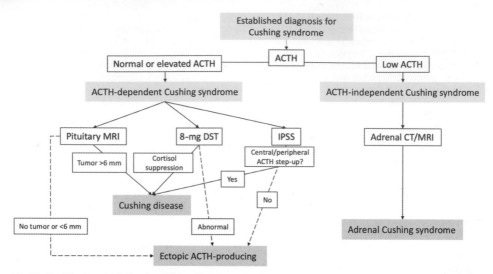

Fig. 9.2 Algorithm for establishing the etiology of Cushing syndrome. In patients with adrenocorticotropic hormone *(ACTH)*-dependent Cushing syndrome, pituitary MRI, 8-mg dexamethasone suppression test *(DST)*, and inferior petrosal sinus sampling *(IPSS)* can be used in conjunction to distinguish between Cushing disease (pituitary adenoma) and ectopic ACTH-producing tumors. *CT,* Computed tomography; *MRI,* magnetic resonance imaging.

Box 9.2 Medical Treatment for Cushing Syndrome	
Adrenal Enzyme Inhibitors • Ketoconazole • Metyrapone **Adrenolytic** • Mitotane	**Glucocorticoid Receptor Inhibitor** • Mifepristone **Others (for Cushing disease only)** • Pasireotide • Cabergoline

12. How is the etiology of Cushing Syndrome established?
    Once endogenous cortisol excess is established as described previously, the next step is to obtain an ACTH, which will guide the subsequent steps in localizing the source of cortisol excess (Fig. 9.2). When ACTH is suppressed, adrenal imaging is obtained. When ACTH is not suppressed, that indicates a pituitary or ectopic ACTH (or, rarely, CRH)-producing tumor. The evaluation of such cases is summarized in Fig. 9.2.

13. What are the treatment options for Cushing syndrome?
    - Surgery is the preferred and only curative treatment for all forms of endogenous Cushing Syndrome:
      - pituitary surgery for Cushing disease;
      - adrenalectomy for cortisol-producing adenomas or carcinomas;
      - resection of the ACTH- or CRH-producing tumor in ectopic Cushing Syndrome;
      - when the primary source of Cushing Syndrome is not found or fully resectable and the clinical manifestations are severe, bilateral adrenalectomy can be done.
    - Radiation therapy is reserved for unresectable or residual Cushing disease or adrenal cortical carcinomas.
    - Medical treatment (Box 9.2) is used to control hypercortisolism and its complications prior to surgery while awaiting the effects of radiation or for occult ectopic Cushing Syndrome.

APPARENT MINERALOCORTICOID EXCESS SYNDROME

14. What is apparent mineralocorticoid excess syndrome?
    Apparent mineralocorticoid excess (AME) syndrome is an autosomal recessive disease characterized by defects in the gene encoding HSD11B2. In these rare inherited HSD11B2 deficiencies, cortisol is not inactivated by target tissues expressing MRs, including the kidneys, allowing physiological concentrations of cortisol to activate MR.

15. **Describe the clinical and laboratory features of AME syndrome.**

    AME syndrome shares several clinical and laboratory features with primary aldosteronism: hypertension, hypokalemia, metabolic alkalosis, and low renin. In contrast with primary aldosteronism, however, plasma aldosterone concentration is low. Affected patients typically present with early-onset severe hypertension accompanied by low birth weight, failure to thrive, renal insufficiency, and hypercalciuria. A milder phenotype occurs in adults with compound heterozygous mutations.

16. **How is AME syndrome diagnosed?**

    When the diagnosis of AME syndrome is suspected based on clinical and initial laboratory features described earlier, a 24-hour urine measurement of cortisol-to-cortisone ratio is useful in making the diagnosis. In the presence of HSD11B2 defects, the normal 24-hour urine cortisol/cortisone of approximately 0.3 to 0.5 is flipped in favor of cortisol, which cannot be appropriately inactivated. Typical 24-hour urinary cortisol-to-cortisone ratios are 5 in children and 18 in adults with AME syndrome. AME syndrome can also be confirmed with commercially available genetic testing.

17. **What treatment options are available for patients with AME syndrome?**

    The primary treatment strategy in AME syndrome is to counteract the MR activation by cortisol. MR antagonists, such as spironolactone and eplerenone, are preferred. Amiloride and triamterene, which block the ENaCs in the distal convoluted tubules and collecting ducts of the nephrons, are other alternatives. Suppression of endogenous cortisol synthesis with low-dose dexamethasone, a synthetic glucocorticoid with negligible mineralocorticoid activity, has also been suggested. Dexamethasone, however, is a potent glucocorticoid with propensity for systemic side effects, including persistence of hypertension and hypokalemia. A thiazide diuretic can be used for patients with AME syndrome and hypercalciuria. Renal transplant has also been reported to cure AME syndrome.

18. **Are there nongenetic forms of HSD11B2 dysfunction?**

    Several exogenous and endogenous compounds can inhibit HSD11B2, leading to hypertension in a similar manner to AME syndrome.

19. **What are the most common inhibitors of HSD11B2?**

    The most recognized HSD11B2 inhibitors are glycyrrhetinic acid, which is a compound found in licorice, and carbenoxolone, a derivative of glycyrrhetinic acid. Licorice extracts are used in sweets, particularly in the Middle East and in parts of Europe and Asia. Chronic consumption of licorice leads to an AME syndrome–like phenotype.

    Several other exogenous and endogenous compounds have HSD11B2-inhibitory effects and collectively are termed *glycyrrhetinic acid–like factors (GALFs)*. Endogenous GALFs might serve as regulators of sodium and blood pressure. Several antifungal agents (itraconazole and posaconazole) and carbenoxolone also inhibit HSD11B2 (see Chapter 13: Drug-Induced Hypertension).

KEY POINTS

1. Cortisol circulates in higher concentrations than aldosterone; whereas cortisol and aldosterone have similar affinity for the MRs, the enzyme HSD11B2 serves as a gatekeeper by inactivating cortisol to cortisone.
2. In Cushing syndrome, supraphysiological concentrations of cortisol lead to activation of both glucocorticoid and MRs due to the saturation of HSD11B2. This leads to sodium and water retention, intravascular volume expansion, and hypokalemia.
3. AME syndrome is a rare inherited disease that displays clinical manifestations similar to primary aldosteronism, except that plasma aldosterone concentrations are low. AME syndrome is caused by defects in the *HSD11B2* gene, which prevent the inactivation of cortisol in target tissues and allow cortisol to overactivate the MRs.
4. Exogenous glucocorticoids and several inhibitors of HSD11B2, including licorice, also lead to MR–mediated hypertension.

BIBLIOGRAPHY

Adamidis A, Cantas-Orsdemir S, Tsirka A, et al. Apparent mineralocorticoid excess in the pediatric population: report of a novel pathogenic variant of the 11β-HSD2 gene and systematic review of the literature. *Pediatr Endocrinol Rev.* 2019;16(3):335–358.

Athimulam S, Lazik N, Bancos I. Low-renin hypertension. *Endocrinol Metab Clin North Am.* 2019;48(4):701–715.

Farese Jr RV, Biglieri EG, Shackleton CH, et al. Licorice-induced hypermineralocorticoidism. *N Engl J Med.* 1991;24(32517):1223–1227.

Isidori AM, Graziadio C, Paragliola RM, et al. The hypertension of Cushing's syndrome: controversies in the pathophysiology and focus on cardiovascular complications. *J Hypertens.* 2015;33(1):44–60.

Ma X, Lian QQ, Dong Q, et al. Environmental inhibitors of 11β-hydroxysteroid dehydrogenase type 2. *Toxicology.* 2011;29(2853):83–89.

Morris DJ, Latif SA, Hardy MP, et al. Endogenous inhibitors (GALFs) of 11beta-hydroxysteroid dehydrogenase isoforms 1 and 2: derivatives of adrenally produced corticosterone and cortisol. *J Steroid Biochem Mol Biol.* 2007;104(3–5):161–168.

Nieman LK, Biller BM, Findling JW, et al. The diagnosis of Cushing's syndrome: an Endocrine Society clinical practice guideline. *J Clin Endocrinol Metab.* 2008;93(5):1526–1540.

Nieman LK, Biller BM, Findling JW, et al. Treatment of Cushing's syndrome: an Endocrine Society clinical practice guideline. *J Clin Endocrinol Metab.* 2015;100(8):2807–2831.

Quinkler M, Stewart PM. Hypertension and the cortisol-cortisone shuttle. *J Clin Endocrinol Metab.* 2003;88(6):2384–2392.

Sharma ST, Nieman LK, Feelders RA. Cushing's syndrome: epidemiology and developments in disease management. *Clin Epidemiol.* 2015;17(7):281–293.

PHEOCHROMOCYTOMA AND PARAGANGLIOMA

CHAPTER 10

Anand Vaidya, MD, MMSc

QUESTIONS

1. **What are pheochromocytoma and paraganglioma?**
   - Pheochromocytomas and paragangliomas are differentiated based on anatomical location.[1]
   - Pheochromocytomas are neuroendocrine tumors that arise from the adrenal medulla.
   - Paragangliomas are neuroendocrine tumors that arise from extraadrenal sympathetic or parasympathetic paraganglia. Therefore paragangliomas can be found anywhere from the base of the skull to the pelvis.

2. **What are the differences between pheochromocytoma and paraganglioma?**
   - Beyond the anatomical differences described earlier, pheochromocytoma and paraganglioma can exhibit biochemical differences.
   - Catecholamines are synthesized from a tyrosine substrate, which is ultimately transformed to produce dopamine, norepinephrine, and epinephrine.
   - Catecholamines typically circulate in low concentrations and have pulsatile and variable levels and short half-lives.
   - Catecholamines are further metabolized to inactive metabolites that have long and stable circulating half-lives. These metabolites are termed "metanephrines." Norepinephrine is metabolized to normetanephrine, and epinephrine is metabolized to metanephrine. Together, these two metabolites are referred to as metanephrines. When ordering testing for metanephrines, the results appear as fractionated concentrations of normetanephrine and metanephrine. This terminology can be confusing as the singular and plural distinctions impart different meanings.
   - Dopamine is metabolized to the inactive metabolite termed "methoxytyramine"; however, the use of this metabolite is not common in clinical care, and this measurement is not widely commercially available.
   - The adrenal medulla expresses the enzymatic machinery to synthesize all the catecholamines. Therefore pheochromocytomas can exhibit a biochemical phenotype that includes elevated normetanephrine and/or elevated metanephrine (i.e., a pheochromocytoma can secrete norepinephrine and/or epinephrine).
   - In contrast, paragangliomas do not express the enzyme that converts norepinephrine to epinephrine and, therefore, do not secrete epinephrine (i.e., paragangliomas can secrete dopamine and/or norepinephrine).
   - Therefore, in practice, elevated normetanephrine levels could signify a pheochromocytoma or a paraganglioma, whereas elevated metanephrine levels could indicate a pheochromocytoma but not a paraganglioma.
   - Finally, it is worth remembering that pheochromocytomas and paragangliomas can be nonfunctional (i.e., neuroendocrine tumors that do not secrete catecholamines or metanephrines).

3. **What causes pheochromocytoma and paraganglioma?**
   - We now understand that 35% to 40% of all pheochromocytoma and paraganglioma are attributed to an inheritable (i.e., germline) pathogenic genetic mutation.[1–4]
   - More than a dozen genetic mutations have been associated with pheochromocytoma-paraganglioma syndromes. Beyond developing these neuroendocrine tumors, some genetic syndromes predispose to developing other tumors and cancers as well.[1,5]
   - For this reason, it is recommended that ***all*** patients with pheochromocytoma and paraganglioma be advised to consider genetic testing. The discovery of a genetic mutation often dictates a tumor surveillance program that involves imaging.
   - The following are genes associated with pheochromocytoma-paraganglioma syndromes:
     - *VHL* (von-Hippel Lindau syndrome)
     - *RET* (multiple endocrine neoplasia type 2)
     - *NF1* (neurofibromatosis type 1)
     - *SDHA* (succinate dehydrogenase subunit A)
     - *SDHB* (succinate dehydrogenase subunit B)
     - *SDHC* (succinate dehydrogenase subunit C)

- *SDHD* (succinate dehydrogenase subunit D)
- *SDHAF2* (succinate dehydrogenase subunit AF2)
- *TMEM127* (transmembrane protein 127)
- *MAX* (myc-associated factor X)
- *FH* (fumarate hydratase)
- *EPAS1* (hypoxia inducible factor 2a)
- It is important to note that the majority of patients with a germline mutation, or hereditary pheochromocytoma-paraganglioma syndrome, do not display specific phenotypic features to help guide genetic testing. Therefore unless there are obvious phenotypic features indicative of a specific genetic syndrome (see Table), genetic testing should be conducted using a comprehensive and unbiased approach (i.e., gene panels).[5]
- For patients who are found to have a pathogenic germline mutation, screening of family members should be recommended. In addition, an imaging and biochemical surveillance program should be recommended to monitor for pheochromocytoma, paraganglioma, and other related tumors.[1,5]
- Patients should be managed by a multidisciplinary team with expertise in genetic testing and imaging surveillance protocols.

4. What other tumors are associated with hereditary pheochromocytoma-paraganglioma syndromes?
   - A list of the most common germline mutations and the tumors that can occur are listed in the following table. Notably, the tumors include both benign and malignant entities.

Gene	Syndrome	Key Features and Associated Tumors
VHL	Von Hippel-Lindau	Pheochromocytoma (PHEO), paraganglioma (PGL), hemangioblastoma, renal cell carcinoma (RCC), renal and pancreatic cysts, endolymphatic sac tumor, neuroendocrine tumors
SDHA	NA	PHEO, PGL, gastrointestinal stromal tumors (GIST), possible pituitary adenoma, and RCC
SDHB	PGL4	PHEO, PGL, GIST, RCC, possible pituitary adenoma
SDHC	PGL3	PHEO, PGL, GIST, RCC, possible pituitary adenoma
SDHD	PGL1	PHEO, PGL, GIST, RCC, possible pituitary adenoma
SDHAF2	PGL2	PHEO, PGL, possibly others
HIF2A	Familial erythrocytosis[3] Zhuang-Pacak syndrome	PHEO, PGL, polycythemia, somatostatinoma
PHD2	Familial erythrocytosis[4]	PHEO, PGL, polycythemia
FH	Hereditary leiomyomatosis and renal cell cancer	PHEO, cutaneous leiomyomata, uterine leiomyomata (fibroids), RCC
NF1	Neurofibromatosis, type 1	PHEO, PGL neurofibromas, optic gliomas, malignant peripheral nerve sheath tumors, astrocytomas, leukemia, breast cancer, boney lesions, short stature, relative macrocephaly, developmental delays in some individuals
RET	Multiple endocrine neoplasia, type 2a	PHEO, PGL, medullary thyroid carcinoma, parathyroid hyperplasia/adenoma
	Multiple endocrine neoplasia, type 2b	PHEO, PGL, medullary thyroid carcinoma, oral mucosal neuromas, marfanoid habitus, distinct facial features with large lips, gastrointestinal ganglioneuromas
TMEM127	NA	PHEO, possible RCC
MAX	NA	PHEO, RCC, possibly others

5. What are the symptoms and signs of pheochromocytoma and paraganglioma?
   - Excessive catecholamine production can induce episodic hyperadrenergic symptoms. Patients may describe episodic palpitations, sweating, headaches, anxiety, or panic attacks. Patients may have pallor (due to vasoconstriction).
   - Flushing is not a symptom or sign of catecholamine excess.
   - Blood pressure may be chronically elevated and, if checked during an episode, may be very elevated. However, it is worth noting that labile blood pressure attributable to causes other than a pheochromocytoma or paraganglioma is far more common. Thus, although pheochromocytoma and paraganglioma are considered "secondary causes of hypertension," it is worth noting that most causes of labile hypertension are not pheochromocytoma or paraganglioma.
   - Hyperglycemia or worsening of glycemic control may be observed.
   - Orthostatic hypotension can be observed. Catecholamine excess can cause a natriuresis and volume depletion, which may result in blood pressure decreases with upright posture. Although orthostatic hypotension may be

seen in more severe cases of pheochromocytoma and is often considered to be a classic finding, most cases in the current era are diagnosed at a relatively early stage (or incidentally) and usually do not have appreciable orthostatic hypotension.

- Importantly, the incidence of asymptomatic pheochromocytoma and paraganglioma is increasing as these tumors are frequently detected incidentally on cross-sectional imaging prior to the development of clinical symptoms.

6. **Which patients should be tested for pheochromocytoma and paraganglioma?**
   - Patients with episodic hyperadrenergic signs or symptoms, described previously.
   - Patients with an adrenal mass that appears lipid-poor (unenhanced Hounsfield units [HU] >10 on computed tomography [CT] or no loss of signal on in-and-out-of-phase magnetic resonance imaging [MRI]).
   - Patients with labile and/or severe hypertension that is not attributable to medication nonadherence or other secondary causes of hypertension.
   - Patients who develop a hypertensive or adrenergic episode triggered by certain medications (induction of anesthesia, opioids, metoclopramide, and others).
   - Patients with a known inheritable syndrome or genetic mutation associated with pheochromocytoma or paraganglioma.

7. **How are pheochromocytoma and paraganglioma diagnosed?**
   - Currently, the majority of pheopchromocytomas are diagnosed incidentally on cross-sectional imaging in asymptomatic individuals. The imaging features are often the most diagnostic in these cases.
   - The diagnostic test of choice in patients who exhibit hyperadrenergic symptoms or episodes is to measure fractionated metanephrines in either the plasma or the urine.[6]
   - Measuring plasma metanephrines or 24-hour urinary metanephrines are both appropriate and have similar diagnostic accuracy. The sensitivity is ~97%, and the specificity is ~90%. Therefore the likelihood of missing a true symptomatic pheochromocytoma or paraganglioma is very low; however, the risk of false-positive testing is not trivial.[6]
   - The negative predictive value of both tests is very high.
   - Plasma catecholamines are not reliable and are not typically recommended.
   - 24-hour urinary fractionated catecholamines can be measured reliably and may provide a useful adjunct when measuring 24-hour urinary metanephrines.
   - In general, measuring plasma metanephrines is the quickest and easiest way to initiate the diagnostic evaluation as it involves only phlebotomy.
   - Metanephrines should ideally be measured by laboratories that use liquid chromatography with tandem mass spectroscopy.

8. **Can false-positive testing results occur?**
   - Yes. False-positive testing is one of the most common pitfalls in the evaluation of pheochromocytoma and paraganglioma.
   - The upper limit of the reference range of metanephrines does not represent a hard and fixed biological boundary of "normal" versus "abnormal;" rather, it must be interpreted in the context of the clinical scenario and expected physiology.
   - A true symptomatic pheochromocytoma or paraganglioma almost always exhibits marked elevations in levels of metanephrines. In most cases, a functional tumor causing symptoms will exhibit fourfold or greater elevations in metanephrine and/or normetanephrine above the upper limit of the reference range. Rarely, a true functional tumor will exhibit twofold or greater elevations.
   - False-positive elevations in metanephrines occur in ~10% to 15% of the population and are generally less than twofold above the upper limit of the reference range. Rarely, false-positive can be seen to rise as high as three- to fourfold the upper limit of the reference range.
   - The most common cause of false-positive elevations in metanephrines are factors that increase sympathoadrenergic activity. These factors can include pain, stress, anxiety, illness (including hospitalization), upright posture (including seated posture during phlebotomy), the use of sympathomimetic agents (including levodopa and vasopressors), and the use of catecholamine-reuptake inhibitors for depression.
   - Medications for depression or anxiety that inhibit the reuptake of catecholamines are a very common cause of false-positive elevations in metanephrines. These include norepinephrine-reuptake inhibitors and selective-serotonin reuptake inhibitors. At times, these medications can cause two- to fourfold elevations in metanephrines. It is important to recognize this potential source of a false-positive before undertaking testing.[7]
   - The negative predictive value of metanephrines is very high. Therefore metanephrine levels that return in the normal reference range provide strong reassurance that the signs and symptoms are not attributable to a functional pheochromocytoma or paraganglioma.
   - Incidentally discovered pheochromocytomas are increasingly common with the use of cross-sectional imaging. Often, incidental pheochromocytomas are detected before the onset of clinical symptoms (i.e., subclinical or nonfunctional). The diagnosis should involve the use of radiographic characteristics (described earlier and later) in combination with metanephrines.

9. **When and how should imaging be used in the evaluation of pheochromocytoma and paraganglioma?**
   - The diagnosis of a symptomatic pheochromocytoma or paraganglioma is biochemical. Imaging should not be pursued until a biochemical diagnosis is confirmed. Therefore, in most instances, imaging should be considered a localization test, not a diagnostic test.
   - Pheochromocytoma and paragangliomas may also be detected incidentally on imaging, in which case biochemical testing should follow. Incidental discovery of these tumors on cross-sectional imaging is steadily increasing.
   - Pheochromocytomas and paragangliomas exhibit high attenuation on unenhanced CT imaging. Typically these tumors will manifest as having greater than 10 HU attenuation on CT done without contrast and will often enhance to greater than 75 HU following intravenous contrast. Low unenhanced attenuation (<10 HU) provides strong evidence against a pheochromocytoma. On MRI, these tumors often exhibit T2 hyperintensity and a lack of signal dropout on in-and-out-of-phase imaging.[8]
   - Pheochromocytomas and paragangliomas are usually fluorodeoxyglucose-avid. However, the most specific tracer and metabolite when positron emission tomography (PET) imaging is used is now DOTATATE, which has the highest sensitivity and specificity for neuroendocrine tumors.[1]
   - When nuclear imaging is needed, metaiodobenzylguanidine has largely been replaced by G^{68}-DOTATATE-PET imaging.

10. **What is the treatment for pheochromocytoma and paraganglioma?**
   - Surgery is the treatment of choice for symptomatic and functional pheochromocytomas and paragangliomas.
   - Given the episodic nature of catecholamine secretion and the risk of intraoperative hemodynamic instability that could induce hypertensive or hypotensive crises, surgery should be coordinated with an experienced team that includes an endocrinologist, a surgeon, and an anesthesiologist. Interdisciplinary teams with large experience bases have lower rates of adverse outcomes.[4]
   - Preoperative alpha- and beta-adrenergic blockade should be implemented, and, when necessary, the use of calcium channel blockers and metyrosine (tyrosine hydroxylase inhibitor) can also be effective.[6]

11. **What should I do if I think I have diagnosed a pheochromocytoma or paraganglioma?**
   - Consult with an experienced endocrinologist and/or adrenal surgeon to ensure that the diagnosis is correct, that the localization procedures are appropriate, and that an adequate medical and surgical treatment plan is developed.
   - Diagnosis and treatment outcomes are optimized when patients are cared for by experienced multidisciplinary teams.

KEY POINTS

- Pheochromocytoma and paraganglioma are neuroendocrine tumors arising from the adrenal medulla or autonomic nervous system, respectively, that are capable of secreting catecholamines.
- The diagnostic test of choice is to measure plasma and/or urinary metanephrines. Symptomatic and functional pheochromocytomas and paragangliomas have substantial elevations in metanephrine levels, often multiple times the upper limit of the reference range. False-positive elevations in metanephrines are common.
- Imaging is used to localize the pheochromocytoma or paraganglioma after biochemical confirmation; however, incidentally discovered tumors are increasing in incidence.

REFERENCES

1. Neumann HPH, Young Jr WF, Eng C. Pheochromocytoma and paraganglioma. *N Engl J Med.* 2019;381:552–565.
2. Crona J, Taïeb D, Pacak K. New perspectives on pheochromocytoma and paraganglioma: toward a molecular classification. *Endocr Rev.* 2017;38:489–515.
3. Dahia PL. Pheochromocytomas and paragangliomas, genetically diverse and minimalist, all at once!. *Cancer Cell.* 2017;31:159–161.
4. Fishbein L, Leshchiner I, Walter V, et al. Comprehensive molecular characterization of pheochromocytoma and paraganglioma. *Cancer Cell.* 2017;31:181–193.
5. Rana HQ, Rainville IR, Vaidya A. Genetic testing in the clinical care of patients with pheochromocytoma and paraganglioma. *Curr Opin Endocrinol Diabetes Obes.* 2014;21:166–176.
6. Lenders JW, Duh QY, Eisenhofer G, et al. Pheochromocytoma and paraganglioma: an endocrine society clinical practice guideline. *J Clin Endocrinol Metab.* 2014;99:1915–1942.
7. Neary NM, King KS, Pacak K. Drugs and pheochromocytoma—don't be fooled by every elevated metanephrine. *N Engl J Med.* 2011;364:2268–2270.
8. Vaidya A, Hamrahian A, Bancos I, Fleseriu M, Ghayee HK. The evaluation of incidentally discovered adrenal masses. *Endocr Pract.* 2019;25:178–192.

CHAPTER 11

OTHER ENDOCRINE CAUSES OF HYPERTENSION

James M. Luther, MD MSCI, and Craig Sussman, MD

QUESTIONS

1. **How does acromegaly cause hypertension, and when should it be suspected?**

   Acromegaly is caused by hypersecretion of growth hormone (GH) usually from the pituitary with peripheral target organ mediation through the excess production of insulin like growth factor 1 (IGF-1). In addition to the classical features of this disease like acral growth, jaw prognathism, and gigantism, IGF-1 causes hypertrophy and growth of multiple other tissues. The heart muscle, adrenal glands, endothelial cell, and kidneys are all targets for excess IGF-1. Pathologically, this results in cardiomyopathy, adrenal hyperplasia (especially aldosterone excess), intravascular volume expansion, and hyperadrenergic vasoconstriction. Hypertension is a prominent feature in one-third of patients presenting with acromegaly.[1] Hypertension is often multifactorial and driven by sodium and water retention, volume expansion, angiotensin II vasoconstriction, increased sympathetic tone, and increased cardiac output. These conditions promote hypertension by the combined increase in stroke volume and peripheral resistance. Other complications of GH excess such as obstructive sleep apnea, diastolic dysfunction, and insulin resistance also contribute to the secondary hypertension of acromegaly.

   The diagnosis of acromegaly can be made by measuring IGF-1 levels especially in patients with acral and facial features. It is very reasonable to screen with IGF-1 levels in the setting of known complications of acromegaly including hypertension, cardiomyopathy, sleep apnea, hyperhidrosis, and polyosteoarthritis. Confirmation can be made by the lack of suppression of GH to less than 1 μg/L following an oral glucose load. Radiographic studies, especially magnetic resonance imaging, can identify a pituitary tumor. Multidisciplinary care involving cardiology and endocrinology is essential for these patients to ensure proper evaluation, treatment, and prevention of cardiovascular complications.

2. **When should testosterone excess be suspected as a cause of hypertension?**

   Common clinical signs and symptoms that should raise suspicion of androgen excess or anabolic steroid abuse are listed in Table 11.1. Virilizing or defeminizing symptoms in women often prompt an evaluation. Androgen excess is more difficult to detect in men and may only be manifest by testicular atrophy and infertility due to decreased spermatogenesis. Testosterone is directly synthesized in the testes in men and in much lesser amounts in the ovaries in women. Testosterone is also derived from the adrenal precursors dehydroepiandrosterone (DHEA), dehydroepiandrosterone sulfate (DHEAS), and androstenedione, which are converted in peripheral tissues (adipose, skin) to testosterone. Testosterone may be converted to the more potent androgen dihydrotestosterone by 5-alpha reductase in peripheral tissues where it activates local androgen receptors, amplifying its local effects.

   Endogenous androgen excess can be seen in prolactinoma or polycystic ovarian syndrome (PCOS) or by secretion from a functional adrenal, testicular, or ovarian tumor. Glucocorticoid resistance or congenital adrenal hyperplasia can also cause androgen excess due to overproduction of adrenal androgens. The rapid development of androgen excess signs and symptoms should prompt the evaluation for an androgen secreting tumor. Adrenocortical carcinomas often secrete multiple steroids including DHEA, DHEAS, and cortisol more often than they are produced by adrenal adenomas. Ovarian or testicular tumors may also secrete androgens. Although total serum testosterone is usually elevated in all of these conditions, increased DHEA and DHEAS suggest an adrenal cause of androgen excess.

   Although synthetic anabolic androgens are often used to enhance athletic performance, supraphysiological doses of transdermal or intramuscular testosterone are increasingly used for low libido, impotence, anorexia, or muscle wasting. When used appropriately to treat true hypoandrogenism, testosterone replacement is associated with little risk and may be associated with reduced blood pressure and cardiovascular risk.

   Anabolic androgen steroids (AAS) derived from testosterone are used by young men (typically aged 20–30) to increase muscle mass or enhance athletic performance, with the vast majority of use by recreational bodybuilders.[2,3] Other anabolic agents (e.g., human growth hormone, insulin like growth factor (IGF-1), and insulin) are often used cyclically with AAS and other drugs to increase pain tolerance (e.g., opiates or nonsteroidal antiinflammatory drugs), promote fat loss (e.g., thyroxine), or prevent adverse effects of testosterone excess (e.g., aromatase inhibitor or estrogen receptor antagonist). Opiates are frequently used with AAS to augment strength training, therefore opiate dependence is more common in AAS users.[3] Additional concern for human immunodeficiency virus, hepatitis C, and hepatitis B is also warranted in users of injectable AAS. Various androgens are available in

Table 11.1 Signs and Symptoms of Other Endocrine Causes of Hypertension

DISORDER	SIGNS AND SYMPTOMS IN ADDITION TO HYPERTENSION	DIAGNOSTIC TESTING
Acromegaly	Enlargement of forehead, nose, jaw, feet, and fingers Sleep apnea, arthritis, carpal tunnel syndrome Headache, visual field deficit	IGF-1 GH after oral glucose tolerance test Pituitary MRI
Testosterone excess	*Men:* Testicular atrophy, male-pattern baldness, breast development *Women:* defeminization (reduction in breast size, hirsutism, facial hair, male-pattern hair loss, menstrual irregularity, clitoral enlargement, voice deepening Acne, irritability, paranoia, delusions, mania, polycythemia, dyslipidemia, kidney failure, liver damage, liver tumors, blood clots	Elevated testosterone/epitestosterone ratio >4 Urine mass spectrometry for AAS Elevated hemoglobin Suppressed LH, FSH, and testosterone Low HDL, increased LDL cholesterol
Hyperthyroidism	Palpitations, tachycardia, anxiety, tremulousness, heat intolerance, fatigue, weight loss, proptosis, dyspnea, edema	TSH, free T4 and T3
Hypothyroidism	Bradycardia, depression, cold intolerance, fatigue, weight gain, edema, dry skin, constipation, loss of eyebrows	TSH, free T4
Hyperparathyroidism	Hypercalcemia, hypophosphatemia, decreased bone density, fractures, kidney stones	Intact PTH, calcium, phosphate, 25-OH vitamin D, urinary calcium excretion, PTH-related protein, serum/urine protein electrophoresis

AAS, Anabolic androgen steroid; *FSH,* follicle-stimulating hormone; *GH,* growth hormone; *HDL,* high-density lipoprotein; *IGF-1,* insulin growth factor 1; *LDL,* low-density lipoprotein; *LH,* luteinizing hormone; *MRI,* magnetic resonance imaging; *PTH,* parathyroid hormone; *T3,* triiodothyronine; *T4,* thyroxine; *TSH,* thyroid-stimulating hormone.

oral, transdermal, or injectable forms depending on the specific compound. Hepatotoxicity is a potential toxicity for several oral AAS (stanazolol, 17-α methyl testosterone, oxandrolone), and therefore intramuscular injection is the preferred route of administration for many weightlifters. The Steroid Control Act of 2004 banned most AAS, but they may still be obtained illicitly, and novel testosterone derivatives continue to surface. In addition to intentional AAS use, patients may unknowingly ingest supplements containing an oral AAS, especially in those marketed as an alternative to anabolic steroids or a supplement for sexual enhancement.

Because of the ethics of providing AAS to healthy volunteers to study their cardiovascular effects, the literature relies on cross-sectional studies of current versus former AAS users or control populations. Adverse cardiovascular and metabolic effects of AAS use may only partially reverse with cessation. Current use of AAS is associated with increased 24-hour ambulatory blood pressure, prevalent hypertension, reduced ventricular function, vascular calcification, and aortic stiffness.[4,5]

Androgen abuse can typically be diagnosed by direct questioning if a trusting patient-physician relationship exists, although many patients are reluctant to offer a history of use. Polycythemia is a frequently observed laboratory clue that should prompt questioning for AAS use. Exogenous testosterone can be detected by an increased urinary testosterone/epitestosterone ratio greater than 4, although common genetic variants in Southeast Asian populations may cause a false negative result. Urinary mass spectrometric assays are performed by specialty laboratories to detect testosterone analogues and derivatives.

3. **How does PCOS cause androgen excess and hypertension, and how should it be treated?**
PCOS is a common condition in young women associated with irregular menstruation, anovulation, and hirsutism due to androgen excess. Androgen excess in PCOS is caused directly by ovarian testosterone secretion and indirectly via ovarian androstenedione secretion and peripheral conversion and excess adrenal DHEAS production and peripheral conversion. Hirsutism or infertility in women often prompts evaluation for PCOS to exclude other clinically important causes of hirsutism. Serum total testosterone is usually only mildly elevated in PCOS. Increased serum DHEAS in the setting of severely elevated testosterone usually indicates a primary adrenal disorder with excess testosterone production, rather than PCOS. Normal serum 17-hydroxy-progesterone excludes nonclassical congenital adrenal hyperplasia due to incomplete loss of 21-hydroxylase activity.

Metabolic complications such as insulin resistance, impaired insulin secretion, glucose intolerance, hyperlipidemia, and hypertension are common in patients with PCOS and contribute to increased risk of cardiovascular complications. Hypertension in PCOS is more closely associated with metabolic complications than with the degree of hyperandrogenism. Treatment for PCOS is intended to reduce hyperandrogenic symptoms, metabolic complications, and cardiovascular risk. Spironolactone is useful for its antiandrogenic and antihypertensive effects and is often used when oral estrogen-progestin therapy is contraindicated. Metformin is commonly used to treat insulin resistance in PCOS.

4. **Do thyroid disorders cause hypertension?**
Hyperthyroidism causes tachycardia and increased cardiac output with pulmonary hypertension and wide pulse pressure.[6,7] Increased beta-adrenergic receptor activity produces symptoms of hyperthyroidism suggestive of catecholamine excess, although circulating catecholamines are not elevated. The renin-angiotensin-aldosterone system is also activated in hyperthyroidism. Hyperthyroidism is associated with increased risk of hypertension, atrial fibrillation, and heart failure. Treatment with beta-blockers can greatly reduce symptoms and should be started soon after diagnosis, but a treatment to reduce thyroid hormone production is typically needed (methimazole, radioiodine, or surgery).

Hypothyroidism is the most common thyroid disorder and is associated with hypercholesterolemia and diastolic hypertension. This is caused by increased peripheral vascular resistance, decreased cardiac output, volume expansion, and a low renin hypertension. It is important to recognize that hypothyroidism in pregnancy is associated with a greater risk of preeclampsia. These abnormalities are reversible with thyroid hormone replacement in many patients.

5. **Does hyperparathyroidism cause hypertension?**
The causative link between primary hyperparathyroidism (PHPT) and hypertension is controversial. Patients with PHPT have a high incidence of hypertension, although confounding effects of age and other comorbidities may contribute. Hyperparathyroidism may also be detected more often in hypertensive patients due to thiazide-provoked hypercalcemia, leading to a selection bias in this population. Approximately 24% of patients with thiazide-associated hypercalcemia are found to have underlying PHPT.[8]

Parathyroid hormone (PTH) directly stimulates renin and aldosterone secretion in animal models, and this has implicated the renin-angiotensin-aldosterone system activation in patients with PHPT and hypertension. Primary aldosteronism is associated with increased PTH, which decreases after adrenalectomy. Parathyroidectomy has inconsistently been shown to reduce renin or improve blood pressure control in patients with PHPT and hypertension.[9]

6. **Does recombinant erythropoietin administration cause hypertension?**
Recombinant erythropoietin (EPO) is used to treat anemia caused by reduced endogenous EPO production most commonly due to chronic kidney disease (CKD). EPO increases blood pressure by angiotensin II type 1 receptor-dependent vasoconstriction and acts independent of effects on hematocrit, blood volume, or blood viscosity.[10] EPO administration doubles the risk of hypertension when compared to placebo administration in CKD patients, and the effect is exacerbated in hemodialysis patients. Although targeting high versus low hemoglobin target does not appear to modify the risk of hypertension, the lower hemoglobin target may be associated with lower risk of hypertensive complications.[10] Studies have demonstrated increased cardiovascular event rates in dialysis patients treated to a higher hemoglobin target, although this risk was independent of blood pressure. Darbepoetin was associated with an increased stroke risk, but this risk was independent of blood pressure and associated with prior stroke, cardiovascular disease, and proteinuria.[11] Recombinant EPO may also increase blood pressure in other populations such as in patients with chronic heart failure and anemia. Notably, EPO use in the absence of CKD does not appear to produce marked hypertension, such as in illicit EPO use (e.g., for athletic performance) or treatment of chemotherapy-associated anemia.[12] The blood pressure effects of drugs that increase endogenous EPO production by stabilizing hypoxia-inducible transcription factors remain to be fully determined. Initial results demonstrate lower blood pressure during the prolyl hydroxylase inhibitor roxadustat versus recombinant EPO in hemodialysis[13] but slightly higher risk of hypertension versus placebo in CKD.[14]

7. **Is there a link between polycythemia and hypertension?**
Common hypertension-related causes of polycythemia are listed in Table 11.2. Polycythemia is a relatively common finding in chronic hypoxic pulmonary conditions (e.g., chronic obstructive pulmonary disease, chronic smoking), including obstructive sleep apnea, which are also associated with resistant hypertension. Polycythemia is associated with multiple cardiovascular risk factors, and the constellation of polycythemia with severe hypertension has been termed *Gaisböck syndrome*.[15] Pressure natriuresis-induced volume contraction in severe hypertension, with a resulting increase in hematocrit, is believed to cause Gaisböck syndrome, which may also be exacerbated by smoking and diuretic use. Angiotensin II infusion or conditions that increase endogenous angiotensin II (e.g., renal artery stenosis or diuretic use) stimulate EPO production, and treatment with an angiotensin-converting enzyme inhibitor or angiotensin II receptor blocker is associated with reduction in hematocrit.[16] Other hypertensive disorders associated with polycythemia include renal artery stenosis, polycystic kidney disease,

Table 11.2 Hypertension-Related Causes of Polycythemia

PATHOPHYSIOLOGY	ASSOCIATED CONDITIONS
Hypoxia-induced EPO production	Sleep apnea Smoking
Ectopic EPO production	Pheochromocytoma
Inappropriately normal or high EPO	Anabolic steroids Androgen excess (adrenal tumor) Glucocorticoid excess Exogenous recombinant EPO Pheochromocytoma
Renal ischemia	Renal artery stenosis: Atherosclerotic disease *JAK2* V617F-positive polycythemia vera Polycystic kidney disease Diuretics
Hemoconcentration or volume contraction	Gaisböck syndrome Diuretics Pheochromocytoma

*This table is not comprehensive for *all* causes of polycythemia.
EPO, Erythropoietin.

pheochromocytoma, anabolic steroid use, Cushing syndrome, and Gaisböck syndrome. Pheochromocytoma could cause polycythemia due to either pressure natriuresis and hemoconcentration or by ectopic EPO production by the tumor. Diseases of the kidney that cause localized tissue ischemia and EPO secretion are common causes of polycythemia, including renal artery stenosis. It should be noted that *JAK2* V6167F-positive polycythemia vera is associated with increased risk of both cardiovascular events and renal artery stenosis.

KEY POINTS

1. Testosterone excess can be caused by steroid use or due to testosterone-secreting tumors of the adrenal, ovary, or testes.
2. Recombinant EPO increases blood pressure in patients with CKD independent of hemoglobin increase but typically responds to non specific antihypertensive medications.
3. Polycythemia is associated with severe hypertension (Gaisböck syndrome) and may be driven by a secondary cause of hypertension.

REFERENCES

1. Pivonello R, Auriemma RS, Grasso LF, et al. Complications of acromegaly: cardiovascular, respiratory and metabolic comorbidities. *Pituitary.* 2017;20:46–62.
2. NIoDA. Steroids and other appearance and performance enhancing drugs (APEDs) research report.
3. Pope Jr HG, Wood RI, Rogol A, Nyberg F, Bowers L, Bhasin S. Adverse health consequences of performance-enhancing drugs: an Endocrine Society scientific statement. *Endocr. Rev.* 2014;35:341–375.
4. Rasmussen JJ, Schou M, Madsen PL, et al. Increased blood pressure and aortic stiffness among abusers of anabolic androgenic steroids: potential effect of suppressed natriuretic peptides in plasma? *J. Hypertens.* 2018;36:277–285.
5. Baggish AL, Weiner RB, Kanayama G, et al. Cardiovascular toxicity of illicit anabolic-androgenic steroid use. *Circulation.* 2017;135:1991–2002.
6. Rivas AM, Pena C, Kopel J, Dennis JA, Nugent K. Hypertension and hyperthyroidism: association and pathogenesis. *Am. J. Med. Sci.* 2021;361:3–7.
7. Berta E, Lengyel I, Halmi S, et al. Hypertension in thyroid disorders. *Front. Endocrinol. (Lausanne).* 2019;10:482.
8. Griebeler ML, Kearns AE, Ryu E, et al. Thiazide-associated hypercalcemia: incidence and association with primary hyperparathyroidism over two decades. *J. Clin. Endocrinol. Metab.* 2016;101:1166–1173.
9. Bernini G, Moretti A, Lonzi S, Bendinelli C, Miccoli P, Salvetti A. Renin-angiotensin-aldosterone system in primary hyperparathyroidism before and after surgery. *Metabolism.* 1999;48:298–300.
10. Krapf R, Hulter HN. Arterial hypertension induced by erythropoietin and erythropoiesis-stimulating agents (ESA). *Clin. J. Am. Soc. Nephrol.* 2009;4:470–480.
11. Skali H, Parving HH, Parfrey PS, et al. Stroke in patients with type 2 diabetes mellitus, chronic kidney disease, and anemia treated with darbepoetin alfa: the trial to reduce cardiovascular events with Aranesp therapy (TREAT) experience. *Circulation.* 2011;124:2903–2908.

12. Agarwal R. Mechanisms and mediators of hypertension induced by erythropoietin and related molecules. *Nephrol. Dial. Transplant.* 2018;33:1690–1698.
13. Chen N, Hao C, Liu BC, et al. Roxadustat treatment for anemia in patients undergoing long-term dialysis. *N. Engl. J. Med.* 2019;381:1011–1022.
14. Fishbane S, El-Shahawy MA, Pecoits-Filho R, et al. Roxadustat for treating anemia in patients with CKD not on dialysis: results from a randomized phase 3 study. *J. Am. Soc. Nephrol.* 2021;32:737–755.
15. Krishnamoorthy P, Gopalakrishnan A, Mittal V, et al. Gaisbock syndrome (polycythemia and hypertension) revisited: results from the national inpatient sample database. *J. Hypertens.* 2018;36:2420–2424.
16. Gossmann J, Burkhardt R, Harder S, Angiotensin II. et al. infusion increases plasma erythropoietin levels via an angiotensin II type 1 receptor-dependent pathway. *Kidney Int.* 2001;60:83–86.

CHAPTER 12

RENOVASCULAR HYPERTENSION

Matthew R. Alexander, MD PhD, James M. Luther, MD MSCI, and Esther S. Kim, MD MPH

QUESTIONS

1. **What is renovascular hypertension?**
   Renovascular hypertension (RVH) is the elevated blood pressures resulting from significant obstruction to renal artery blood flow and decreased renal perfusion pressure.[1]

2. **What is the prevalence of RVH?**
   RVH accounts for 1% to 2% of all hypertension (HTN) in the general population and up to 6.8% of those older than 65 years old with greater than 60% renal artery stenosis (RAS) on imaging. The prevalence is 11% to 18% in those with known coronary artery disease, using a greater than 50% stenosis cutoff. The prevalence is up to 24% in some selected populations with resistant HTN.[1–3]

3. **What are the common and uncommon causes of RVH?**
   Common causes include atherosclerosis (90%) and fibromuscular dysplasia (FMD) (10%). Atherosclerotic plaques are typically found at the ostium of the renal artery and are associated with typical risk factors including age, dyslipidemia, smoking, diabetes mellitus, and atherosclerosis in other vascular beds. FMD more commonly involves the mid to distal two-thirds of the renal artery and is associated with distinct risk factors including female sex, age younger than 50 years old, and family history of FMD or arterial dissection/aneurysm.

   Uncommon causes include iatrogenic dissection, aortic stent graft occlusion, renal artery stent branch vessel occlusion, trauma, Takayasu arteritis, aortic dissection, and arterial embolus. Microvascular disease caused by small and medium vessel vasculitis (e.g., polyarteritis nodosa, scleroderma renal crisis) can also produce renin-dependent HTN.[4,5]

4. **What is FMD?**
   FMD is an idiopathic, segmental, nonatherosclerotic and noninflammatory disease of the musculature of the arterial walls, leading to stenosis of small and medium-sized arteries. FMD lesions are characterized by their angiographic appearance as either focal or multifocal. The most common type of FMD (90% of lesions) is the multifocal type in which there are alternating areas of stenosis and aneurysmal dilatation, usually in the mid to distal portion of the artery, resulting in a "string-of-beads" appearance (Fig. 12.1A). Focal FMD may occur in any portion of the artery and appears as a single concentric lesion or a smooth tapered lesion (see Fig. 12.1B). Both types of FMD are important causes of RVH.[4]

5. **Why does renal artery obstruction cause HTN?**
   RASs produce minimal hemodynamic effects and are clinically silent until they cross a critical level of stenosis. Beyond approximately 70% stenosis, a 10 to 20 mm Hg reduction in perfusion pressure can result, causing decreased perfusion to the kidney. The pathophysiological effects of renal artery obstruction were experimentally determined in the 1930s by Goldblatt and Loesch. Their model of kidney clipping in animals led to understanding of the important role of the kidneys and the renin angiotensin system in HTN. The two-kidney-one-clip model mimics unilateral renal artery obstructive disease with a contralateral normal kidney. This causes high renin production from the abnormal kidney, resulting in blood pressure elevation. In this setting pressure natriuresis also occurs, which enhances sodium excretion in the contralateral functional kidney to help reduce pressures and prevent volume overload. In the one-kidney-one-clip model, which mimics stenosis to a solitary functioning kidney or bilateral RAS, HTN occurs with systemic volume overload due to reduced glomerular filtration rate (GFR) from diminished kidney function. This pathophysiology results in low renin levels due to renin suppression from elevated blood volume. Of note, bilateral RAS is associated with higher rates of progressive renal dysfunction, including with the initiation of angiotensin converting enzyme inhibitor (ACEi) or angiotensin II, type 1 receptor blocker (ARB).[1,2,6]

6. **What clinical signs suggest RVH and may prompt further testing?**
   Clinical signs, which should prompt the consideration of RVH, are listed in Box 12.1.

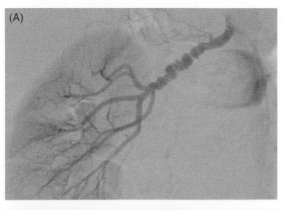

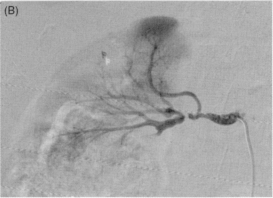

Fig. 12.1 Angiographic images of multifocal (A) and focal (B) fibromuscular dysplasia of the right renal artery.

Box 12.1 Clinical Findings Suggestive of Renovascular Hypertension

Onset of hypertension at <30 years of age (FMD) or severe hypertension at >55 years of age (atherosclerotic RVH)
Accelerated, resistant, or malignant hypertension
Unexplained atrophic kidney or size discrepancy >1.5 cm between kidneys
Sudden, unexplained pulmonary edema
Unexplained renal dysfunction, including individuals starting renal replacement therapy
Development of new azotemia or worsening renal function after administration of an ACEi or ARB agent
Unexplained congestive heart failure or refractory angina
Presence of systolic and/or diastolic abdominal bruit

ACEi, Angiotensin converting enzyme inhibitor; *ARB,* angiotensin II, type I receptor blocker; *FMD,* fibromuscular dysplasia; *RVH,* renovascular hypertension.
Adapted from Hirsch AT, Haskal ZJ, Hertzer NR, et al, ACC/AHA Guidelines for the management of patients with peripheral vascular disease. *Circulation.* 2006;113(11):e463-e654.

---

7. **What testing should be performed for evaluation of RVH?**

Renovascular disease is typically assessed by imaging of the renal arteries by renal duplex ultrasound, computed tomographic angiography (CTA), magnetic resonance angiography (MRA), or digital subtraction angiography. Renal duplex doppler ultrasound is often used as the initial diagnostic test, because it is noninvasive and does not expose the patient to radiation. Although it has a reported high specificity and sensitivity (reported sensitivity of 84% to 98% and specificity of 62% to 99%) and ability to provide both anatomical and functional information on blood flow, it is operator dependent and quality can be diminished in obesity.

In the absence of availability or institutional expertise with renal doppler ultrasound, MRA or CTA can be performed. MRA has the advantage of providing functional information on blood flow in addition to anatomic information but carries some risk of nephrogenic systemic fibrosis in patients with kidney disease

GFR <30 mL/min/1.73m^2). CTA has higher spatial and temporal resolution than MRA but exposes the patient to the risks of ionizing radiation and iodinated contrast.

Renal angiography remains the definitive diagnostic study and provides direct access for pressure monitoring and possible intervention, but this test is invasive with attendant increased risks.

Laboratory testing such as plasma renin activity cannot reliably diagnose RAS. Renin is elevated in 15% of those with essential HTN, and, with bilateral RAS or stenosis of a solitary functional kidney, renin levels are often normal or low. Renin levels may be elevated with unilateral RAS, but this is not diagnostic of renal artery obstruction, and anatomical and/or functional imaging studies are required to make the diagnosis of RVH.[2,6,7]

8. **What increase in creatinine with ACEi/ARB initiation is suggestive of RVH?**
Blockade of the renin-angiotensin-aldosterone system with either an ACEi or ARB relieves angiotensin II-induced efferent arteriolar constriction, resulting in decreased intraglomerular pressure and GFR. This can cause an increase in serum creatinine up to 30%. Markedly increased creatinine can suggest bilateral RAS, particularly in the setting of volume contraction. Bilateral RAS is a contraindication for ACEi/ARB use due to the risk of precipitating severe kidney failure and is an indication to perform further evaluation with possible intervention in appropriately selected patients.[1,8]

9. **What additional testing is helpful after making a diagnosis of RVH?**
Renal function should also be assessed with serum creatinine, urinalysis for proteinuria, and kidney size assessment with renal ultrasound or abdominal computed tomography.

For those with FMD as the cause of RVH, all vessels from the brain to the pelvis should be screened (usually with CTA or contrast-enhanced MRA) to identify other areas of FMD and to identify occult aneurysms and dissections. This practice is recommended out of the recognition that FMD is a systemic arterial disorder involving multiple arterial beds and associated with aneurysms and dissections.[4]

10. **What is the most appropriate initial treatment for RVH?**
In addition to HTN control, treatment of RVH focuses on cardiovascular risk reduction. This increased cardiovascular risk (e.g., stroke and heart failure) associated with atherosclerotic RVH is much greater than the risk of kidney failure in patients with RAS. Lifestyle changes and medical therapy are indicated in patients, with three primary goals:

- **Control hypertension** – ACEi or ARBs directly target the pathogenesis of RVH and should be offered as first-line antihypertensive therapy to every patient in the absence of contraindications. With unilateral RAS, exercise and the Dietary Approaches to Stop Hypertension diet provide additional benefit to reduce hyperfiltration in the functional contralateral kidney and decrease proteinuria.
- **Reduce atherosclerotic cardiovascular disease risk** – All applicable interventions should be aggressively pursued, including exercise, smoking cessation, statin therapy, low-dose aspirin, and glycemic control.
- **Preserve kidney function** – In addition to BP control, ACEi or ARBs are first-line therapy to preserve renal function.[1,3,7] In bilateral RAS, revascularization may be required to preserve kidney function.

11. **What are the indications for revascularization in atherosclerotic RVH?**
Intervention is not indicated in most cases. If the RAS is clinically significant with clinical indicators (see Box 12.1), Fig. 12.2 presents conditions in which revascularization should be considered. If revascularization is pursued, percutaneous angioplasty and stenting is used when possible, although no studies have clearly demonstrated its effectiveness over surgical intervention.

Of note, percutaneous revascularization in addition to medical therapy failed to preserve kidney function or reduce cardiovascular events in two recent randomized clinical trials of atherosclerotic RAS (CORAL and ASTRAL). However, in both studies a significant proportion of patients had, at most, a moderate degree of stenosis (<70%), and neither study measured hemodynamic significance of the lesions. In addition, CORAL participants were enrolled without HTN at baseline if they had chronic kidney disease. Results of these trials may not extend to patients with poorly controlled RVH with severe and hemodynamically significant stenoses.[3,5–7,9]

12. **When should revascularization be performed with FMD?**
Revascularization for FMD should be considered in cases of HTN refractory to medical treatment, HTN of short duration with goal of cure, and preservation of renal function in patients with severe stenosis. In contrast to atherosclerotic RAS, revascularization for FMD can usually be achieved with angioplasty alone, without the need for stenting. Cure of HTN after angioplasty for FMD has been associated with younger patient age at the time of renal angioplasty and shorter duration of HTN. An accurate visual assessment of stenosis severity is not possible in multifocal FMD. For this reason, a consensus-based protocol of catheter-based angiography and angioplasty for patients with renal artery FMD recommends that simultaneous, unstimulated, translesional pressure gradient be measured to determine severity of RAS in patients with FMD lesions. In experienced centers, intravascular ultrasound or optical coherence tomography may also be used to determine stenosis severity.[4]

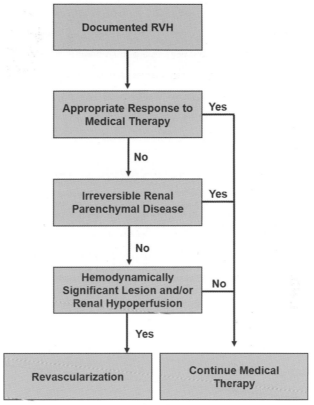

Fig. 12.2 Indications for revascularization in atherosclerotic renovascular hypertension. In the presence of documented renovascular hypertension *(RVH)*, lack of appropriate response to medical therapy including inability to control blood pressure, worsening of renal dysfunction, repeated flash pulmonary edema, and/or intractable heart failure should prompt evaluation for irreversible renal parenchymal disease. In the absence of evident irreversible injury including proteinuria >1 g/24 hours or renal length <6 cm, objective evidence of renal hypoperfusion with nuclear scintigraphy or elevated translesional pressure gradients (systolic gradient >20 mm Hg or mean gradient >10 mm Hg) or renal fractional flow reserve <0.8 with invasive pressure wires should prompt consideration for revascularization.[1,3]

13. **When should surgical revascularization be performed?**

   Surgical revascularization should be considered in patients who fail percutaneous revascularization, who have anatomy that limits percutaneous access, or who have aortic surgical disease. Clinical scenarios include rapid loss of kidney function, uncontrollable HTN despite optimal medical therapy, and recurrent hospitalization for pulmonary edema or hypertensive crises. Surgical options include aortorenal or splenorenal bypass, renal artery thromboendarterectomy, and renal artery reimplantation. Surgical nephrectomy should also be considered for an atrophic kidney contributing minimal renal function as assessed by nuclear renogram. If renal vein renin testing is performed, a ratio greater than 2 would suggest near-total occlusion and benefit from nephrectomy to eliminate the source of elevated renin levels contributing to blood pressure elevation.[10,11]

KEY POINTS

1. RVH is a relatively common condition in those with resistant HTN and is primarily due to renal artery atherosclerosis (90%) or FMD (10%).
2. In those suspected of RVH, renal duplex ultrasound, CTA, or MRA are typical first-line imaging modalities for diagnosis.
3. Lifestyle changes and medical therapy to control blood pressure, reduce atherosclerotic cardiovascular disease risk, and protect kidney function are the most appropriate initial therapies for RVH, with revascularization reserved for those who do not respond to medical therapy with potentially reversible renal dysfunction and hemodynamically significant lesions.
4. RVH due to FMD should be considered in patients without traditional atherosclerotic risk factors, particularly young to middle-aged women. FMD is a systemic arterial disorder associated with aneurysm and dissection in other vascular beds.

REFERENCES

1. Herrmann SM, Textor SC. Current concepts in the treatment of renovascular hypertension. *Am J Hypertens*. 2018;31(2):139–149.
2. Carey RM, Calhoun DA, Bakris GL, et al. Resistant hypertension: detection, evaluation, and management: a scientific statement from the American Heart Association. *Hypertension*. 2018;72(5):e53–e90.
3. Creager MA, Beckman JA, Loscalzo J. *Vascular Medicine: a Companion to Braunwald's Heart Disease*. 2nd ed. Philadelphia, PA: Elsevier/Saunders; 2013.
4. Gornik HL, Persu A, Adlam D, et al. First international consensus on the diagnosis and management of fibromuscular dysplasia. *Vasc Med*. 2019;24(2):164–189.
5. Textor SC, Taler SJ. Rediscovering renovascular hypertension. *Hypertension*. 2019;74(6):1297–1299.
6. Prince M, Gupta A, Bob-Manuel T, Tafur J. Renal revascularization in resistant hypertension. *Prog Cardiovasc Dis*. 2020;63(1):58–63.
7. Whelton PK, Carey RM, Aronow WS, et al. 2017 ACC/AHA/AAPA/ABC/ACPM/AGS/APhA/ASH/ASPC/NMA/PCNA Guideline for the prevention, detection, evaluation, and management of high blood pressure in adults: executive summary: a report of the American College of Cardiology/American Heart Association task force on clinical practice guidelines. *Circulation*. 2018;138(17):e426–e483.
8. Ohkuma T, Jun M, Rodgers A, et al. Acute increases in serum creatinine after starting angiotensin-converting enzyme inhibitor-based therapy and effects of its continuation on major clinical outcomes in type 2 diabetes mellitus. *Hypertension*. 2019;73(1):84–91.
9. Courand PY, Dinic M, Lorthioir A, et al. Resistant hypertension and atherosclerotic renal artery stenosis: effects of angioplasty on ambulatory blood pressure: a retrospective uncontrolled single-center study. *Hypertension*. 2019;74(6):1516–1523.
10. Hirsch AT, Haskal ZJ, Hertzer NR, et al. ACC/AHA 2005 Practice guidelines for the management of patients with peripheral arterial disease (lower extremity, renal, mesenteric, and abdominal aortic): a collaborative report from the American Association for Vascular Surgery/Society for Vascular Surgery, Society for Cardiovascular Angiography and Interventions, Society for Vascular Medicine and Biology, Society of Interventional Radiology, and the ACC/AHA Task Force on Practice Guidelines (Writing Committee to Develop Guidelines for the Management of Patients With Peripheral Arterial Disease): endorsed by the American Association of Cardiovascular and Pulmonary Rehabilitation; National Heart, Lung, and Blood Institute; Society for Vascular Nursing; TransAtlantic Inter-Society Consensus; and Vascular Disease Foundation. *Circulation*. 2006;113(11):e463–e654.
11. Rossi GP, Cesari M, Chiesura-Corona M, Miotto D, Semplicini A, Pessina AC. Renal vein renin measurements accurately identify renovascular hypertension caused by total occlusion of the renal artery. *J Hypertens*. 2002;20(5):975–984.

CHAPTER 13

DRUG-INDUCED HYPERTENSION

Jiun-Ruey Hu, MD, MPH, and J. Matt Luther, MD, MSCI

1. **What are the four main mechanisms by which drug-induced hypertension may occur?**
   See Fig. 13.1:
   - Sympathomimetic activation
   - Volume retention via mineralocorticoid activation
   - Direct vasoconstriction via increased vasoconstrictors, decreased vasodilators, or upregulation of the angiotensin II receptor type 1 (AT_1)
   - Drug withdrawal

2. **What drug classes cause hypertension by sympathomimetic activation?**
   - See Fig. 13.1

3. **What drug classes cause hypertension by mineralocorticoid activation?**
   - See Fig. 13.1

4. **What drug classes cause hypertension by direct vasoconstriction?**
   - See Fig. 13.1

5. **What drug classes cause hypertension as a withdrawal syndrome?**
   - See Fig. 13.1

6. **What hypertension-producing drugs do patients routinely omit from their medication list?**
   Patients unintentionally omit over-the-counter medications (e.g., nonsteroidal antiinflammatory drugs [NSAIDs], nasal decongestants), herbal medications, and nutritional supplements from their medication list (Table 13.1). Alcohol or recreational drug use may be withheld due to social stigma or for legal reasons. Unless specifically asked, patients may not report recent cessation or intermittent use of a drug that may cause withdrawal or rebound effects.

7. **Which drugs of abuse cause or worsen hypertension and how?**
   3,4-Methylenedioxy methamphetamine (MDMA), also known as ecstasy or molly, acts at the vesicular monoamine transporter 2 and trace amine-associated receptor 1 (TAAR1) to stimulate release of serotonin, norepinephrine, and dopamine, resulting in increased sympathetic activation.

   Phencyclidine (PCP), or angel dust, is an *N*-methyl-D-aspartate (NMDA) receptor antagonist that also inhibits synaptic uptake of dopamine and norepinephrine, resulting in increased sympathetic activation.

   Cocaine blocks the dopamine transporter protein, causing synaptic accumulation of dopamine and norepinephrine, which results in increased sympathetic activation. Dopamine stimulation of the ventral tegmental area increases blood pressure. Moreover, cocaine's primary vasoactive metabolite, benzoylmethylecgonine, blocks sodium channels, resulting in enhanced sympathetic activity. Finally, chronic cocaine use increases levels of vascular cell adhesion molecules and intracellular adhesion molecules, increasing arterial wall stiffness and peripheral vascular resistance.

8. **How do stimulants cause or worsen hypertension?**
   Agents used to stimulate wakefulness, such as modafinil, adrafanil, and armodafinil, block the dopamine transporter and prevent dopamine reuptake, potentiating noradrenergic neurotransmission and increasing sympathetic activation. Similarly, agents used to treat attention deficit/hyperactivity disorder, such as dextroamphetamine and methylphenidate, are norepinephrine-dopamine reuptake inhibitors and thus potentiate noradrenergic neurotransmission and increase sympathetic activation.

9. **Which antidepressants can cause or worsen hypertension and how?**
   Selective-serotonin norepinephrine reuptake inhibitors (SNRIs), such as venlafaxine and duloxetine, are used to treat depression and a range of other psychiatric conditions. They cause increased sympathetic activity by increasing norepinephrine and potentiating noradrenergic neurotransmission.

   Tricyclic antidepressants (TCAs), such as amitriptyline, were previously used to treat depression but are now more commonly used to treat chronic pain conditions such as fibromyalgia and neuralgia. They act similarly to SNRIs by blocking the serotonin transporter and norepinephrine transporter, thereby potentiating noradrenergic neurotransmission and increasing sympathetic activation.

Drug-Induced Hypertension

Increased Sympathetic activation:

DA/NE reuptake inhibitors:

Illicit drugs: Amphetamine, MDMA('Ecstasy'), Cocaine
Stimulants: Modafinil, Adrafanil, Armodafinil,
   Dextroamphetamine, Methylphenidate, Solriamfetol
SNRIs: Venlafaxine, Sibutramine, Duloxetine
NRIs: Atomoxetine, Reboxetine
Tricyclic antidepressants: Amitriptyline, Nortriptyline
DA/NE agonists: Ergotamine, Dihydroergotamine

α1-stimulants:

Nasal decongestants: Pseudoephedrine, oxymetazoline
Weigh loss supplements: Ephedra (*ma huang*)
Weight loss agents: Phenylpropanolamine, Phentermine,
   Dexfenfluramine
α₂-antagonists: Yohimbine (erectile dysfunction supplement)
Intravenous α₂-agonist (acute phase): Xylazine, Clonidine,
   Dexmedetomidine

Increased Mineralocorticoid activity

Glucocorticoids: Prednisone, Methylprednisolone
Mineralocorticoids: Fludrocortisone

Estrogens: oral contraceptives (↑renin)
Anabolic steroids: Stanazolol, nandrolene
11bHSD-2 inhibitors: Glycyrrhizic acid (licorice, tobacco),
   Itraconazole, Posaconazole
Cortisol synthesis inhibition: CYP11B1 inhibition
   (Fluconazole, Posaconazole) or CYP17 inhibition
   (Abiraterone)

Drug withdrawal syndromes

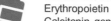

Ethanol, Opioid, or Benzodiazepine withdrawal
Opioid antagonist-induced: Naloxone, Pentazocine
Central α₂-agonist withdrawal: Clonidine, Tizanidine,
   Methyldopa
Beta-blocker withdrawal: Atenolol, Metoprolol

Miscellaneous

Non-steroidal anti-inflammatory drugs: Ibuprofen, Naproxen.
Angiogenesis Inhibitors: Bevacizumab, Sunitinib, Sorafenib
Calcineurin inhibitors: Tacrolimus, Cyclosporine
Erythropoietin
Calcitonin gene-related peptide receptor antagonist :
   Erenumab
Metabolism induction of antihypertensive agents: Rifampin

Fig. 13.1 Etiologies of drug-induced hypertension by mechanism of action. *DA/NE,* Dopamine/norepinephrine; *Epi,* epinephrine; *MDMA,* 3,4-methylenedioxymethamphetamine (ecstasy or molly); *NO,* nitric oxide; *NRI,* norepinephrine reuptake inhibitor; *PGE2,* prostaglandin E2; *SNRI,* selective serotonin-norepinephrine reuptake inhibitor; *TCA,* tricyclic antidepressant; *VEGF,* vascular endothelial growth factor. HSD11B2, 11β-hydroxysteroid dehydrogenase type 2

10. **Which headache treatments can cause or worsen hypertension and how?**
Ergot alkaloids, such as ergotamine and dihydroergotamine, are used in the treatment of migraine headaches and cluster headaches. Ergot alkaloids share structural similarity with serotonin, dopamine, and epinephrine, and thus act as agonists of these neurotransmitters, leading to increased sympathetic activation. The new monoclonal antibody against calcitonin gene-related peptide receptor erenumab, has been associated with worsening or new hypertension, although the precise mechanism is undetermined. NSAIDs also can cause hypertension (see later question).

11. **What commonly used over-the-counter medication can cause or worsen hypertension?**
Sympathomimetic amines, such as pseudoephedrine, phenylpropanolamine, and oxymetazoline, are packaged as cough decongestants available over the counter. They stimulate alpha-1 receptors and cause vasoconstriction.

Table 13.1 Hypertension-Inducing Drugs to Consider in Association with Specific Patient Populations

IF UNEXPLAINED HYPERTENSION OCCURS IN:	RULE OUT DRUG-INDUCED HYPERTENSION FROM:
Patient currently using recreational substances	Amphetamine, MDMA, cocaine
Patient recently using recreational substances	Withdrawal from opioids, benzodiazepines, or ethanol
Patient being treated for pain	NSAIDs (ibuprofen, naproxen), TCAs (amitriptyline, nortriptyline)
Patient being treated for muscle spasms	Withdrawal from alpha-2 agonists (tizanidine)
Patient being treated for a cold	Alpha-1 agonists for nasal congestion (pseudoephedrine, oxymetazoline), SNRIs for cough suppression (dextromethorphan)
Patient being treated for cancer	VEGF inhibitors (bevacizumab), calcineurin inhibitors (tacrolimus, cyclosporine), receptor tyrosine kinase inhibitors (sunitinib, sorafenib), CYP17 inhibitors (abiraterone)
Patient being treated for anemia	Exogenous erythropoietin
Patient being treated for fungal infection	CYP11B1 inhibitors (posaconazole, fluconazole), HSD11B2 inhibitors (itraconazole, posaconazole)
Reproductive-aged woman	Estrogen-containing oral contraceptives
Patient attempting to build muscle mass	Anabolic steroids (stanozolol, nandrolone decanoate)
Patient being treated for depression or anxiety	SNRIs (venlafaxine, sibutramine, duloxetine)
Patient being treated for ADHD	Stimulants (methylphenidate, dextroamphetamine)
Patient being treated for trouble staying awake	Stimulants (modafinil, adrafinil, armodafinil)
Patient attempting to lose weight	Weight loss supplements (sibutramine, ephedra)
Patient using eye drops	Alpha-1 agonists (phenylephrine)
Patient being treated for vasculitis or other systemic inflammatory disorder	Glucocorticoids (prednisone, methylprednisolone)
Patient being treated for opioid overdose	Opioid antagonists (naloxone)
Patient who drinks caffeine	Caffeine
Patient who smokes	Tobacco
Patient who eats licorice	Glycyrrhizzic acid
Patient recently taken off an antihypertensive	Withdrawal from clonidine, methyldopa, or atenolol

HSD11B2, 11-β-H-hydroxysteroid dehydrogenase type 2; *ADHD,* attention deficit/hyperactivity disorder; *CYP17,* cytochrome P450 17α-hydroxy/17,20-lyase; *CYP11B1,* cytochrome P450 11β-hydroxylase; *MDMA,* 3,4-methylenedioxymethamphetamine (ecstasy, molly); *NSAIDs,* nonsteroidal antiinflammatory drugs; *SNRI,* serotonin-norepinephrine reuptake inhibitor; *TCA,* tricyclic antidepressant; *VEGF,* vascular endothelial growth factor.

The blood pressure–raising effect of pseudoephedrine is augmented when coadministered with acetaminophen, which increases the bioavailability of pseudoephedrine.

Cough suppressants, such as dextromethorphan, which is a sigma-1 receptor agonist and NMDA receptor antagonist, also act as an SNRI, thus potentiating noradrenergic neurotransmission and increasing sympathetic activation.

NSAIDs also can cause hypertension (see later question).

12. **What supplements can cause or worsen hypertension?**

Appetite suppressants for weight loss contain ephedra-like compounds, which have alpha-1 agonist activity, thus increasing sympathetic activation. Ephedra-containing drugs were removed from the market by the US Food and Drug Administration (FDA) beginning in 2004.

Appetite suppressants for weight loss often contain sibutramine, which blocks reuptake of noradrenaline and dopamine (and serotonin), potentiating noradrenergic neurotransmission and increasing sympathetic activity. Sibutramine-containing drugs were removed from the market by the FDA in 2010, but this drug is a common adulterant, leading to supplement withdrawal from the market.

The appetite suppressants for weight loss, phentermine (Adipex-P) and dexfenfluramine (Redux), are better known for their effects causing pulmonary hypertension than systemic hypertension. Phentermine, similar to amphetamine, is an antagonist of TAAR1, increasing the release of norepinephrine, dopamine, and serotonin into the synapse. Dexfenfluramine is a serotonin reuptake inhibitor.

Anabolic steroids used in muscle building come in oral forms such as stanozolol (Winstrol) and oxymetholone (Anadrol) as well as injectable forms such as nandrolone decanoate (Deca-Durabolin) and boldenone undecylenate (Equipoise). This occurs through water-sodium retention via activation of the renin-angiotensin-aldosterone system (reversible hypertension) and plaque formation leading to atherosclerosis (irreversible hypertension).

Supplements for erectile dysfunction such as yohimbine are alpha-2 antagonists with actions effectively opposite of clonidine. Yohimbine thus raises blood pressure by removing the central feedback inhibition of sympathetic activity.

13. How does caffeine cause or worsen hypertension?
Caffeine is a xanthine that antagonizes adenosine receptors in vascular tissue, resulting in vasoconstriction. Caffeine also increases sympathetic activity.

14. What does it mean for a corticosteroid to have glucocorticoid activity or mineralocorticoid activity?
Corticosteroids, which are synthesized in the adrenal cortex, can have selectivity for glucocorticoid receptors or mineralocorticoid receptors. Glucocorticoids are responsible for regulating glucose metabolism and reducing inflammation, whereas mineralocorticoids are responsible for regulating the retention of sodium and thus water. Cortisol, the natural glucocorticoid, is released in a circadian diurnal pattern, meaning that it peaks at 8:00 a.m. and nadirs around midnight under the regulation of adrenocorticotropic hormone (ACTH). Compared to cortisol, fludrocortisone and aldosterone have significantly elevated mineralocorticoid activity, at 125 times and 3000 times higher than that of cortisol, respectively. On the other hand, prednisone, methylprednisolone, and dexamethasone have 0.8, 0.5, and 0 times the mineralocorticoid activity of cortisol, thus making them glucocorticoids.

15. How do glucocorticoids cause or worsen hypertension?
Even though glucocorticoids, such as prednisone and methylprednisolone, act primarily on glucocorticoid receptors, they may also activate mineralocorticoid receptors and promote sodium and fluid retention. Glucocorticoids can also act on vascular smooth muscle glucocorticoid receptors to upregulate AT_1 receptors, which increase influx of sodium and calcium, thus increasing the tone of smooth muscle cells.

16. How do mineralocorticoids cause or worsen hypertension?
Mineralocorticoids such as fludrocortisone and aldosterone are highly selective for the mineralocorticoid receptor. Activation of the mineralocorticoid receptor increases expression of the epithelial sodium channel as well as the Na/K-ATPase, resulting in increased reabsorption of sodium. This increases extracellular volume and, consequently, blood pressure.

17. How do oral contraceptives cause or worsen hypertension?
The estrogen component of oral contraceptives increases renin levels, stimulating the renin angiotensin aldosterone system, acting on the mineralocorticoid receptor and thus causing salt and fluid retention and vasoconstriction. This effect is opposed by aldosterone antagonism from the natural progesterone produced by ovulating women but not synthetic progesterone.

18. How do antifungals cause or worsen hypertension?
Azole antifungals may interfere with cortisol synthesis, metabolism, or both. CYP11B1 (also known as 11β-hydroxylase) catalyzes the conversion of 11-deoxycortisol to the potent glucocorticoid cortisol (Fig. 13.2). Posaconazole and fluconazole can inhibit CYP11B1, impairing synthesis of cortisol, which produces a compensatory ACTH response and mineralocorticoid excess. Hypertension can be prevented by glucocorticoid supplementation with 2.5 to 5 mg prednisone twice daily, providing more effective suppression than lower doses.

HSD11B2 catalyzes the conversion of the active cortisol to the inert cortisone. Itraconazole and posaconazole inhibit HSD11B2, causing an accumulation of the active cortisol, which acts on the mineralocorticoid receptors to retain sodium and on glucocorticoid receptors on smooth muscle cells to upregulate AT_1 receptors.

19. How does licorice cause or worsen hypertension?
The active ingredient in licorice is glycyrrhizic acid, which inhibits HSD11B2, an enzyme that converts the active cortisol to the inert cortisone. Inhibition of HSD11B2 causes an excess of cortisol, which acts on mineralocorticoid receptors to retain sodium and on glucocorticoid receptors on smooth muscle cells to upregulate AT_1 receptors.

20. How do NSAIDs cause or worsen hypertension?
NSAIDs inhibit cyclooxygenase (COX) 1 and 2, which reduce prostaglandin AT_2 (PGE_2), an eicosanoid that mediates natriuresis, thus reducing urine sodium excretion and retaining volume. COX inhibition also reduces prostaglandin

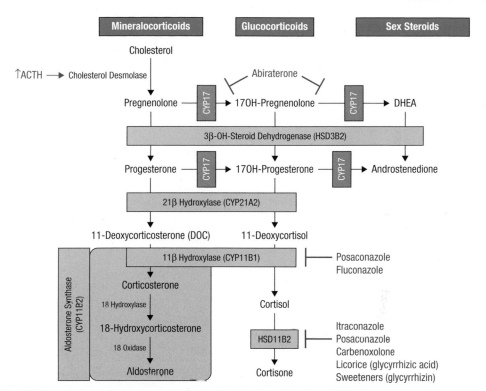

Fig. 13.2 Drugs that cause hypertension by interfering with the steroidogenic pathway. *ACTH,* Adrenocorticotropic hormone; *DHEA,* dihydroxyepiandrosterone HSD11B2, 11β-hydroxysteroid dehydrogenase type 2.

I$_2$ (PGI$_2$), a potent vasodilator of smooth muscle, thus raising peripheral vascular resistance. NSAIDs also inhibit the glucuronidation of aldosterone, thus accumulating intrarenal levels of the mineralocorticoid and retaining volume. Patients with underlying kidney disease are especially susceptible to these effects as they are unable to upregulate renal sodium excretion to compensate for the above mechanisms.

21. What cancer agents produce hypertension and how?

Vascular endothelial growth factor (VEGF) inhibitors, such as bevacizumab, are used in the treatment of many cancers. They antagonize VEGF receptor-2, decreasing production of nitric oxide (NO), a vasodilator, and increasing production of ET-1, a vasoconstrictor.

Tyrosine kinase inhibitors, such as sorafenib and sunitinib, inhibit the tyrosine kinase on the intracellular end of the VEGF receptor-2, thus also decreasing production of NO, a vasodilator, and increasing production of ET-1, a vasoconstrictor.

CYP17 inhibitors, such as abiraterone, are used in the treatment of prostate cancer. CYP17 is responsible for four reactions in two parallel pathways: the conversion of pregnenolone to 17α-hydroxypregnenolone and progesterone to 17α-hydroxyprogesterone; and the conversion of 17α-hydroxypregnenolone to dihydroepiandrosterone and 17α–hydroxyprogesterone to androstenedione. As a result of 17α-hydroxylase inhibition, cortisol levels decline, causing a reactive rise in ACTH secretion. Therefore abiraterone therapy is usually coadministered with prednisone or methylprednisolone to counteract adrenal insufficiency and mineralocorticoid excess to prevent drug-induced hypertension.

22. What immunosuppressive agents produce hypertension and how?

Calcineurin inhibitors, such as cyclosporine and tacrolimus, are used to treat autoimmune disease and to achieve posttransplant immunosuppression. They cause renal vasoconstriction by increased ET-1 production and decreased NO production in preglomerular vessels. In addition, tacrolimus increases lysine-deficient protein kinase (WNK) activity, stimulates the thiazide-sensitive sodium-chloride cotransporter and inhibits renal outer medullary potassium channel activity. Cyclosporine also increases sympathetic activity by glutaminergic-mediated postsynaptic excitation.

23. **Abrupt discontinuation of which recreational drugs may result in hypertension?**

    Rebound hypertension can arise from abrupt cessation of use of opioids, ethanol, and benzodiazepines. Note that naloxone, which is an opioid antagonist used to treat opioid overdose, also causes hypertension.

24. **Abrupt discontinuation of which medications may result in hypertension?**

    Rebound hypertension can arise from abrupt discontinuation of alpha-2 agonists, especially clonidine and tizanidine, and less likely with longer acting agents such as guanfacine and methyldopa. Rebound hypertension occurs due to a rapid increase of catecholamines (leading to sympathetic activity) or increased receptor sensitivity developed during the low norepinephrine accompanying long-term alpha-2 agonist use. Unlike other antihypertensive agents, the rebound hypertension that occurs from alpha-2 agonists occurs within a day and causes blood pressure to overshoot pretreatment levels. Therefore alpha-2 agonists should be tapered over a 6- to 10-day interval. Similarly, inappropriately intermittent dosing of alpha-2 agonists (e.g., every other day) can iatrogenically cause recurrent rebound hypertension. Please refer to Chapter 38 for further details.

    Dexmedetomidine is an alpha-2 agonist frequently used as a sedative and analgesic in the ICU that can be associated with hypotension. Dexmedetomidine can provoke rebound hypertension after long-term use.

    Rebound hypertension also can arise from abrupt discontinuation of beta-blockers, such as atenolol or metoprolol, but is less pronounced.

25. **What drug-drug interactions can cause or worsen hypertension?**

    The combination of monoamine oxidase inhibitors (e.g., phenelzine, selegiline) used for depression and tyramine-containing foods (e.g., aged cheese, cured meats, wine) can result in hypertension.

    The combination of norepinephrine reuptake inhibitors (NRIs; e.g., atomoxetine) or SNRIs (e.g., venlafaxine) used for mood and alpha-2 antagonists used in erectile dysfunction (e.g., yohimbine) can result in hypertension.

    The use of a beta-blocker during clonidine withdrawal, pheochromocytoma, or a hyperadrenergic state can lead to unopposed alpha activation and result in hypertension.

    The combination of cough suppressants (e.g., dextromethorphan), which is itself an SNRI, with other SNRIs for depression (e.g., venlafaxine, duloxetine) can result in hypertension.

    The combination of a sympathomimetic with caffeine can result in hypertension.

KEY POINTS

1. NSAIDs, nasal decongestants (e.g., pseudoephedrine), cough suppressants (e.g., dextromethorphan), herbal medications, and nutritional supplements are hypertension-causing drugs that patients commonly omit from their medication lists.
2. Oral contraceptives and caffeine can cause or worsen hypertension.
3. Stimulants, SNRIs, NRIs, and TCAs are psychiatric drugs that can cause or worsen hypertension.
4. MDMA, PCP, and cocaine are drugs of abuse that can cause or worsen hypertension.
5. Hypertension can arise from abrupt discontinuation of alpha-2 agonists (e.g., clonidine), benzodiazepines, opioids, and ethanol.

CHAPTER 14

OBSTRUCTIVE SLEEP APNEA AND HYPERTENSION

Marcel Ruzicka, MD, PhD, FRCPC

QUESTIONS

1. **What is obstructive sleep apnea?**
   Obstructive sleep apnea (OSA) is a sleep disorder characterized by recurrent episodes of upper airway inspiratory collapse during sleep causing hypopnea and apnea leading to oxygen desaturation and arousals from sleep.

2. **How common is OSA?**
   It has been estimated that 2% to 5% of the adult population in Western countries have symptomatic OSA. Prevalence of asymptomatic or minimally symptomatic OSA without daytime sleepiness and fatigue is likely underestimated but has been reported to be as high as 30% among middle-aged adults. The prevalence of OSA is increased in patients with chronic kidney disease (30%), in patients with type 2 diabetes (25%), and in obese patients (30%) as compared with the general age-matched population. OSA is even more prevalent in patients with hypertension (HTN) resistant to treatment. For example, Logan et al. reported a prevalence of OSA of over 80% among nondiabetic patients with a blood pressure of 140/90 mm Hg or higher treated with three or more antihypertensive drugs.

3. **What is the relevance of OSA in HTN?**
   As mentioned previously, the prevalence of OSA is higher in patients with HTN and particularly in those with HTN resistant to pharmacotherapy. Similarly, the prevalence of HTN among those with moderate to severe OSA is as high as 53%. Data from the large, prospective, longitudinal observational study, the Wisconsin Sleep Cohort Study, suggest that moderate to severe OSA is the independent cause of HTN. Several national professional organizations including the American Heart Association, European Society of Hypertension, and Hypertension Canada, to name just a few, recognize OSA as an independent secondary cause of HTN.

4. **What are the humoral and hemodynamic effects of OSA?**
   Non–rapid eye movement sleep is a period of cardiovascular quiescence with a fall in heart rate, cardiac output, blood pressure, and peripheral vascular resistance due to a decrease in sympathetic activity and an increase in efferent vagal tone. OSA is characterized by repeated upper airway obstructions during sleep that lead to hypopneic and apneic episodes, causing hypoxemia and hypercapnia and triggering brain arousal and restoration of upper airway tone and airflow. Arousal from sleep, which terminates the obstructive episode, is associated with a surge in central sympathetic outflow and is followed by hyperpnea, an increase in heart rate, peripheral vascular resistance, and blood pressure. Intermittent sympathetic activation by nocturnal hypoxemia and hypercapnia out-lasts the triggering mechanism, as indicated by increased levels of urinary norepinephrine at all hours. Similarly, resting muscle sympathetic nerve activity is elevated in patients with OSA. Patients with OSA are therefore exposed to increased adrenergic drive over a 24-hour period.
   OSA is also characterized by increased activity of the renin-angiotensin-aldosterone system, an increase in endothelin-1, decrease in nitric oxide bioavailability, and increased markers of chronic inflammation including C-reactive protein and proinflammatory cytokines. Increased availability of angiotensin II, catecholamines, and endothelin-1 may contribute to the development and maintenance of HTN in patients with OSA via their direct hemodynamic effects on heart rate, cardiac output, and peripheral vascular resistance as well as vascular trophic effects (leading to vascular remodeling and an increase in vascular resistance). An excess of aldosterone may lead to sodium and fluid retention, which, in turn, may aggravate rostral fluid shift during the sleep and aggravate the severity of OSA.
   Decreased nitric oxide production may promote vasoconstriction via central sympathoexcitatory effects as well as via loss of vasodilator tone at vascular smooth muscle cells.
   A persistent increase of prohypertensive factors such as sympathetic activity, renin-angiotensin-aldosterone system, and plasma endothelin-1, along with decreased nitric oxide production, appear to contribute to the development and maintenance of elevated blood pressure beyond the postapneic period of OSA. It is important to acknowledge that the exact role and interplay among these factors in the development and maintenance of HTN in patients with OSA is unclear. Similarly, although the prevalence of HTN in patients with OSA is high, not all patients with OSA develop HTN, suggesting genetic factors may play a role as well.

5. **How should patients with suspected OSA in the setting of HTN undergo evaluation?**
Polysomnography is the gold standard to diagnose the presence and the severity of OSA in patients with HTN. However, it is a time-, infrastructure-, and labor-intensive test, limiting its availability. Hence it is endorsed for patients demonstrating symptoms of OSA such as snoring and daytime fatigue and sleepiness. Furthermore, given the high prevalence of OSA in patients with resistant HTN, polysomnography is reasonable to rule out OSA as the cause or contributing factor to HTN resistance to pharmacotherapy. The same also applies to patients with primary hyperaldosteronism who have a higher prevalence of OSA.

   Given the effect of OSA on blood pressure, particularly during sleep, 24-hour ambulatory blood pressure monitoring (ABPM) is the modality of choice as it is the only method that detects nocturnal HTN, the absence of nocturnal dipping in blood pressure, and masked HTN. A 24-hour ABPM test may also help stratify patients with regards to future blood pressure response to continuous positive airway pressure (CPAP) as data from prospective studies indicate significant blood pressure decreases in those with (masked) HTN, nocturnal HTN, and non-dippers but minimal to no changes in normotensive patients with a normal nocturnal dipping pattern of blood pressure.

6. **What are the treatment modalities for OSA in patients with HTN?**
Treatment options for OSA include surgical procedures such as tonsillectomy and adenoidectomy (particularly in children), uvulopalatopharyngoplasty (in adults), and noninvasive measures such as CPAP, oral appliances, and lifestyle modifications.

   CPAP is the treatment of choice for OSA as it eliminates apneic and hypopneic episodes in the majority of patients. Although CPAP prevents airway obstruction, it is, however, not well tolerated by up to 30% of patients for whom it is prescribed. Hence, the assessment of adherence to the device is crucial.

   Oral appliances may offer an effective alternative to CPAP therapy in patients with OSA, particularly in those who do not tolerate chronic CPAP treatment. Lifestyle modifications include weight loss and elimination of alcohol prior to sleep, which may reduce the severity of OSA.

7. **What are the effects of treatment of OSA on blood pressure in patients with HTN?**
There is significant heterogeneity with regards to the effect of CPAP on blood pressure. Whereas some studies showed significant decreases in blood pressure during sleep as well as during the awake period, others reported decreases in blood pressure only during sleep period or no decreases in blood pressure at all. These discordant results likely reflect differences in subjects studied such as:
   - inclusion of patients with normal blood pressure,
   - large variability in the severity of OSA among subjects studied,
   - methods of blood pressure assessment (office blood pressure versus 24-hour ABPM),
   - adherence (or lack thereof) with CPAP,
   - treatment of control group (e.g., standard care versus sham CPAP), and
   - duration of follow up.

   Results from metaanalyses of clinical trials indicate decreases in blood pressure by about 2 mm Hg. For example, Haentjens et al. reported that in 572 patients from 12 randomized clinical trials, mean 24-hour blood pressure decreased by 1.69 mm Hg (95% confidence interval [CI]: -2.69 to -0.69; $P < .001$). Decrease in blood pressure was more pronounced during the sleep period (-1.92; 95% CI: -2.83 to -1.01; $P = .002$) as compared with the awake period (-1.31; 95% CI: -2.19 to -0.43; $P = .03$). Metaanalyses by Bazanno et al. and Alajmi et al. reported similar decreases in blood pressure by -2.2 and -1.5 mm Hg, respectively. In contrast, metaanalysis of 4 randomized controlled trials by Bratton et al., which included 1206 patients, reported a slight increase in systolic blood pressure (1.1 mm Hg; 95% CI: -0.2 to 2.3; $P = .086$) and a slight reduction in diastolic blood pressure (-0.8 mm Hg; 95% CI: -1.6 to 0.1; $P = .083$). In contrast to the other metaanalyses, the metaanalysis by Bratton et al. only included patients with minimally symptomatic OSA (Epworth Sleepiness Score ≤ 10). Data from these metaanalyses indicate a minimal effect on blood pressure not only in those with minimally symptomatic OSA, but also in those with normal blood pressure at baseline, low adherence to CPAP (<4 hours per night), and patients with mild OSA (apnea-hypopnea index [AHI] <15).

   Furthermore, results of two recent studies suggest that blood pressure response could be predicted from patients' baseline clinical characteristics. Firstly, Castro-Grattoni et al. reported that in 60 male patients with severe OSA (AHI = 42.5; range 29.9–58.9) and Epworth Sleepiness Score of 10.7 ± 5.02, treatment with CPAP for 6 months resulted in significantly different blood pressure outcomes based on results of the baseline 24-hour ABPM. Nocturnal blood pressure decreased in those with nocturnal HTN and in non-dippers but actually increased in dippers and patients nonadherent to CPAP (<4 hours per night). Similarly, in the study by Sapina-Beltran et al., 131 normotensive patients (based on office blood pressure readings) with moderate OSA (AHI >15) underwent 24-hour ABPM at baseline and after treatment with CPAP for 6 months. Although the treatment with CPAP showed overall decrease in mean 24-hour blood pressure by 1.80 mm Hg (95% CI: -3.16 to -0.44; $P < .05$), the blood pressure response was quite heterogenic with regards to baseline blood pressure characteristics derived from 24-hour ABPM. Mean 24-hour blood pressure showed no change in true normotensive patients, but it decreased significantly by -3.65 mm Hg (95% CI: -6.76 to -0.54; $P = .021$). Similarly, nocturnal blood pressure actually increased in dippers by 2.61 mm Hg (95% CI: 0.60 to 4.62) but significantly decreased in non-dippers by 4.75 mm Hg (95% CI: -7.39 to -2.06; $P = .044$ for adjusted difference between the groups).

These data suggest that blood pressure response to CPAP is highly variable, ranging from no to minimal blood pressure–lowering effect in those with mild OSA, minimal symptoms, and normal blood pressure with preserved nocturnal dipping to significant and clinically meaningful blood pressure decreases, in particular during nighttime, in hypertensive patients with symptomatic moderate to severe OSA, and with impaired blood pressure pattern during the sleep period (nocturnal HTN and non-dipping). Assessment of blood pressure by 24-hour ABPM in patients with OSA appears highly desirable for decision making regarding the initiation of therapy with CPAP and/or blood pressure–lowering drugs.

Data on the effect of oral appliances on blood pressure in patients with OSA are limited to mostly observational studies. Metaanalysis of seven studies including 399 patients with OSA found decrease in mean blood pressure (-2.40 mm Hg [95% CI: -4.00 to -0.80; $P = .003$]) comparable to that of CPAP. The net effect of an oral appliance on blood pressure in patients with OSA is, however, limited by the fact that even in this metaanalysis, the majority of studies were observational.

8. **What is the effect of treatment of OSA on blood pressure in patients with resistant HTN?**
Findings from prospective randomized control trials (RCTs) reported significant heterogeneity with regard to the effect of CPAP on blood pressure (as assessed from 24-hour ABPM). In a metaanalysis of five RCTs by Liu et al., the pooled difference in systolic blood pressure on 24-hour ABPM was 4.78 mm Hg (95% CI: -7.95, -1.61) and the study level mean difference in systolic blood pressure lowering ranged from +2.89 to -9.20 mm Hg. Two RCTs reported no decreases in blood pressure in response to CPAP. The largest RCT, the Hipertension Arterial Resistente Control con CPAP trial (HIPARCO) reported a decrease in diastolic blood pressure but no change in systolic blood pressure. The other two trials reported decreases in systolic blood pressure by 10.0 and 6.5 mm Hg, respectively. Furthermore, two trials included in this metaanalysis that showed no change in blood pressure in response to CPAP also share in common the lowest pretreatment blood pressure (129.9 and 129 mm Hg, respectively). On the other hand, the largest decreases in blood pressure were observed in those with the highest pretreatment blood pressure (148 mm Hg). Although this metaanalysis did not demonstrate statistical heterogeneity, from this discussion, there is clearly a significant clinical heterogeneity with regards to the population studied as well as the study design among trials on CPAP in patients with OSA and resistant HTN.

9. **What are important aspects of pharmacotherapy of HTN in patients with OSA?**
Although the data suggest a modest decrease in blood pressure in response to CPAP in hypertensive patients with OSA, the majority of patients with HTN and OSA will require blood pressure–lowering drugs to control their HTN. Careful attention should be paid to clinical evaluation and management of sodium retention, which may be contributory in some cases. Otherwise, there is no evidence indicating the superiority of specific blood pressure–lowering drug classes concerning the effect on blood pressure in patients with OSA.

KEY POINTS

1. HTN is highly prevalent among patients with OSA.
2. Prevalence of OSA is increased in patients with obesity, diabetes mellitus, and chronic kidney disease.
3. Prevalence of OSA appears very high among patients with resistant HTN.
4. OSA is now recognized as a cause of secondary HTN.
5. Polysomnography is the method of choice for diagnosis of OSA.
6. 24-Hour ABPM should be considered in those with suspected as well as diagnosed OSA.
7. Treatment with CPAP causes a modest decrease in blood pressure in hypertensive patients with impaired nocturnal blood pressure pattern (non-dippers) and symptomatic OSA and in patients with HTN resistant to pharmacotherapy.
8. CPAP may cause no changes in blood pressure in minimally symptomatic patients with OSA.
9. The majority of hypertensive patients with OSA will require blood pressure–lowering drugs to control their HTN.

BIBLIOGRAPHY

Alajmi M, Mulgrew AT, Fox Jet al. *Impact of continuous positive airway pressure therapy on blood pressure in patients with obstructive sleep apnea/hypopnea: a meta-analysis of randomized controlled trials.* 2007;185:67–72.

Bazzano LA, Khan Z, Reynolds K, He J. Effect of nocturnal nasal continuous positive airway pressure on blood pressure in obstructive sleep apnea. *Hypertension.* 2007;50:417–423.

Bratton DJ, Stradling JR, Barbe F, Kohler M. Effect of CPAP on blood pressure in patients with minimally symptomatic obstructive sleep apnoea: a meta-analysis using individual patient data from four randomized controlled trials. *Thorax.* 2014;69:1128–1135.

Castro-Grattoni AL, Torres G, Martinez-Alonso, et al. Blood pressure response to CPAP treatment in subjects with obstructive sleep apnoea: the predictive value of 24-h ambulatory blood pressure monitoring. *Eur Respir J.* 2017;50:1700651. doi: 10.1183/13993003.00651-2017.

de Oliveira AC, Martinez D, Massierer D, et al. The antihypertensive effect of positive airway pressure on resistant hypertension of patients with obstructive sleep apnea: a randomized, double-blind, clinical trial. *Am J Respir Crit Care Med.* 2014;190:345–347.

Fava C, Dorigoni S, Vedove D, et al. Effect of CPAP on blood pressure in patients with OSA/hypopnea a systematic review and meta-analysis. *Chest.* 2014;154:762–771.

Ficker JH, Dertinger SH, Siegfried W, et al. Obstructive sleep apnoea and diabetes mellitus: the role of cardiovascular autonomic neuropathy. *Eur Respir J.* 1998;11:14–19.

Friedman O, Bradley TD, Logan AG. Influence of lower body positive pressure on upper airway cross-sectional area in drug-resistant hypertension. *Hypertension.* 2013;61:240–245.

Grassi G, Facchini A, Trevano FQ, et al. Obstructive sleep apnea-dependent and -independent adrenergic activation in obesity. *Hypertension.* 2005;46:321–325.

Haentjens P, Van Meerhaeghe A, Moscariello Am De Weerdt S, Poppe K, Dupont A, Velkeniers B. The impact of continuous positive airway pressure on blood pressure in patients with obstructive sleep apnea syndrome. *Evidence from meta-analysis of placebo-controlled randomized trials. Arch Intern Med.* 2007;167:757–765.

Iftikhar IH, Hays ER, Iverson MA, Magalang UJ, Maas AK. Effect of oral appliances on blood pressure in obstructive sleep apnea: a systematic review and meta-analysis. *J Clin Sleep Med.* 2013;9:165–174.

Lavie P, Ben-Yosef R, Rubin AE. Prevalence of sleep apnea syndrome among patients with essential hypertension. *Am Heart J.* 1984;108:373–376.

Liu L, Cao Q, Guo Z, Dai Q. Continuous positive airway pressure in patients with obstructive sleep apnea and resistant hypertension: a meta-analysis of randomized controlled trials. *J Clin Hypertens.* 2016;18:153–158.

Logan AG, Perlikowski SM, Mente A, et al. High prevalence of unrecognized sleep apnea in drug-resistant hypertension. *J Hypertens.* 2001;19:2271–2277.

Logan AG, Tkacova R, Perlikowski SM, et al. Refractory hypertension and sleep apnoea: effect of CPAP on blood pressure and baroreflex. *Eur Respir J.* 2003;21:241–247.

Lozano L, Tovar JL, Sampol G, et al. Continuous positive airway pressure treatment in sleep apnea patients with resistant hypertension: a randomized, controlled trial. *J Hypertens.* 2010;28:2161–2168.

Martínez-García MA, Capote F, Campos-Rodríguez F, et al. Effect of CPAP on blood pressure in patients with obstructive sleep apnea and resistant hypertension: the HIPARCO randomized clinical trial. *JAMA.* 2013;310:2407–2415.

Mo L, He QY. Effect of long-term continuous positive airway pressure ventilation on blood pressure in patients with obstructive sleep apnea hypopnea syndrome: a meta-analysis of clinical trials. *Zhonghua Yi Xue Za Zhi.* 2007;87:1177–1180.

Muxfeldt ES, Margallo V, Costa LM, et al. Effects of continuous positive airway pressure treatment on clinic and ambulatory blood pressures in patients with obstructive sleep apnea and resistant hypertension: a randomized controlled trial. *Hypertension.* 2015;65:736–742.

Narkiewicz K, Kato M, Phillips BG, Pesek CA, Davison DE, Somers VK. *Nocturnal continuous positive airway pressure decreases daytime sympathetic traffic in obstructive sleep apnea.* 1999;100:2332–2335.

Pedrosa RP, Drager LF, de Paula LKG, Amaro ACS, Bortolotto LA, Lorenzi-Filho G. Effects of OSA treatment on BP in patients with resistant hypertension: a randomized trial. *Chest.* 2013;144:1487–1494.

Peppard PE, Young T, Barnet JH, Palta M, Hagen EW, Hla KM. Increased prevalence of sleep-disordered breathing in adults. *Am J Epidemiol.* 2013;177:1006–1014.

Peppard PE, Young T, Palta M, Skatrud J. Prospective study of the association between sleep-disordered breathing and hypertension. *N Engl J Med.* 2000;342:1378–1384.

Pratt-Ubunama MN, Nishizaka MK, Boedefeld RL, Cofield SS, Harding SM, Calhoun DA. Plasma aldosterone is related to severity of obstructive sleep apnea in subjects with resistant hypertension. *Chest.* 2007;131:453–459.

Rosas SE. Sleep apnea in individuals with chronic kidney disease: a wake-up call. *Clin J Am Soc Nephrol.* 2011;6:954–956.

Sapina-Beltran E, Santamaria-Martos F, Benitez I, et al. Normotensive patient with obstructive sleep apnoea: changes in 24-h ambulatory blood pressure monitoring with continuous positive airway pressure treatment. *J Hypertens.* 2019;37:720–727.

Somers VK, Dyken ME, Clary MP, Aboud FM. Sympathetic neural mechanisms in obstructive sleep apnea. *J Clin Invest.* 1995;96:1897–1904.

West SD, Nicoll DJ, Stradling JR. Prevalence of obstructive sleep apnoea in men with type 2 diabetes. *Thorax.* 2006;61:945–950.

Worsnop CJ, Naughton MT, Barter CE, Morgan TO, Anderson A, Pierce RJ. The prevalence of obstructive sleep apnea in hypertensives. *Am J Respir Crit Care Med.* 1998;157:111–115.

Zoccali C, Mallamaci F, Tripepi G. Sleep apnea in renal patients. *J Am Soc Nephrol.* 2001;12:2854–2859.

CHAPTER 15

HEREDITARY CAUSES OF HYPERTENSION

Eric Judd, MD

QUESTIONS

1. **How common are hereditary forms of hypertension?**
   Evidence from family studies, including monozygotic and dizygotic twins, reveal that up to 50% of hypertension is heritable. However, the collective effect of all the known monogenic causes of hypertension and blood pressure (BP) loci identified through genome-wide association and exome sequencing studies explain only ~2% of BP heritability.[1] Monogenic causes of hypertension are rare, with fewer than 100 families identified per cause. For example, the occurrence of Liddle syndrome in the general population is too infrequent to calculate an accurate prevalence. In select populations (e.g., among teenagers and young adults with difficult-to-control hypertension in which primary aldosteronism and renovascular disease have been excluded) the prevalence of Liddle syndrome by genetic testing was 1.5%.[2]

2. **When should genetic testing be pursued?**
   Guideline recommendations for the evaluation of hypertension and resistant hypertension do not include genetic testing.[3] A hypertension specialist may undertake specific genetic testing in patients with difficult-to-control hypertension presenting early in life and in those who have had negative screening studies for primary aldosteronism, fibromuscular dysplasia, aortic coarctation, cortisol excess, and pheochromocytoma. Clinical presentation of monogenetic causes of hypertension typically includes a low plasma renin activity, a family history of resistant hypertension or a family member with a stroke before age 50 years old, and abnormal serum electrolyte values (Table 15.1).

3. **Which hereditary causes of hypertension present in pediatric populations?**
   Although severe phenotypes manifest during infancy, the majority of monogenic causes of hypertension do not become clinically identifiable until late childhood or early adulthood. One exception to delayed presentation is **congenital adrenal hyperplasia**. The two subtypes of congenital adrenal hyperplasia that result in hypertension present during infancy. Defects in 11β-hydroxylase (loss of function mutations of *CYP11B1*) result in an increased sex hormone with androgenic action causing virilization in girls and precocious puberty in boys.[4] Defects in 17α-hydroxylase result in primary amenorrhea and delayed sexual development in girls and ambiguous genitalia in boys.[4]

   Recessive missense mutations in *HSD11B2*, which encodes the 11β-hydroxysteroid dehydrogenase type 2 enzyme, cause the **syndrome of apparent mineralocorticoid excess** (AME). Without *HSD11B2* enzyme activity, intracellular cortisol binds and activates the mineralocorticoid receptor (MR). Individuals with the inherited form of AME syndrome present with severe and early-onset hypertension during infancy and childhood.[5] AME syndrome can also be acquired later in life by consuming natural licorice (or licorice-flavored chewing tobacco) that inhibits the activity of *HSD11B2*, resulting in resistant hypertension with low levels of aldosterone and suppressed renin activity.

   Chimeric fusion of the 11β-hydroxylase gene *(CYP11B1)* with the coding sequences of aldosterone synthase *(CYP11B2)* results in the release of aldosterone by adrenocorticotropic hormone, which is named **glucocorticoid-remedial aldosteronism**.[6] Glucocorticoid-remedial aldosteronism (also known as familial hyperaldosteronism type 1) presents as resistant hypertension in childhood and is associated with stroke before age 45 years old.[7]

   An **activating mutation in the MR** presents as severe hypertension in childhood with 100% of cases having hypertension before age 20.[8] In vitro study of MR with the activating mutation showed normal activation from binding with aldosterone but basal activity in the absence of hormonal binding. In addition, mutated MR was activated by progesterone at high levels and by the MR antagonist spironolactone. Females with an activating MR mutation experience severe hypertension during pregnancy, when progesterone levels reach 100 times normal.[8]

4. **Why do the majority of hereditary causes of hypertension tend toward hypokalemia?**
   Maintaining potassium homeostasis requires matching dietary intake with kidney excretion (gastrointestinal losses account for less than 10% of total excretion). Most urinary potassium can be accounted for by electrogenic potassium secretion in the collecting duct.[9] Reabsorption of sodium in the principal cell generates a negative

Table 15.1 Monogenic Causes of Hypertension

SYNDROME	GENE INVOLVED	INHERITANCE	MECHANISM RESULTING IN HYPERTENSION	CLINICAL PRESENTATION	TYPICAL LABORATORY FINDINGS	TREATMENT
Familial hyperkalemic hypertension[c]	CUL3[a] KLHL3[b] WNK1[a] WNK4[b]	AD and AR	Increased activity of sodium-chloride cotransporter in distal convoluted tubule	Salt-sensitive hypertension that is resistant to antihypertensive medications other than thiazide diuretics	↓ Aldo ↑ Renin ↑ Potassium ↓ Bicarbonate	Long-acting thiazide diuretic
Glucocorticoid remedial aldosteronism[d]	CYP11B1 chimeric fusion with CYP11B2	AD	Adrenocorticotropic hormone (ACTH) results in release of aldosterone from adrenal cortex	Resistant hypertension in childhood with a family history of early-onset stroke; not identified in Black populations	↑↑ Aldo ↓ Renin ↓/N Potassium ↑/N Bicarbonate	Glucocorticoids amiloride
Familial hyperaldosteronism type II	CLCN2	AD	Increased aldosterone secretion from adrenal gland	Early-onset primary aldosteronism or bilateral adrenal hyperplasia	↑↑ Aldo ↓ Renin ↓/N Potassium ↑/N Bicarbonate	MR antagonist, amiloride
Familial hyperaldosteronism type III	KCNJ5[a]	AD	Increased aldosterone secretion from adrenal gland	Early-onset primary aldosteronism with massive bilateral adrenal hyperplasia and poor response to MR antagonists	↑↑ Aldo ↓ Renin ↓ Potassium ↑ Bicarbonate	MR antagonist, adrenalectomy (often bilateral)
Familial hyperaldosteronism type IV	CACNA1H[a]	AD	Increased aldosterone secretion from adrenal gland	Early-onset primary aldosteronism	↑↑ Aldo ↓ Renin ↓/N Potassium ↑/N Bicarbonate	MR antagonist, amiloride
Sporadic aldosterone-producing adenoma	ATP1A1 ATP2B3 CACNA1D CACNA1H KCNJ5	Somatic	Aldosterone-producing adenoma	Resistant hypertension in adulthood	↑ Aldo ↓ Renin ↓ Potassium ↑ Bicarbonate	MR antagonist, adrenalectomy (unilateral)
Liddle syndrome	SCNN1B[a] SCNN1G[a]	AD	Increased activity of epithelial sodium channel (ENaC) in collecting tubule/duct	Blood pressure (BP) unresponsive to antihypertensive medications except for ENaC-blocking agents	↓ Aldo ↓ Renin ↓/N Potassium ↑/N Bicarbonate	Amiloride
Apparent mineralocorticoid excess	HSD11B2[b]	AR	Cortisol binds MR due to lack of enzyme activity to degrade cortisol intracellularly	Severe phenotype presents during infancy with low birth weight and failure to thrive with severe hypertension	↓ Aldo ↓ Renin ↓ Potassium ↑ Bicarbonate	MR antagonist, kidney transplant curative
Hypertension with brachydactyly type E	PDE3A[a]	AD	Salt-resistant form of hypertension without clear mechanism	Neurovascular contact at the rostral ventrolateral medulla, brachydactyly, family history of death from stroke before age 50 years	N Aldo N Renin	Not yet defined
Activating MR mutation	NR3C2[a]	AD	Progesterone activates MR receptor	Severe HTN during pregnancy; BP rises with spironolactone	↓ Aldo ↓ Renin ↓ Potassium N Bicarbonate	Amiloride, delivery of fetus
Congenital adrenal hyperplasia	CYP11B1[b] CYP17A1[b]	AR	Overproduction of 21-hydroxylated steroids that activate the MR	Virilization in girls and precocious puberty in boys (CYP11B1); primary amenorrhea and delayed sexual development in girls and ambiguous genitalia in boys (CYP17A1)	↓ Aldo ↓ Renin ↓/N Potassium	MR antagonist

[a]Gain of function mutation.

[b]Loss of function mutation.

[c]Also known as pseudohypoaldosteronism type II and Gordon syndrome.

[d]Also known as familial hyperaldosteronism type I.

Aldo, Aldosterone; AD, autosomal dominant; AR, autosomal recessive; HTN, hypertension; MR, mineralocorticoid receptor; N, normal.

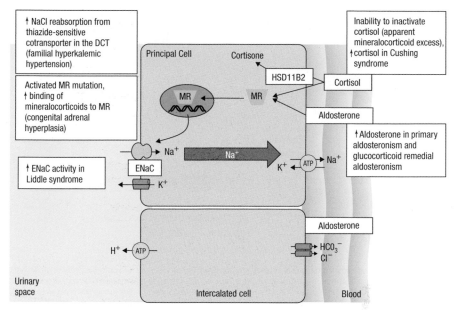

Fig. 15.1 Electrogenic link between potassium and sodium in the distal nephron. *ATP,* Adenosine triphosphate; *DCT,* distal convoluted tubule; *ENaC,* epithelial sodium channel; *MR,* mineralocorticoid receptor; *NaCl,* sodium chloride.

transepithelial voltage that draws potassium into the lumen through the leaky renal outer medullary potassium channel (ROMK). The majority of the identified monogenic causes of hypertension result in increased sodium reabsorption in the collecting duct (Figs. 15.1 and 15.2). For example, in familial hyperaldosteronisms, the excess aldosterone increases basolateral sodium-potassium ATPase activity in the principal cell, which provides the driving force to pull sodium through the epithelial sodium channel (ENaC).

The negative luminal charge caused by the reabsorption of sodium can be mitigated by accompanied chloride reabsorption or secretion of protons in the distal nephron. Upregulating proton secretion from alpha intercalated cells would tend toward metabolic alkalosis, which often accompanies hypokalemia in monogenic hypertensive syndromes.

5. **How does familial hyperkalemic hypertension cause hyperkalemia?**
   Familial hyperkalemic hypertension (FHH) was originally identified as Gordon syndrome and later termed *pseudo-hypoaldosteronism type II* due to the seemingly confusing combination of adrenal insufficiency by laboratory testing and hypertension. Abnormally increased sodium-chloride cotransporter activity (the thiazide-sensitive cotransporter) in the distal convoluted tubule explains the FHH phenotype. However, the genetic mutations associated with FHH are not in the sodium-chloride cotransporter but in the pathways that regulated its activity. With-no-lysine kinase (WNK) 1 and 4 regulate sodium-chloride cotransporter phosphorylation, and WNK signaling is physiologically regulated by Kelch-like 3 (KLHL3)- and Cullin 3 (CUL3)-mediated ubiquitination.[10] Mutations in *WNK1, WNK4, KLHL3,* and *CUL3* genes all have been linked to FHH (see Table 15.1 and Fig. 15.2).
   FHH tends toward hyperkalemia by two complementary mechanisms: (1) Supraphysiological salt reabsorption in the distal convoluted tubule creates a positive total body salt balance, which acts to suppress aldosterone. Urinary potassium excretion is limited in the absence of aldosterone. (2) Aggressive sodium uptake in the distal convoluted tubule leaves little sodium for electrogenic exchange with potassium in the collecting tubule/duct. In order to satisfy the body's acid-base balance, reabsorbed sodium after the distal convoluted tubule would favor proton secretion over potassium (see Fig. 15.1).

6. **Which monogenic cause of hypertension is not directly associated with renal salt handling?**
   Individuals with autosomal hypertension with type E brachydactyly underwent formal salt sensitivity testing and were found to be salt resistant. The causal genetic mutation identified in hypertension with brachydactyly type E is a gain-of-function mutation in *PDE3A,* which encodes for phosphodiesterase 3A.[11] Increased protein kinase A–mediated PDE3A phosphorylation increases cyclic adenosine monophosphate hydrolytic activity and enhanced cell proliferation.[6] Hypertension with type E brachydactyly is associated with vascular smooth muscle cell proliferation, altered baroreflex BP regulation, and abnormal fingertip development.

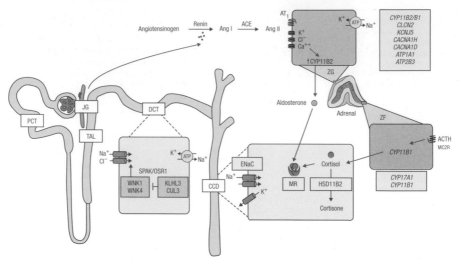

Fig. 15.2 Location of monogenic mutations in the kidney and adrenal gland. *ACE,* Angiotensin converting enzyme; *ACTH,* adreno-corticotropic hormone; *Ang,* angiotensin; *AT_1,* angiotensin II type 1 receptor; *ATP,* adenosine triphosphate; *CCD,* cortical collecting duct; *DCT,* distal convoluted tubule; *ENaC,* epithelial sodium channel; *JG,* juxtaglomerular apparatus; *MR,* mineralocorticoid receptor; *PCT,* proximal convoluted tubule; *TAL,* thick ascending limb; *ZF,* zona fasciculata; *ZG,* zona glomerulosa.

7. **Why is amiloride the ideal treatment for Liddle syndrome?**
    Liddle syndrome results from mutations in the beta (encoded by *SCNN1B*) or gamma (encoded by *SCNN1G*) subunits of the ENaC. The gain-of-function mutations prevent ENaC internalization by impairing its ubiquitination. Therapy necessitates directly blocking ENaC, which is active independent of MR signaling. Of the available ENaC blocking medication, amiloride is preferred over triamterene because the liver metabolizes triamterene in a first-pass effect and amiloride has a longer half-life, resulting in sustained ENaC blockade.

8. **What genetic disorders are associated with pheochromocytoma/paraganglioma?**
    The majority of neuroendocrine tumors associated with hypertension occur within the adrenal medulla (e.g., pheochromocytoma) as opposed to arising in the extraadrenal sympathetic paraganglia (e.g., paraganglioma). Pheochromocytomas and catecholamine-producing paragangliomas often occur sporadically, but germline muta-tions or mutations in inherited susceptibility genes are found in 30% to 60% of cases.[5,6] Germline mutations in neurofibromatosis type 1 lead to pheochromocytoma in up to 5% of patients. Pheochromocytomas arise in ~50% of individuals with missense mutations in the proto-oncogene, RET, seen in multiple endocrine neoplasia type 2. Pheochromocytomas are among the tumors typically seen in von Hippel-Lindau disease. Due to the frequent as-sociation between genetic syndromes and pheochromocytomas, any patient with a pheochromocytoma should be considered for further genetic evaluation.

9. **What secondary cause of hypertension is associated with Turner syndrome?**
    Turner syndrome, also known as 45,X syndrome, is characterized by partial or complete loss of one of the second sex chromosomes in females. Affected individuals typically have short stature and ovarian dysgenesis resulting in lack of puberty and infertility. Other characteristics like webbed neck, broad chest with widely spaced nipples, and low hairline have variable penetrance. Approximately 5% to 10% of individuals with Turner syndrome have coarctation of the aorta, which leads to hypertension and may go undiagnosed until adulthood.

10. **What somatic mutations are associated with hypertension?**
    Somatic mutations are acquired mutations in nongermline cells that cannot be inherited. Primary aldosteronism, which can be identified in 8% to 20% of individuals with hypertension, may result from either adrenal adenomas or bilateral adrenal hyperplasia.[12] Heterozygous somatic mutations in the *KCNJ5* gene account for up to 40% of aldosterone-producing adenomas.[5] *KCNJ5* encodes a G protein–coupled, inwardly rectifying potassium channel in the cortex of the adrenal gland. Mutations that alter permeability of this channel make the cell membrane susceptible to depolarization and subsequent increase in aldosterone production.[5] Other genes encoding proteins associated with cell membrane depolarization in the adrenal cortex (e.g., *CACNA1D, ATP1A1,* and *ATPT2B3*) are associated with aldosterone-producing adenomas (see Table 15.1).

KEY POINTS

1. Consider a hereditary cause of hypertension when (1) BP is elevated early in life, (2) BP appears resistant to antihypertensive therapy, (3) there are accompanying electrolyte disorders, and/or (4) there is a pattern in the family history.
2. Hereditary causes of hypertension are rare, and more common causes of secondary hypertension like primary aldosteronism or renal artery stenosis should be considered before embarking on genetic testing.
3. Salt sensitivity with suppressed plasma renin activity commonly accompany monogenic causes of hypertension; however, both salt sensitivity and suppressed renin activity are also common in the absence of a monogenic cause of hypertension.

REFERENCES

1. Padmanabhan S, Caulfield M, Dominiczak AF. Genetic and molecular aspects of hypertension. *Circ Res.* 2015;116:937–959.
2. Wang L-P, Yang K-Q, Jiang X-J, et al. Prevalence of Liddle syndrome among young hypertension patients of undetermined cause in a Chinese population. *J Clin Hypertens (Greenwich).* 2015;17:902–907.
3. Carey RM, Calhoun DA, Bakris GL, et al. Resistant hypertension: detection, evaluation, and management: a scientific statement from the American Heart Association. *Hypertension.* 2018;72:e53–e90.
4. Simonetti GD, Mohaupt MG, Bianchetti MG. Monogenic forms of hypertension. *Eur J Pediatr.* 2012;171:1433–1439.
5. Seidel E, Scholl Ul. Genetic mechanisms of human hypertension and their implications for blood pressure physiology. *Physiol Genomics.* 2017;49:630–652.
6. Luft FC. What have we learned from the genetics of hypertension? *Med Clin North Am.* 2017;101:195–206.
7. Lifton RP, Dluhy RG, Powers M, et al. A chimaeric 11 beta-hydroxylase/aldosterone synthase gene causes glucocorticoid-remediable aldosteronism and human hypertension. *Nature.* 1992;355:262–265.
8. Geller DS, Farhi A, Pinkerton N, et al. Activating mineralocorticoid receptor mutation in hypertension exacerbated by pregnancy. *Science.* 2000;289:119–123.
9. Palmer BF. Regulation of potassium homeostasis. *Clin J Am Soc Nephrol.* 2015;10:1050–1060.
10. Sohara E, Uchida S. Kelch-like 3/Cullin 3 ubiquitin ligase complex and WNK signaling in salt-sensitive hypertension and electrolyte disorder. *Nephrol Dial Transplant.* 2016;31:1417–1424.
11. Maass PG, Aydin A, Luft FC, et al. PDE3A mutations cause autosomal dominant hypertension with brachydactyly. *Nat Genet.* 2015;47:647–653.
12. Whelton PK, Carey RM, Aronow WS, et al. 2017 ACC/AHA/AAPA/ABC/ACPM/AGS/APhA/ASH/ASPC/NMA/PCNA Guideline for the prevention, detection, evaluation, and management of high blood pressure in adults: a report of the American College of Cardiology/American Heart Association task force on clinical practice guidelines. *Hypertension.* 2018;71:e13–e115.

CHAPTER 16

HYPERTENSION IN CHILDREN AND ADOLESCENTS

Joseph T. Flynn

QUESTIONS

1. **How is hypertension defined in children and adolescents?**
   The definition of hypertension in adults is based on data from large clinical trials, which show that as blood pressure (BP) rises, the risk of cardiovascular endpoints such as stroke, myocardial infarction, and mortality increases. As these events are rare in the pediatric age group, a statistical definition has been adopted that is based upon the distribution of BPs in healthy children, with BP values at the upper end of the distribution ($\geq$90th percentile) considered abnormal. In 2017 the American Academy of Pediatrics (AAP) issued an updated clinical practice guideline for the evaluation and management of childhood hypertension. This new guideline included new normative BP data based only upon children of normal weight, as well as revised BP categories. The new normative BP values (available at https://pediatrics.aappublications.org/content/140/3/e20171904.long) are generally 2 to 3 mm Hg lower than the values previously in use. This guideline for the first time also adopted adult BP categories for adolescents at least 13 years of age. The categories can be summarized as follows:
   - **Normal BP:** BP <90th percentile for age, sex, and height; or <120/<80 mm Hg for adolescents $\geq$13 years old;
   - **Elevated BP:** BP $\geq$90th percentile and <95th percentile for age, sex, and height; or 120 to 129/<80 mm Hg for adolescents $\geq$13 years old;
   - **Hypertension:** BP >95th percentile for age, sex, and height; or $\geq$130/80 mm Hg for adolescents $\geq$13 years old. Hypertensive-level BP is further staged as follows:
     - **Stage 1 hypertension:** BP >95th percentile for age, sex, and height up to the 95th percentile + 11 mm Hg; or 130 to 139/80 to 89 mm Hg for adolescents $\geq$13 years of age; and
     - **Stage 2 hypertension:** BP $\geq$95th percentile +12 mm Hg for age, sex, and height; or >140/90 mm Hg for adolescents $\geq$13 years of age.

   Other organizations, including Hypertension Canada and the European Society of Hypertension (ESH), have also issued guidelines for evaluation of children and adolescents with high BP; their definitions of the different BP categories are roughly similar to those in the AAP guideline. The major differences are that these other guidelines were issued prior to the availability of the revised American normative BP data and used different static cut-points for adolescents.

2. **How common is hypertension in children and adolescents?**
   Initially, the thresholds used for defining hypertension in the young were the same as those used in adults. Unsurprisingly, hypertension was found to be exceedingly rare in young children but could affect up to 2% of adolescents. Later screening studies applied population-based percentiles of BP as the threshold for diagnosis (see earlier) and confirmed that less than 2% of children had hypertension. These screening programs also demonstrated the importance of performing repeated measures of BP before diagnosing hypertension: studies that used just one BP determination found significantly higher "prevalences" of hypertension than studies in which repeated measurements were obtained.

   Over the past decade, however, the childhood obesity epidemic has resulted in an increased prevalence of hypertension in the young. Multiple studies have demonstrated an increased prevalence of hypertension among obese children—as high as 4.5%—compared with nonobese children. Indeed, it is now generally accepted that the prevalence of elevated BP has reached 10%, and the overall prevalence of hypertension is nearly 4%. Of significant concern in the United States is that this increase has been much greater in non-Hispanic Black and Mexican American children than in White children. Similar findings have been seen in screening studies performed in other countries, including China, the Seychelles, and Iceland. Finally, with the publication of the new normative data in the AAP guideline, recent studies have shown even greater rates of elevated BP and hypertension both in the United States and abroad.

3. **What are the causes of hypertension in children and adolescents?**
   Historically, hypertension in children and adolescents was considered secondary in origin, and the diagnosis of primary hypertension was made only after an exhaustive diagnostic evaluation. As discussed previously, this

may have been related to the lack of normative childhood BP data, which required the use of adult hypertension cut-points to identify high BP in children as well. If an 8-year-old child was only diagnosed with hypertension if their BP was greater than 140/90, then of course secondary causes would be commonly found given that 140/90 is now known to be well above the normal distribution of BP in 8-year-old children. This began to change in the late 1970s as large-scale population-based screening studies began to elucidate what constitutes normal and high BPs among children and adolescents. Further refinement of the normative data as described in question 1 has established much different—and lower—thresholds for diagnosing hypertension in the young, resulting in a larger number of children identified with high BP and reducing the proportion with severe hypertension likely to be secondary in origin.

The other major change since the earliest efforts to understand childhood hypertension has been the rapid increase in childhood obesity (see later). Given this, it is now clear that the predominant form of hypertension in children, at least those older than 6 years of age, is primary hypertension with secondary causes accounting for a smaller proportion of all hypertension. In fact, at least one recent multicenter study conducted in the United States demonstrated that primary hypertension was found in 90% of all children and adolescents referred to tertiary pediatric centers. This means that most children and adolescents with hypertension do not need the exhaustive evaluation for secondary forms of hypertension that was previously recommended. As discussed further in question 7, only children with characteristic findings on history and physical examination, or with markedly abnormal screening test results, should be evaluated for secondary causes.

4. What factors contribute to the development of childhood primary hypertension?

The two factors that appear to be most influential in children and adolescents with primary hypertension are family history and obesity. In multiple cases series, the majority of children with primary hypertension had a parent or grandparent with hypertension. Twin studies have also confirmed the familial tendency toward hypertension, with heritability estimates of around 50% to 60%.

Obesity is well-known to contribute to the development of hypertension via a variety of mechanisms, including activation of the sympathetic nervous system, activation of the renin-angiotensin-aldosterone system, and impaired renal sodium handling. Screening studies conducted over the past two decades in the United States and elsewhere have shown that the prevalence of hypertension in children with body mass index at the 95th percentile or above is several times higher than among children with normal weight. Most alarmingly, the steady increase in obesity rates among children in the United States, Mexico, Chile, India, China, and many other countries has been accompanied by increases in the prevalence of elevated BP and hypertension in youth, which is likely to be followed by increased rates of adult cardiovascular disease.

Recently, another important factor has emerged as a likely contributor to the development of primary hypertension in the young—premature birth. It has become increasingly clear that hypertension occurs more commonly among children born early compared with those born at term. Mechanisms are unclear but likely include reduced nephron endowment and epigenetic changes in DNA function induced by an adverse intrauterine environment. With the increased survival of premature infants as young as 24 weeks' gestation, the importance of prematurity as a contributing factor to pediatric hypertension is likely to increase. Given this, it is important to obtain a full birth history when evaluating children and adolescents with suspected hypertension (see later).

5. What is the best approach for identifying children and adolescents with high BP?

Routine BP measurement beginning at 3 years of age during well-child care is recommended by both the AAP and ESH as an appropriate approach to identifying children and adolescents with abnormal BP. BP should also be routinely measured in children younger than 3 years of age known to have conditions associated with hypertension such as diabetes or kidney disease. This universal screening strategy is not without its detractors. The United States Preventive Services Task Force, for example, conducted an evidence review in 2013 and concluded that there was insufficient evidence to warrant universal BP screening in childhood (an updated evidence review was in progress at the time this chapter was written). This recommendation was based on the absence of clinical trials linking childhood BP to adult cardiovascular disease, even though such clinical trials could probably never be conducted. Thus most experts in childhood hypertension concur with the AAP and ESH and endorse universal screening.

Correct identification of abnormal BP obviously requires proper BP measurement technique, and this point has been appropriately emphasized in the AAP, Canadian, and ESH pediatric hypertension guidelines. As the normative data for childhood BP are derived from screening studies that used auscultation, auscultation is the recommended method of measuring BP in children and adolescents. The correct technique is described in the 2017 AAP Clinical Practice Guideline. Not unexpectedly, it is important to have a wide variety of cuff sizes available, especially larger sizes given the increased arm circumferences seen in adolescents with obesity.

Oscillometric devices, although not recommended in the AAP guideline for diagnosis of hypertension in childhood, may be employed for screening and are typically used to measure BP in infants given the difficulties with auscultation in this age group. If an oscillometric device is used, it is important to choose a device that has been validated in children and adolescents. Lists of devices with pediatric validation can be found at www.dableducational.org and www.stridebp.org.

6. **How is the diagnosis of hypertension confirmed in children and adolescents?**
   All current pediatric hypertension guidelines require that abnormal office BP readings be documented on three occasions before the diagnosis of hypertension is made. This is because BP in childhood is known to be labile; older studies document that even in children with known secondary hypertension, BP can be normal at times. Other studies have demonstrated that children with a high office BP reading at the beginning of a clinical encounter can have a normal reading at the end of that encounter. Thus multiple readings are needed, typically obtained over a period of several weeks with shorter intervals between repeat readings for children and adolescents with BPs at the stage 2 hypertension level than for those with readings at the elevated BP level.

   However, even repeated office BP readings may not completely eliminate the white coat effect, which can be seen in up to 40% of children referred to tertiary pediatric hypertension clinics for evaluation of office hypertension. Ambulatory blood pressure monitoring (ABPM) has therefore found an increasingly important role in management of hypertension in the young—all major pediatric hypertension guidelines advocate use of ABPM to confirm the diagnosis of hypertension. It is important to note, however, that ABPM is not required to make the diagnosis of hypertension in children and adolescents; diagnosis is based on office BP, and ABPM is used for confirmation and/or to rule out white coat hypertension. As with office BP, correct cuff size and other technique-related issues are important in obtaining a valid ABPM study in the young, and there are age- and sex-specific normative data that should be used when interpreting ABPM in pediatric patients.

7. **How should hypertension in a child or adolescent be evaluated?**
   As with any patient, evaluation of the child or adolescent with hypertension begins with obtaining a careful history, then moving on to the physical examination and targeted laboratory testing and imaging. In pediatrics, it is important to include a thorough birth and family history in addition to eliciting a complete personal medical history. Perinatal events have been shown to influence BP beginning in childhood, and a positive family history of hypertension or conditions that increase the risk of hypertension can be influential on the child's BP. When performing a systems review, keep in mind that one of the goals of the evaluation is to identify potential underlying secondary causes of hypertension, so questions should be geared toward uncovering symptoms of kidney, cardiac, endocrine disorders, etc. Finally, as many medications and other ingested substances can affect BP, a thorough medication/substance use history is also important.

   In most youth with hypertension, especially those with primary hypertension, the physical examination will be normal (except for the BP of course!). However, the examination may uncover previously unknown conditions such as chronic kidney disease (CKD), especially in younger children (see earlier). Comprehensive tables of physical findings suggestive of specific underlying causes of hypertension are available elsewhere and should be consulted if necessary. Table 16.1 provides a brief summary of history and physical examination findings that may help differentiate between primary and secondary forms of hypertension in the young.

   All children and adolescents with hypertension warrant a basic battery of diagnostic studies as summarized in Table 16.2. These are designed to uncover secondary causes of hypertension and comorbidities such as dyslipidemia or impaired glucose tolerance. Other testing should be guided by the results of the history, physical

Table 16.1 Primary vs. Secondary Hypertension in Children and Adolescents

FEATURES SUGGESTIVE OF PRIMARY HYPERTENSION	FEATURES SUGGESTIVE OF SECONDARY HYPERTENSION
History • Age >6 years old • Hypertension in a parent or grandparent • Premature birth	History • Age <6 years old • No family history of hypertension • Failure to thrive • Frequent urinary tract infections • New-onset enuresis • Solid organ or bone marrow transplant
Physical examination • Isolated systolic hypertension • Overweight or obesity • Lack of abnormal findings	Physical examination • Diastolic hypertension • Severe hypertension (30 mm Hg >95th percentile) • Short stature • Absent/diminished femoral pulses • Elfin facies (Williams syndrome) • Shield chest, webbed neck (Turner syndrome) • Café-au-lait spots (neurofibromatosis) • Abdominal bruit • Abdominal or flank mass • Edema (kidney disease)

Table 16.2 Laboratory and Imaging Evaluation

PATIENT CATEGORY	RECOMMENDED STUDIES
All patients	Urinalysis Electrolytes, BUN, creatinine, lipid panel
Patients with overweight/obesity	Studies for all patients, plus ALT, AST Glycosylated hemoglobin Consider fasting glucose
Children <6 years of age or with abdominal/flank mass	Studies for all patients, plus Renal ultrasound
Children with reduced/absent femoral pulses, girls with Turner syndrome	Studies for all patients, plus Echocardiography
Children with abdominal bruit, significant diastolic hypertension, Williams syndrome, neurofibromatosis	Studies for all patients, plus CT or MR angiogram
Children with hypokalemia on screening laboratory tests	Renin, aldosterone Monogenic hypertension testing

ALT, Alanine transaminase; *AST,* aspartate transaminase; *BUN,* blood urea nitrogen; *CT,* computed tomographic; *MR,* magnetic resonance.

examination, and basic laboratory studies. For example, thyroid studies should be obtained if symptoms or examination findings suggestive of thyroid disease are elicited. With respect to imaging, there are two important points to emphasize:
- Renal ultrasonography is warranted only in those younger than 6 years old or those with stage 2 hypertension; when an ultrasound is indicated, do not order Doppler studies because the sensitivity and specificity of renal Doppler to detect renovascular disease in the pediatric age group is poor.
- Echocardiography is no longer recommended at time of diagnosis of hypertension in the 2017 AAP guideline; echocardiography is now only recommended at the time of initiation of antihypertensive medications.

8. **What is the recommended initial treatment for hypertension in children and adolescents?**
Treatment of the child or adolescent with hypertension should begin with lifestyle modification. Increased physical activity, dietary changes, and weight loss have all been shown to reduce BP in the young. Children and adolescents with hypertension should be encouraged to participate in at least 30 to 40 minutes of vigorous physical activity 4 to 5 days per week. Research studies have shown that this can reduce systolic BP by 6 to 7 mm Hg and may also improve vascular function. Concomitantly, they should be encouraged to reduce screen time, which has been on the rise with the widespread use of smart phones and other devices.

Sodium restriction has been the mainstay of dietary recommendations for the treatment of hypertension in adults and has been shown to be useful in children with hypertension as well. However, a more comprehensive approach to dietary change such as the Dietary Approaches to Stop Hypertension (DASH) diet may have even greater benefits, especially when combined with advice from a pediatric dietitian on other aspects of nutrition such as reducing portion sizes. A recent systematic review showed that a DASH-style diet can reduce BP and improve body composition in adolescents with hypertension. Although there have not been studies of the DASH diet in younger children, fruit, vegetable, and whole-grain consumption is generally low in most children, so it is logical to assume that implementation of the DASH eating plan in children of all ages will have health benefits.

As in adults, lifestyle changes need to be sustained to be effective—numerous studies have shown that once stopped, BP will rise to pretreatment levels. Furthermore, given the strong role of environment and family history on BP in childhood, lifestyle changes should be implemented among the entire family to have the greatest chances of success.

9. **When should antihypertensive medications be used in a child or adolescent with hypertension?**
Lifestyle measures do not result in immediate reduction of BP and may not reduce BP sufficiently in children and adolescents with more severe hypertension. Additionally, there may be other considerations such as the presence of underlying conditions or symptoms or hypertensive target-organ damage that may justify starting an antihypertensive medication early. Thus all current pediatric hypertension guidelines recommend initiating antihypertensive medications in the following circumstances:
- Symptomatic or stage 2 hypertension
- Hypertension associated with diabetes, CKD, or coarctation of the aorta
- Hypertension with known target-organ damage such as left ventricular hypertrophy
- Persistent hypertension despite a trial of lifestyle changes (generally at least 6 months)

10. What medications can be used in children with hypertension?

Historically, drugs prescribed for children were not studied rigorously to assess for efficacy, safety, or appropriate dosing regimens. The passage of the US Food and Drug Administration (FDA) Modernization Act in 1997 heralded an era of increased rigor with respect to pediatric drug development by providing financial incentives to industry sponsors for conducting pharmaceutical trials in children. Subsequent legislative efforts have facilitated ongoing attention to this area. Antihypertensive drugs represent one of the largest groups of medications impacted by these efforts. Consequently, a growing number of antihypertensive medications from different classes have been studied in children and adolescents, resulting in more of these agents receiving FDA-approved labeling for use in children and adolescents. Recent pediatric guidelines, including those from the AAP and the ESH, have taken advantage of this new information in their recommendations for antihypertensive medication prescribing in children and include detailed dosing recommendations, many derived from the recent clinical trials.

First-line agents recommended by the AAP include long-acting calcium channel blockers, angiotensin-converting enzyme inhibitors (ACEIs), angiotensin receptor blockers (ARBs), and thiazide diuretics. Other classes of agents, including beta- and alpha-adrenergic blockers, are generally reserved for second- or third-line use, given their known side effects. Although some experts recommend using a pathophysiologic approach to the use of antihypertensive medications in children and adolescents, in general the choice of agent is left up to the individual prescriber. Consideration should be given to special conditions such as CKD or the concurrent presence of migraine headache when choosing a medication, similar to the "compelling indications" approach recommended in the past for adults.

Antihypertensive drugs in children and adolescents are generally prescribed in a stepped-care manner: The child is initially started on the lowest recommended dose, then the dose is increased until the highest recommended dose is reached or until the child experiences adverse effects from the medication, at which point a second drug from a different class should be added, and so on, until the desired goal BP is reached. Pediatric dosing recommendations for selected antihypertensive medications can be found in Table 16.3.

11. How should children with hypertension be followed after treatment has been started?

Once treatment has been started, it is important to ensure that BP goals are reached and maintained. Children and adolescents treated with lifestyle measures only should be seen every 3 to 6 months to monitor the effect of treatment and to encourage continued adherence. Those started on antihypertensive medications should be seen frequently at first, perhaps every 6 to 8 weeks, so that drugs can be titrated and then less often once a stable regimen and the goal BP is attained. We utilize home BP monitoring to help determine response to medication

Table 16.3 Selected Antihypertensive Medications Commonly Used in Children and Adolescents[a]

CLASS	DRUG	DOSING[a,b]
Angiotensin receptor blocker	Candesartan	Start: 0.2 mg/kg/d up to 8 mg/d; Max: 0.4 mg/kg/d up to 32 mg/d (32 mg)
	Losartan	Start: 0.7 mg/kg/d *divided BID*; Max: 1.4 mg/kg/d divided BID; (100 mg)
	Olmesartan	Start: 10–20 mg/d; Max: 20–40 mg/d (40 mg)
	Valsartan	Start: 1.3 mg/kg/d up to 40 mg/d; Max: 2.7 mg/kg/d up to 160 mg/d (320 mg)
Angiotensin-converting enzyme inhibitor	Enalapril[c]	Start: 0.08 mg/kg/d *divided BID*; Max: 0.6 mg/kg/d divided BID (40 mg)
	Lisinopril[c]	Start: 0.07 mg/kg/d; Max: 0.6 mg/kg/d (40 mg)
Beta-adrenergic blocker	Atenolol	Start: 0.5 mg/kg/d *divided BID*; Max: 2 mg/kg/d divided BID (100 mg)
	Propranolol[c]	Start: 1 mg/kg/d *divided BID-TID*; Max: 8 mg/kg/d (640 mg)
	Metoprolol succinate	Start: 1 mg/kg/d up to 50 mg; Max: 2 mg/kg/d up to 200 mg/d (200 mg)
Calcium channel blocker	Amlodipine[c]	Start: 0.1 mg/kg/d; Max: 0.6 mg/kg/d (10 mg)
	Extended-release nifedipine	Start: 0.2 mg/kg/d; Max: 3 mg/kg/d (120 mg)
Thiazide diuretic	Hydrochlorothiazide	Start: 1 mg/kg/d; Max: 2 mg/kg/d (50 mg)
	Chlorthalidone	Start: 0.3 mg/kg/d; Max: 2 mg/kg/d (50 mg)

[a]Starting and maximal doses given either as absolute dose or as weight-based ranges. Maximum adult dose in parentheses. Always consult updated US Food and Drug Administration–approved prescribing information.
[b]All drugs should be administered once-daily except as otherwise indicated.
[c]Suspension preparation commercially available.
BID, Twice-daily; *d*, day; *kg*, kilogram; *mg*, milligram; *TID*, three times daily.

treatment; repeat ABPM may also be used and is mandatory in certain children with hypertension (see later). Finally, children treated with specific medication classes—ACEIs, ARBs, and diuretics—require periodic laboratory monitoring to assess for electrolyte disturbances and other medication-related toxicities.

12. **What about sports participation?**
As physical activity is an essential component of hypertension treatment, children and adolescents with hypertension who wish to participate in sports should be allowed to do so. The AAP guideline contains two specific recommendations with respect to participation in competitive athletics:
- Athletes with hypertension should be evaluated for cardiovascular risk and hypertensive target-organ damage, and
- BP should be lowered to below the stage 2 hypertension level.

Once these conditions have been met, the child or adolescent with hypertension may be allowed to compete without further restriction. Of course, they should be carefully followed to ensure that goal BP has been reached as detailed previously.

13. **Are there specific forms of childhood hypertension that require special consideration?**
Although less common than primary hypertension, secondary forms of hypertension in children and adolescents have unique aspects that warrant enhanced diagnostic testing, intensified treatment, or both. The most prominent of these is hypertension associated with CKD. Uncontrolled hypertension in persons with CKD can hasten the progression toward end-stage kidney disease. It is also well-known to be associated with blunted nocturnal BP dipping on ABPM and is more likely to be masked than in primary hypertension. Therefore ABPM should be performed at the outset in the evaluation of hypertension in children and adolescents with CKD and should be performed periodically after initiation of treatment to ensure adequate BP control. Hypertension in persons with CKD should preferentially be treated with an ACEI or ARBs, with diuretics, calcium channel blockers, and beta-adrenergic blockers added as needed to reach goal BP.

Children with repaired aortic coarctation also warrant special consideration. A significant percentage of these children will be found to be hypertensive years after repair, many with masked hypertension detected only by ABPM. The etiology of recurrent hypertension is unknown but probably is related to an underlying vasculopathy; recurrent hypertension probably explains the increased late mortality in adults with a history of coarctation. Periodic ABPM should therefore be part of the routine follow-up of these children, and if hypertension is present, antihypertensive medications should be prescribed. We typically use either ARBs or beta-adrenergic blockers both of which have been shown to improve vascular stiffness.

Children with several other underlying diagnoses also merit routine use of ABPM for diagnosis, including those with diabetes (increased prevalence of nocturnal hypertension), genetic syndromes such as Turner syndrome (increased prevalence of aortic coarctation), and neurofibromatosis (increased prevalence of renovascular hypertension). With respect to treatment, it may be advisable to avoid using beta-adrenergic blockers or thiazide diuretics in children with hypertension and obesity or type 2 diabetes (impaired glucose tolerance). This discussion is by no means exhaustive and the interested reader should consult more comprehensive references.

14. **Does hypertension in childhood have implications for future cardiovascular health?**
Although there is a lack of clinical trial evidence demonstrating long-term adverse consequences of high BP in children and adolescents, other sources of evidence can be examined to ascertain the immediate and future effects of high BP in youth. Examples of such data include cross-sectional studies that demonstrate associations between high BP and target-organ effects such as left ventricular hypertrophy and studies that demonstrate tracking of BP levels from childhood into adulthood. Longitudinal cohort studies such as the Bogalusa Heart Study and Cardiovascular Risk in Young Finns Study constitute yet another body of evidence that can be examined to determine the long-term cardiovascular risk of BP measured in childhood. Data from these cohorts have linked childhood BP levels with intermediate markers of adult cardiovascular disease, including left ventricular hypertrophy, metabolic syndrome, increased pulse wave velocity, and increased carotid intima-media thickness. Although additional data are needed, especially data linking childhood BP to "hard" cardiovascular endpoints, there is already sufficient information available to support the concept that childhood BP matters and should be considered a predictor of adult cardiovascular disease.

KEY POINTS

1. Since cardiovascular events are rare in the pediatric age group, a statistical definition for hypertension has been adopted, based upon the distribution of BPs in healthy children, with BP values at the upper end of the distribution ($\geq 90^{th}$ percentile) considered abnormal.
2. Over the past decade, with the childhood obesity epidemic has resulted in an increased prevalence of hypertension in the young with a prevalence of hypertension as high as 4.5% among obese children as compared to less than 2% in non-obese children.
3. White coat effect is common in children, and ambulatory blood pressure monitoring is recommended to establish the diagnosis of hypertension.

BIBLIOGRAPHY

Baracco R, Kapur G, Mattoo T, et al. Prediction of primary vs secondary hypertension in children. *J Clin Hypertens (Greenwich)*. 2012;14:316–321.

Davis ML, Ferguson MA, Zachariah JP. Clinical predictors and impact of ambulatory blood pressure monitoring in pediatric hypertension referrals. *J Am Soc Hypertens*. 2014;8:660–667.

Dionne JM, Harris KC, Benoit G, et al. Hypertension Canada's 2017 guidelines for the diagnosis, assessment, prevention and treatment of pediatric hypertension. *Can J Cardiol*. 2017;33:577–585.

Falkner B. Recent clinical and translational advances in pediatric hypertension. *Hypertension*. 2015;65:926–931.

Falkner B. Maternal and gestational influences on childhood blood pressure. *Pediatr Nephrol*. 2020;35(8):1409–1418. doi: 10.1007/s00467-019-4201-x.

Ferguson M, Flynn JT. Rational use of antihypertensive medications in children. *Pediatr Nephrol*. 2014;29:979–988.

Flynn JT, Daniels SR, Hayman LL, et al. American Heart Association Atherosclerosis, Hypertension and Obesity in Youth Committee of the Council on Cardiovascular Disease in the Young. Update: ambulatory blood pressure monitoring in children and adolescents: a scientific statement from the American Heart Association. *Hypertension*. 2014;63:1116–1135.

Flynn JT, Kaelber DC, Baker-Smith CM, et al. Clinical practice guideline for screening and management of high blood pressure in children and adolescents. *Pediatrics*. 2017;140:e20171904.

Hanevold CD. White coat hypertension in children and adolescents. *Hypertension*. 2019;73:24–30.

Juhola J, Magnussen CG, Viikari JS, et al. Tracking of serum lipid levels, blood pressure, and body mass index from childhood to adulthood: the Cardiovascular Risk in Young Finns Study. *J Pediatr*. 2011;159:584–590.

Lurbe E, Agabiti-Rosei E, Cruickshank JK, et al. 2016 European Society of Hypertension guidelines for the management of high blood pressure in children and adolescents. *J Hypertens*. 2016;34:1887–1920.

Maahs DM, Daniels SR, de Ferranti SD, et al. American Heart Association Atherosclerosis, Hypertension and Obesity in Youth Committee of the Council on Cardiovascular Disease in the Young; Council on Clinical Cardiology; Council on Cardiovascular and Stroke Nursing; Council for High Blood Pressure Research; Council on Lifestyle and Cardiometabolic Health. Cardiovascular disease risk factors in youth with diabetes mellitus: a scientific statement from the American Heart Association. *Circulation*. 2014;130:1532–1558.

O'Sullivan J. Late hypertension in patients with repaired aortic coarctation. *Curr Hypertens Rep*. 2014;16:421.

Wilson AC, Flynn JT. Blood pressure in children with chronic kidney disease: lessons learned from the Chronic Kidney Disease in Children Cohort Study. *Pediatr Nephrol*. 2020;35(7):1203–1209. doi: 10.1007/s00467-019-04288-6.

CHAPTER 17

HYPERTENSION IN CHRONIC KIDNEY DISEASE AND END-STAGE KIDNEY DISEASE

Nishigandha Pradhan, MD, and Mahboob Rahman, MD

QUESTIONS

HYPERTENSION IN CHRONIC KIDNEY DISEASE

1. **What is the prevalence of hypertension in chronic kidney disease?**
   Hypertension is common in patients with chronic kidney disease (CKD). In the 2015–16 National Health and Nutrition Examination survey, 61.4% of patients with CKD had hypertension; 37.4% of patients had controlled blood pressure (BP).

2. **How should BP be measured in the office in patients with CKD?**
   BP measurement in the office should follow standard guidelines for accuracy including avoidance of caffeine, exercise, and smoking for at least 30 minutes prior to measurement, appropriate positioning, and using the proper sized cuff. Two or more readings should be averaged for each visit. Automated oscillometric BP monitors are preferred.

3. **What is the role of ambulatory blood pressure monitoring and home BP monitoring in CKD?**
   Indications for ambulatory blood pressure monitoring (ABPM) include:
   - To evaluate white coat or masked hypertension
   - To monitor antihypertensive medication efficacy in treated patients
   - To evaluate postural, postprandial, and medication-induced hypotension
   - To assess hypotension from autonomic dysfunction

   Home BP monitoring is less cumbersome than ABPM and is a valuable adjunct in the management of hypertension. Patient education regarding proper technique of BP measurement and periodic assessment of home BP devices for accuracy is essential. An average of two morning and two nightly readings over 7 days should be used to assess BP control.

4. **What is the pathophysiology of hypertension in CKD?**
   The pathophysiology of hypertension in CKD is complex and multifactorial. Reduction in the glomerular filtration rate (GFR) leads to sodium and water retention. This, along with endothelial dysfunction, nitric oxide inactivation, and activation of intrarenal renin-angiotensin-aldosterone system (RAAS) leads to central sympathetic activation, vasoconstriction, and increased peripheral resistance, eventually resulting in elevated BP (Fig. 17.1).

5. **What are the consequences of untreated hypertension in patients with CKD?**
   Hypertension contributes to ongoing decline in kidney function regardless of the underlying cause of CKD. Normally, afferent arteriolar contraction in response to elevated BP protects the glomerular capillaries from elevated systemic pressures. Chronically elevated systemic arterial pressures impair the ability of afferent arterioles to respond to systemic BP, leading to higher intraglomerular pressure, nephrosclerosis, and progressive loss of kidney function.
   Hypertension also adds to the high risk of cardiovascular disease in patients with CKD.

6. **What is the target BP in CKD?**
   The 2017 American College of Cardiology/American Heart Association guidelines recommend a target BP less than 130/80 mm Hg for all CKD patients with hypertension. This has been shown to reduce risk of cardiovascular events and mortality, although, interestingly, it does not reduce the rate of progression of CKD. Of note, the 2018 European Society of Cardiology/European Society of Hypertension guidelines recommend lowering BP to less than 140/90 mm Hg, with systolic BP in the 130- to 139-mm Hg range.

7. **What are some of the nonpharmacologic treatment strategies that can be used in the treatment of hypertension in CKD?**
   Nonpharmacologic interventions are important in the management for the treatment of hypertension and are summarized in Table 17.1.

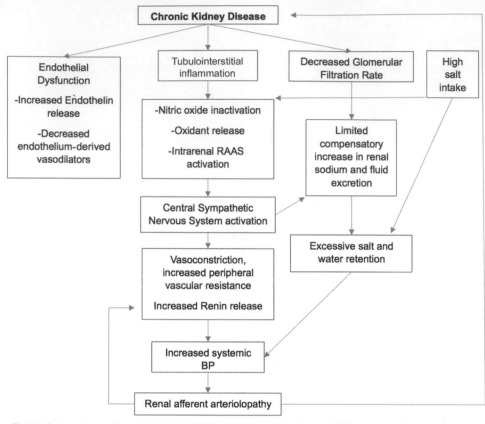

Fig. 17.1 Pathophysiology of hypertension in chronic kidney disease. *BP,* Blood pressure; *RAAS,* renin-angiotensin-aldosterone system.

Table 17.1	Impact of Nonpharmacologic Measures on Systolic Blood Pressure	
INTERVENTION	**GOAL**	**APPROXIMATE IMPACT ON SBP**
Achieving and/or maintaining a healthy weight	Body mass index 20–25	Mean −9 mm Hg in nonsurgical weight loss Mean −22.6 mm Hg in surgical weight loss
Lower salt intake	<2 g sodium intake per day	SBP −4.7 mm Hg
Aerobic exercise	At least 30 minutes 5 times per week	SBP −6.1 mm Hg
Limit alcohol intake	No more than two "standard drinks (8–19.7 g of alcohol)" for men and one for women	SBP −3.8 mm Hg

SBP, Systolic blood pressure.
Adapted from Kidney Disease: Improving Global Outcomes (KDIGO) Blood Pressure Work Group. KDIGO clinical practice guideline for the management of blood pressure in chronic kidney disease. *Kidney Inter.* 2012;2:337-414.

Potassium and magnesium supplementation and fish oil supplements are not recommended due to absence of specific evidence of benefit in hypertensive CKD patients and the risk of hyperkalemia and hypermagnesemia.

8. **Why is it important to restrict sodium intake in hypertensive patients with CKD?**
Salt and water retention are the key drivers of elevated BP in CKD. High dietary sodium intake raises the BP and worsens proteinuria, induces glomerular hyperfiltration, and blunts the effects of RAAS blockade. Lowering sodium intake reduces both the BP and the albuminuria in CKD.

9. **What is the drug of choice for treatment of hypertension in patients with CKD and proteinuria?**
RAAS inhibitors such as angiotensin-converting enzyme inhibitors (ACEIs) and angiotensin receptor blockers (ARBs) are the drugs of first choice in treating proteinuric CKD as they have been shown to slow decline in renal function and to lower proteinuria.
     Combination of two RAAS inhibitors should not be used due to a greater risk of hyperkalemia, worsened renal function, and possible increase in mortality.

10. **On initiation of treatment with an ACEI/ARB, a rise in serum creatinine is often noted. Why does this occur, and what should the provider do when this happens?**
ACEIs and ARBs cause efferent arteriolar vasodilation, thus reducing the intraglomerular pressure, resulting in hemodynamically mediated reduction in GFR and a higher creatinine. Increased intraglomerular pressure often reflects hyperfiltration that may play a role in the progression of CKD; it is possible that the increase in creatinine after initiation of an ACEI/ARB represents blockade of hyperfiltration and may be beneficial in the long run. In most patients, the rise in creatinine is less than 30% from baseline; in these patients, the RAAS inhibitor should be continued with periodic monitoring of renal function and potassium level. If the rise in creatinine exceeds 30% from baseline and is sustained, other causes such as volume contraction, nephrotoxic drugs, or renovascular disease should be considered.

11. **Describe the role of diuretics in the treatment of hypertension in CKD.**
Diuretics reduce BP by inducing negative sodium and fluid balance in the short term and by possibly causing direct or indirect vasodilation on chronic use. As expanded intravascular volume is an important contributor to hypertension in CKD, diuretics are often needed to achieve and maintain BP control. Of the thiazide and "thiazide-like" diuretics, chlorthalidone is preferred due to its longer action and greater potency. These drugs are generally less effective in advanced CKD when loop diuretics are preferred for control of volume overload; however, recent data demonstrate that chlorthalidone effectively reduces blood pressure in stage 4 CKD. Diuretics are effective in combination with most antihypertensive drugs, especially RAAS inhibitors.

12. **What other antihypertensive drugs can be used in patients with CKD?**
Most patients with hypertension and CKD will require multiple medications to control BP. Most antihypertensives can be used, and salient features are summarized in Table 17.2.

HYPERTENSION IN END-STAGE KIDNEY DISEASE

13. **What is the prevalence of hypertension in end-stage kidney disease?**
Hypertension is highly prevalent in patients with end-stage kidney disease (ESKD). It is seen in about 88% to 90% of patients on peritoneal dialysis (PD) and 90% to 95% of patients on incident hemodialysis (HD), decreasing to 85% 30 to 36 months after onset of dialysis.

14. **What is the optimal timing of measurement of BP in patients on HD?**
BP readings measured before, during, and after HD are often not obtained in a standardized manner and have weak prognostic relationship with mortality. In contrast, mean 44-hour interdialytic BP correlates well with target-organ damage and is more predictive of cardiovascular and all-cause mortality. If ABPM is not available, home BP measured in the morning and at night on six consecutive non dialysis days or an average of three interdialysis office BP readings should be used. Lastly, if none of the above is feasible, then a median intradialytic BP reading on a midweek dialysis day may be used to diagnose and treat hypertension.

15. **How is hypertension defined in patients with ESKD using the different methods of BP measurement?**
Thresholds and methods for definition of hypertension in ESKD as proposed by the American Society of Hypertension/American Society of Nephrology, European and Renal Cardiovascular medicine working group of European Renal Association/European Dialysis and Transplant Association and European Society of Hypertension Guidelines can be summarized as seen in Table 17.3.
     The National Kidney Foundation guidelines recommend aiming for pre-HD BP less than 140/90 mm Hg and post-HD BP less than 130/80 mm Hg.

16. **What is the pathophysiology of hypertension in ESKD?**
Inability to regulate volume with sodium and fluid retention is the primary cause of hypertension in ESKD. Other contributing factors are listed in Table 17.4.

17. **Describe the relationship between BP and the risk for cardiovascular events and death in patients on HD.**
There is unclear association between peridialytic BP and all-cause and cardiovascular mortality. In fact, a paradoxical relationship is seen in many studies in which lower rather than higher BP is related to increased

Table 17.2 Antihypertensive Medications in Chronic Kidney Disease

ANTIHYPERTENSIVE CLASS	MECHANISM OF ACTION	PERTINENT ADVERSE EVENTS	POSSIBLE ROLE IN CKD PATIENTS
Calcium channel blockers: Dihydropyridine (e.g., amlodipine), Nondihydropyridine (e.g., Diltiazem and Verapamil)	Vasodilation by blocking L and T type calcium channels	• Peripheral edema • Dihydropyridine calcium channel blockers can worsen proteinuria if used without concomitant RAAS inhibitors	• Nondihydropyridine calcium channel blockers have additional antiproteinuric action with RAAS inhibitors, possible first-line drugs in proteinuric patients intolerant of ACEI/ARB
Aldosterone antagonists (spironolactone, eplerenone)	Block aldosterone action	• Hyperkalemia	• Useful in resistant hypertension • Avoid or use with caution in advanced CKD
Centrally acting alpha agonists (Clonidine, guanfacine)	Reduce central sympathetic outflow→vasodilation	• Sedation • Bradycardia • Rebound hypertension	
Alpha-blockers (terazosin, prazosin)	Peripheral vasodilation	• Postural hypotension • Not recommended as first-line agents	• Useful in benign prostatic hypertrophy and intolerance to other medications
Beta-blockers (metoprolol, carvedilol)	Variable alpha- and beta-adrenergic receptor blockade	• Renally excreted beta-blockers can accumulate, exacerbating bradycardia and other side effects	• Not preferred except in case of specific indications like recent myocardial infarction, heart failure with reduced ejection fraction
Direct vasodilators (hydralazine, minoxidil)	Smooth muscle relaxation→vasodilation	• Fluid retention, headaches, tachycardia	• Minoxidil useful in resistant hypertension

ACEI, Angiotensin-converting enzyme inhibitor; *ARB,* angiotensin receptor blocker; *CKD,* chronic kidney disease; *RAAS,* renin-angiotensin-aldosterone system.

Table 17.3 Definition and Method of Measurement of Blood Pressure in Patients with End-Stage Kidney Disease

	HEMODIALYSIS	PERITONEAL DIALYSIS
Ambulatory blood pressure (BP) monitoring	≥130/80 (44 hours) during midweek dialysis-free interval	≥130/80 (24 hours)
Home BP	≥135/85 (a.m. and p.m. readings over 6 consecutive nondialysis days)	≥135/85 (a.m. and p.m. readings over 7 consecutive days)
Office BP	>140/90 (average of 3 appropriately measured readings on a midweek dialysis-free day)	>140/90

Table 17.4 Mechanisms of Hypertension in End-Stage Kidney Disease

- Sodium and volume overload
- Arterial stiffness
- Sympathetic hyperactivity
- Renin-angiotensin system activation
- Endothelial dysfunction with reduced nitric oxide synthesis
- Sleep apnea
- Use of erythropoietin stimulating agents
- Secondary causes (e.g., thyroid disease, pheochromocytoma, renin-secreting tumors, etc.)

Adapted from K/DOQI clinical practice guidelines for cardiovascular disease in dialysis patients. *Am J Kid Dis.* 2005;45(3):16-153.

mortality. This likely reflects confounding due to comorbid conditions such as advanced heart failure. In contrast, interdialytic BP measured at home or by ABPM is associated with all-cause and cardiovascular mortality in a linear manner.

18. **What are the nonpharmacologic interventions to control BP in patients with ESKD?**
As sodium and water retention is the primary mechanism driving hypertension in ESKD, achievement of each patient's "dry weight" and restricting intra- and interdialytic sodium gain form the cornerstone of therapy. "Dry weight" is the lowest tolerated post dialysis weight at which patients experience minimal symptoms of hypervolemia or hypovolemia. Dry weight is most often achieved by "probing" (i.e., gradual reduction in target weight while assessing patient response).

In patients on PD, in addition to dietary sodium restriction, use of icodextrin to increase ultrafiltration, use of diuretics, and preservation of residual renal function all play an important role in controlling BP.

Table 17.5 Role of Different Antihypertensive Drug Classes in Treatment of Hypertension in Patients with End-Stage Kidney Disease

DRUG CLASS	DATA ON CARDIOVASCULAR/ MORTALITY OUTCOMES IN CLINICAL TRIALS	PHARMACOKINETIC CONSIDERATIONS	OTHER COMMENTS
Beta-blockers	• Reduced mortality vs. placebo in cardiomyopathy • Thrice weekly atenolol reduced cardiovascular events as compared to thrice-weekly lisinopril in patients with left ventricular hypertrophy	• Variable removal by dialysis	• Nondialyzable agents preferred to avoid intradialytic arrhythmias • Carvedilol may help control intradialytic hypertension
RAAS inhibitors	• Fosinopril did not reduce cardiovascular (CV) events and mortality compared to placebo • Losartan/candesartan/valsartan reduced CV events and mortality compared to treatment with no ACEI/ARB	• ARBs are not dialyzable but most ACEIs except Fosinopril are dialyzable	• ACEIs and ARBs not interchangeable due to different pharmacokinetics • Clear superiority over other drug classes not demonstrated
Calcium channel blockers (CCBs)	• Amlodipine reduced CV events compared to placebo	• All CCBs are not removed during dialysis and can be dosed once daily	
Mineralocorticoid receptor antagonists		• Unknown removal with dialysis	• May be useful in resistant hypertension • Risk of hyperkalemia
Loop diuretics	• None	• Ineffective with loss of residual renal function with longer HD vintage	• May have a role in controlling volume overload and BP in patients on PD with preserved residual renal function
Central alpha agonists	• None	• Variably removed by HD	• Clonidine may be used to treat refractory hypertension, patch is preferable to pills for sustained action
Vasodilators	• None	• Hydralazine is 25%–40% removed, whereas Minoxidil is not removed at all by HD	• Minoxidil used as a "last line" therapy; may cause pericardial effusion
Alpha 1 blockers	• None	• Not removed by dialysis	• Useful in patients with BPH and residual renal function

ACEI, Angiotensin-converting enzyme inhibitor; *ARB,* angiotensin receptor blocker; *BP,* blood pressure; *BPH,* benign prostatic hyperplasia; *ESKD,* end-stage kidney disease; *HD,* hemodialysis; *PD,* peritoneal dialysis; *RAAS,* renin-angiotensin-aldosterone system.

19. **Discuss the role of antihypertensive medications in patients with ESKD.**
Despite utmost efforts to control sodium and volume overload, most patients with ESKD require pharmacotherapy for BP control. All major classes of antihypertensive drugs except thiazides are useful in lowering BP in patients with ESKD.
    The role of different classes of antihypertensives in ESKD is summarized in Table 17.5.

20. **How do you choose antihypertensive agents in patients with ESKD?**
There is paucity of data showing benefit of one class of antihypertensives over others in terms of cardiovascular and mortality outcomes. Thus the choice of antihypertensive drug is based on patient's other comorbidities, intra- and interdialytic pharmacokinetics of the drug, efficacy of BP reduction, side effect profile, independent cardio-protective effects, noncardiovascular effects, and drug interactions with other medications. The timing, duration, etiology, and severity of intradialytic BP changes, as well as BP in the interdialytic period, should be considered.

KEY POINTS

1. Hypertension is highly prevalent in patients with CKD and ESKD patients and contributes to the high burden of cardiovascular disease in this population.
2. Sodium and fluid retention coupled with RAAS and sympathetic system activation, as well as endothelial dysfunction, are the main pathogenic mechanisms leading to hypertension.
3. RAAS inhibitors are the first drugs of choice in patients who are proteinuric and also have CKD.
4. The choice and timing of antihypertensive drugs in patients with ESKD is determined by their comorbidities and the pharmacokinetics of the drug in the absence of definitive evidence of superiority of one class over another.

BIBLIOGRAPHY

Hypertension in CKD

Andersen MJ, Agarwal R. Etiology and management of hypertension in chronic kidney disease. *Med Clin N Am*. 2005;89:525–547.
Campese VM. Pathophysiology of resistant hypertension in chronic kidney disease. *Sem in Nephrol*. 2014;34(5):571–576.
Dorans KS, Mills KT, Liu Y, He J. Trends in prevalence and control of hypertension according to the 2017 American College of Cardiology/ American Heart Association (ACC/AHA) guideline. *J Am Heart Assoc*. 2018;7(11):e008888. doi: 10.1161/JAHA.118.008888. Published 2018 Jun 1.
Kidney DiseaseImproving Global Outcomes (KDIGO) Blood Pressure Work Group. KDIGO clinical practice guideline for the management of blood pressure in chronic kidney disease. Kidney Inter. 2012;2:337–414.
Muntner P, Shimbo D, Carey RM, et al. Measurement of blood pressure in humans: a scientific statement from the American Heart Association. *Hypertension*. 2019;73:e35–e66. doi: 10.1161/HYP.0000000000000087.
Sinha A, Agarwal R. The complex relationship between CKD and ambulatory blood pressure patterns. *Adv in Chronic Kidney Dis*. 2015;22(2):102–107.
Whelton PK, Carey RM, Aronow WS, et al. 2017 ACC/AHA/AAPA/ABC/ACPM/AGS/APhA/ASH/ASPC/NMA/PCNA guideline for the prevention, detection, evaluation, and management of high blood pressure in adults: a report of the American College of Cardiology/American Heart Association Task Force on Clinical Practice Guidelines. *J Am Coll Cardiol*. 2018;71:e127–248.

Goal blood pressure in adults with hypertension

Williams B, Mancia G, Spiering W, et al. ESC Scientific Document Group, 2018. ESC/ESH Guidelines for the management of arterial hypertension: the task force for the management of arterial hypertension of the European Society of Cardiology (ESC) and the European Society of Hypertension (ESH). *European Heart Journal*. 2018;39(33):3021–3104.

Hypertension in ESKD

Gosmanova EO, Kovesdy CP. Patient centered approach for hypertension management in end-stage kidney disease: art or science? *Semin in Nephrol*. 2018;38(4):355–368.
K/DOQI clinical practice guidelines for cardiovascular disease in dialysis patients. *Am J Kid Dis*. 2005;45(3):16-153.
Levin NW, Kotanko P, Eckardt U, et al. Blood pressure in chronic kidney disease stage 5D-report from a Kidney Disease: Improving Global Outcomes controversies conference. *Kidney International*. 2010;77:273–284.
Sarafidis PA, Persu A, Agarwal R, et al. Hypertension in dialysis patients: a consensus document by the European Renal and Cardiovascular medicine (EURECA-m) working group of the European Renal Association-European Dialysis and Transplant Association (ERA-EDTA) and the Hypertension and the Kidney working group of the European Society of Hypertension (ESH). *Nephrol Dial Transplant*. 2017;32:620–640.

CHAPTER 18

HYPERTENSION IN DIABETES

Fabian Bock, MD, PhD, and Julia B. Lewis, MD

QUESTIONS

1. **Is hypertension common in patients with diabetes?**
   Diabetes and hypertension share pathophysiologic mechanisms of vascular dysfunction, so they commonly coexist, and hypertension is an important contributor to diabetes-associated vascular complications including kidney disease. According to the Centers for Disease Control and Prevention, about 74% of those with type 2 diabetes mellitus (T2DM) have hypertension, and in the San Antonio Heart Study, 85% of participants with T2DM had hypertension by the fifth decade of life. Interestingly, compared to hypertension, hyperglycemia itself in T2DM is a weak modifiable risk factor for cardiovascular disease (CVD), underscoring the importance of blood pressure (BP) control. The prevalence of hypertension in type 1 diabetes mellitus (T1DM) is significantly less, at 30% to 40% by the third decade of life after around 20 years diabetes duration. The following questions will focus on systolic blood pressure (SBP in mm Hg) as the SBP represents a stronger cardiovascular risk factor, especially with increasing age, than diastolic BP.

2. **What are the current guideline-oriented BP goals in patients with hypertension and diabetes?**
   In 2014 the Eighth Joint National Committee (JNC) on the Prevention, Detection, Evaluation, and Treatment of High Blood Pressure recommended a target SBP of less than 140 mm Hg for patients with T2DM because many trials had demonstrated a benefit. The 2017 American College of Cardiology/American Heart Association (ACC/AHA) guidelines broadly recommend a target of SBP less than 130 mm Hg. It is important to note that many other guidelines did not follow this recommendation and continue to recommend a target SBP of less than 140 mm Hg in patients with diabetes, including the American Diabetes Association (ADA), the American Academy of Family Physicians, the Australian National Heart Foundation, and the National Institute for Health and Clinical Excellence.

3. **What is the main evidence for current BP goals in patients with T2DM?**
   Numerous studies randomizing subjects, including patients with T2DM, to different BP regimens but not specific BP targets demonstrated a strong association between lower achieved BP and reduced cardiovascular risk, particularly stroke. This led to the recommendation of lowering SBP to less than 140 mm Hg. The UK Prospective Diabetes Study Substudy 38 (UKPDS 38) randomly assigned hypertensive diabetic patients to tight or less tight BP control and assessed the impact on micro- and macrovascular complications of diabetes. The tight group achieved a mean SBP of 144 mm Hg versus 154 mm Hg in the less tight group. In the group with tight control, all diabetes-related complications and the microvascular composite were significantly reduced, laying the foundation for the importance of BP control in T2DM. The Action to Control Cardiovascular Risk in Diabetes (ACCORD-BP) trial randomized 4733 participants with T2DM and a high CVD risk to either intensive control (SBP <120 mm Hg) or standard therapy (SBP <140 mm Hg). The mean achieved SBPs in the intensive group and standard group were 119.3 and 133.5, respectively. There was no difference in the primary composite endpoint of nonfatal myocardial infarction (MI), nonfatal stroke or cardiovascular mortality. The intensive group required on average 3.4 antihypertensives compared to 2.1 medications in the standard group. There were more adverse events with more creatinine elevations and electrolyte abnormalities in the intensive group. The Systolic Blood Pressure Intervention Trial (SPRINT), which randomized 9361 participants at high CVD risk to either intensive (SBP <120 mm Hg) or standard (SBP <140 mm Hg) goals, achieved a good separation between the intensive (121.4 with 2.8 drugs) and standard (136.2 with 1.8 drugs) arm with a significant reduction in the primary composite of MI, other acute coronary syndrome, stroke, heart failure, or cardiovascular mortality in the intensive group. Most importantly, the trial excluded patients with diabetes. The differing results between these trial results are unexplained but may reflect differences in the trials such as sample size or true differences in response to BP lowering of patients with T2DM. Thus the main evidence for BP targets in patients with diabetes supporting much lower targets (than the current SBP <140 mm Hg) is derived from trials reporting achieved BP and trials with randomized BP goals that excluded patients with diabetes. The current recommendations all include an individualized approach to BP control for the patient with diabetes and an SBP goal of at least 140 mm Hg or less. Table 18.1 summarizes current guidelines, and Table 18.2 summarizes major BP goal trials.

Table 18.1 Summarizing Current Guidelines

GUIDELINE GROUP	TARGET BP	COMMENTS
American College of Cardiology/American Heart Association (2017)	<130/80	Mainly driven by SPRINT results.
European Society of Cardiology and the European Society of Hypertension (2018)	<140/90	If tolerated, consider lower target of SBP 130 or less. In patients <65 years of age SBP should be lowered to 120–129 in most patients.
American Diabetes Association Standards of Medical Care (2019)	<140/90	Consider SBP <130 if high cardiovascular risk and further lowering is safe.
American Academy of Family Physicians (2014)	<140/90	In a 2017 update with the ACP for patients older than 60 years, the individualization of BP goals was emphasized.
Australian National Heart Foundation (2016)	<140/90	Consider lower targets in select high cardiovascular risk populations.
National Institute for Health and Clinical Excellence Draft (2019)	<140/90	For patients ≥80 years old, target SBP <150.

ACP, American College of Physicians; BP, blood pressure; SBP, systolic blood pressure; SPRINT, Systolic Blood Pressure Intervention Trial.

Table 18.2 Summarizing UKPDS, ACCORD-BP, and SPRINT

TRIAL	POPULATION	N	INTERVENTION	CONCLUSION	COMMENTS
UKPDS 38	Hypertensive patients with newly diagnosed T2DM	1148	Tight (SBP <150) or less tight (SBP <180) BP control	Significant reduction in all diabetes-related and microvascular endpoints in the tight compared to the less tight group.	The tight group achieved a SBP of 144 vs. 154 in the less tight group. Tight group required ≥3 BP medications.
ACCORD-BP	T2DM patients with CVD or CVD risk factors	4733	Intensive therapy (goal SBP <120) or standard therapy (goal SBP <140)	No difference in primary cardiovascular composite outcome.	Achieved SBP in intensive group of 119 and in standard group 134. More adverse events in intensive group.
SPRINT	Nondiabetic patients with SBP >130 and at increased cardiovascular risk	9631	Intensive therapy (goal SBP <120) or standard therapy (goal SBP <140)	Significant reduction of primary cardiovascular composite in the intensive compared to standard group.	Achieved SBP in intensive group of 121 and in standard group 136. More adverse events in intensive group. The intensive group required, on average, 3 BP medications.

ACCORD-BP, Action to Control Cardiovascular Risk in Diabetes-Blood Pressure; BP, blood pressure; N, number; SBP, systolic blood pressure; SPRINT, Systolic Blood Pressure Intervention Trial; T2DM, type 2 diabetes mellitus; UKPDS 38, UK Prospective Diabetes Study Substudy 38.

4. **What is the evidence for BP goals in patients with T1DM?**
No large randomized trials have specifically studied BP targets for CVD risk reduction in T1DM. The strong association between achieved BP and micro- and macrovascular events observed in T2DM is also true for T1DM. Guidelines mostly extrapolate from ACCORD-BP and SPRINT, and the ADA 2017 guidelines recommend a target SBP less than 140 mm Hg in T1DM. Similar to tight glycemic control, which is better tolerated in young patients, the ADA recommends considering lower individualized BP targets for young patients with T1DM as they may derive the most benefit.

5. **How is hypertension treated in patients with diabetes?**
Nonpharmacologic lifestyle interventions including weight loss; physical activity (at least 30–45 minutes of brisk walking on most days of the week); sodium reduction (<100 mmol, or 2.3 g); a diet rich in fruits, vegetables, and low-fat dairy; smoking cessation; and avoidance of excessive alcohol intake are all recommended to lower BP. Over-the-counter nonsteroidal antiinflammatory agents (NSAIDs) should be avoided or used with caution because they can raise BP and adversely affect renal function.

Based on the data presented, most patients with diabetes will need at least two antihypertensive drugs to achieve the recommended goal SBP of less than 140 mm Hg, especially if the initial SBP is greater than 160 mm Hg. Long-term follow-up of UKPDS showed that the "glycemic memory" phenomenon (sustained benefits from initial intense glycemic control regardless of follow-up HbA1c levels) observed in the Diabetes Control and Complications Trial (DCCT)/Epidemiology of Diabetes Interventions and Complications (EDIC) trials in T1DM does not apply to BP, and BP control with antihypertensive medications needs to be continued to maintain cardiovascular benefits. The Antihypertensive and Lipid-Lowering Treatment to Prevent Heart Attack Trial (ALLHAT) tested the efficacy of first-line antihypertensive agents (chlorthalidone, amlodipine, lisinopril) in preventing CVD. About one third of the ALLHAT study population had diabetes. There were no differences in the primary cardiovascular outcome or all-cause mortality between subjects randomized to any of the three antihypertensive agents. Thus any first-line agent can lower BP effectively, and a combination of two or three first-line agents of different classes may be needed to achieve the BP goal. Supportive cardiovascular outcome data for a combination of antihypertensives in patients with T2DM comes from The Action in Diabetes and Vascular disease: Preterax and Diamicron-MR Controlled Evaluation-BP (ADVANCE-BP) and the diabetic subpopulation of the Avoiding Cardiovascular Events through Combination Therapy in Patients Living with Systolic Hypertension (ACCOMPLISH) trial, both of which demonstrated the efficacy in reducing cardiovascular events of a fixed angiotensin-converting enzyme (ACE) inhibitor, calcium channel blocker or ACE inhibitor, thiazide diuretic combination, respectively. Whereas most antihypertensive classes (mainly ACE inhibitors, angiotensin receptor blockers (ARBs), thiazide-like diuretics, and dihydropyridine calcium channel blockers) can be effective alone or in combination in lowering BP, comorbidities play a major role when choosing drug therapy. Diabetes commonly leads to kidney disease and renin-angiotensin-aldosterone system (RAAS) inhibitor use at maximum tolerated dose is recommended as first-line treatment for hypertension in the presence of any kidney disease, including microalbuminuria, macroalbuminuria, and decreased estimated glomerular filtration rate (eGFR). Some studies even support their use in the normoalbuminuric patient with diabetes and preserved eGFR. RAAS inhibitors hereafter refer to ACE inhibitors or ARBs.

6. **How does diabetes cause diabetic nephropathy?**
Diabetes leads to kidney disease in ~40% of patients with diabetes and is the most common cause of end-stage renal disease (ESRD) in the world. Approximately 80% of patients with diabetes and kidney disease will have hypertension. The cause of kidney disease in diabetes is multifactorial including hyperglycemia-induced diffuse endothelial cell damage, increased inflammation, the accumulation of advanced glycosylation end products, dyslipidemia, and increases in reactive oxygen species. There are changes in multiple circulating factors including angiotensin II, insulin-like growth factor, atrial natriuretic factor, growth hormone, connective tissue growth factor, and transforming growth factor beta (TGF-β). These changes lead to increased glomerular pressures (intraglomerular hypertension), glomerular hyperfiltration, and altered glomerular composition with increased matrix production and alterations in the glomerular basement membrane. Clinical manifestations are renal hypertrophy and albuminuria. This microvascular injury further triggers RAAS activation and hypertension, which, in turn, further exacerbate the renal injury leading to a vicious cycle. RAAS activation and angiotensin II play a key role in the pathogenesis of diabetic kidney disease with angiotensin II increasing intraglomerular pressure and causing podocyte damage. Elegant microperfusion studies and large clinical trials demonstrated that RAAS inhibition is a crucial intervention for renoprotection and lowering blood pressure in patients with diabetes and kidney disease. The recommendation for these patients is to first treat hypertension with a RAAS inhibitor.

7. **What is the evidence for efficacy of RAAS inhibition in diabetic nephropathy?**
RAAS inhibition has been demonstrated in multiple clinical trials to be an effective intervention to lower BP and to slow the progression of kidney disease in patients with diabetic nephropathy, hypertensive nephrosclerosis, and other glomerular diseases. RAAS inhibition has been tested in multiple stages of diabetic nephropathy as well as before disease onset. The Bergamo Nephrologic Diabetes Complications Trial (BENEDICT) conducted in individuals with T2DM and hypertension, normal renal function, and normoalbuminuria demonstrated that the ACE inhibitor trandolapril decreased the incidence of microalbuminuria compared to placebo or a calcium channel blocker and this effect was independent of BP. The Randomized Olmesartan and Diabetes Microalbuminuria Prevention (ROADMAP) study followed 4449 patients with T2DM, normal renal function, and normoalbuminuria randomized to the ARB olmesartan (at a maximum dose of 40 mg daily) or placebo with the primary outcome time to first onset of microalbuminuria. The trial found a 23% increase in the time to microalbuminuria onset with olmesartan. The achieved BPs were lower in the olmesartan group compared to placebo. The Irbesartan in Patients with Type 2 Diabetes and Microalbuminuria Study (IRMA 2) showed that irbesartan (in a dose-dependent fashion) reduced the risk of overt proteinuria in patients with microalbuminuric hypertensive T2DM. The first clinical trial to demonstrate

the efficacy of RAAS inhibition in slowing the rate of decline of renal function was done in patients with T1DM and overt proteinuria (>500 mg/day), and randomization to the ACE inhibitor captopril demonstrated a 48% reduction in the risk for doubling of serum creatinine concentration and a 50% reduction in the composite endpoint of death, dialysis, or transplantation compared to placebo. The irbesartan diabetic nephropathy (IDNT) trial randomized patients with T2DM, hypertension, and proteinuria to one of three groups: the ARB irbesartan, amlodipine, or placebo. IDNT demonstrated a statistically significant reduction in the primary composite outcome of doubling of serum creatinine, ESRD, or death in the irbesartan group compared to placebo and to the amlodipine group after a mean follow-up duration of only 2.6 years. There was identically achieved BP control in the subjects randomized to either amlodipine or irbesartan, demonstrating the benefit of RAAS inhibition was independent of lowering BP. Similarly, the Reduction of Endpoints in NIDDM with the Angiotensin II Antagonist Losartan (RENAAL) study showed that, in patients with T2DM (96.5% also had hypertension) and proteinuria, the ARB losartan significantly reduced the same primary composite by 16%. At the end of the study there was a small but significant BP difference (SBP 140 mm Hg vs. 142 mm Hg in the losartan and the placebo group, respectively) but the losartan benefit was independent of BP reduction. Together the trials show that the renoprotection of RAAS-blocking agents in T2DM with hypertension is likely a class effect that is independent of BP reduction. It is important to note that in both trials the ARB dose for maximum renoprotection was the maximum dose of 300 mg daily for irbesartan and 100 mg daily for losartan.

Taken together, the evidence supports the use of ACE inhibitors and ARBs across the continuum of diabetic nephropathy. Other RAAS-blocking agents, including aldosterone receptor antagonists (such as spironolactone) and renin inhibitors (aliskiren), have been shown to reduce albuminuria and thus likely have renal benefits beyond BP reduction, but, unlike ACE inhibitors or ARBs, they have not been demonstrated to preserve renal function. Table 18.3 summarizes major RAAS inhibitor trials on diabetes and kidney disease.

8. **Do all patients with diabetes and chronic kidney disease have diabetic nephropathy?**
In classically observed diabetic nephropathy, patients progress over years from microalbuminuria to frank proteinuria to declining GFR and, if not censored by cardiovascular death, to ESRD. Prospective renal biopsy studies in these patients reveal diabetic nephropathy often with hypertensive nephrosclerosis. However, a subset of about 25% of patients with diabetes and decreased GFR who have little or no albuminuria have been described. It is not clear if they have an altered form of diabetic nephropathy or a different mechanism of disease because biopsy studies have not been done in these patients. They are described as having diabetic kidney disease in contrast to diabetic nephropathy. As discussed previously, RAAS inhibition has been shown to slow the progression of diabetic nephropathy in all stages. RAAS inhibitors have been shown to be beneficial in many other renal diseases including chronic kidney disease due to hypertensive nephrosclerosis in Blacks. Although not studied, it is thus prudent to treat diabetic kidney disease first line with RAAS inhibitors as well. As even in normoalbuminuric patients with diabetes RAAS inhibitors prevent the development of microalbuminuria, one might consider RAAS inhibitors as first line in all diabetic patients with hypertension. Of note, 25% of patients randomized to captopril in the captopril trial described earlier were not hypertensive but nevertheless had a slower rate of decline of renal function, indicating that RAAS inhibition may also be a good option for diabetic patients even in the absence of hypertension.

9. **How does one manage the side effects of RAAS inhibitors?**
Because RAAS inhibition is proven to be beneficial in diabetes, efforts to continue these medications long term must be continuously reassessed, especially by adjusting treatment in response to side effects. A common side effect of ACE inhibitors is nonproductive cough in 15% of patients, which is more common in Asians. This is likely due to bradykinin accumulation in the pulmonary vasculature as a consequence of local ACE inhibition. In agreement with this mechanism, patients can safely be switched to ARBs, which specifically do not lead to bradykinin accumulation in the lung. ACE inhibitors and ARBs are contraindicated during pregnancy because of their teratogenic effects, including cardiovascular and central nervous system malformations, and their negative effect on fetal renal hemodynamics to cause anuria, oligohydramnios, and renal failure after delivery.

Other side effects of RAAS inhibition are hyperkalemia and transient deterioration of kidney function. Hyperkalemia is the result of decreased angiotensin II generation resulting in aldosterone inhibition and impaired renal potassium excretion. The renoprotective effect of decreased angiotensin II–dependent efferent arteriolar resistance resulting in lower intraglomerular pressure can be detrimental in situations in which the kidney is depending on increased efferent arteriole constriction to maintain glomerular perfusion such as in renal artery stenosis and decreased intravascular volume. In the setting of volume depletion and decreased renal perfusion, the decreased GFR and decreased distal sodium delivery for exchange with potassium may further exacerbate hyperkalemia. Elderly patients with T2DM with low renal function at baseline, significant vascular disease, or patients on NSAIDs (that reduce glomerular perfusion by abolishing prostaglandin-mediated afferent arteriolar vasodilation) are especially at risk for these side effects. A creatinine increase greater than 30% above baseline within 6 weeks of initiating RAAS inhibition or hyperkalemia that cannot be controlled warrants discontinuation of RAAS inhibition. It is prudent to check serum potassium and creatinine levels within 10 to 14 days of starting RAAS inhibitors. If no other cause for a greater than 30% serum creatinine increase, such as volume depletion,

Table 18.3 Summarizing Select Pivotal RAAS Inhibitor Trials

TRIAL	POPULATION	N	INTERVENTION	CONCLUSION	COMMENTS
BENEDICT	Hypertensive patients with T2DM and without microalbuminuria	1204	Trandolapril plus verapamil vs. each alone vs. placebo	Trandolapril significantly delayed the onset of microalbuminuria by a factor of 2.1	
ROADMAP	T2DM patients without microalbuminuria	4449	Olmesartan vs. placebo	Significant delay in onset of microalbuminuria with olmesartan	The olmesartan group achieved a lower BP compared to placebo
IRMA 2	Hypertensive T2DM patients with microalbuminuria	590	Irbesartan 150 mg vs. irbesartan 300 mg vs. placebo	Irbesartan significantly decreased the time to onset of overt proteinuria	Likely dose-dependent effect
Captopril trial	T1DM patients with proteinuria >500 mg/day and sCr ≤ 2.5 mg/dL 1.0–3.0 (men) and 1.2–3.0 mg/dL (women)	409	Captopril vs. placebo	Captopril significantly reduced the primary outcome (doubling of sCr) and secondary outcome (death, dialysis, transplant)	76% had hypertension at baseline
IDNT	Hypertensive T2DM patients with proteinuria and reduced kidney function (sCr 1.2–3.0 for men and 1.0–3.0 mg/dL for women)	1715	Irbesartan vs. amlodipine vs. placebo	Irbesartan significantly reduced the primary composite outcome of doubling of sCr, ESRD, or death	
RENAAL	T2DM patients with proteinuria and reduced kidney function (sCr 1.3–3.0 and 1.5–3.0 for men >60 kg BW)	1513	Losartan vs. placebo	Losartan significantly reduced the primary composite outcome of doubling of serum creatinine, ESRD or death	96.5% had hypertension at baseline

BENEDICT, Bergamo Nephrologic Diabetes Complications Trial; *BW,* body weight; *ESRD,* end-stage renal disease; *IDNT,* Irbesartan Diabetic Nephropathy Trial; *IRMA 2,* IRbesartan in MicroAlbuminuria, Type 2 Diabetic Nephropathy Trial; *RAAS,* renin-angiotensin-aldosterone system; *RENAAL,* Reduction of Endpoints in NIDDM with the Angiotensin Antagonist Losartan; *ROADMAP,* Randomized Olmesartan and Diabetes Microalbuminuria Prevention; *sCr,* serum creatinine; *T1DM,* type 1 diabetes mellitus; *T2DM,* type 2 diabetes mellitus.

is found, evaluation for renal artery stenosis should be considered. Maintaining background RAAS inhibition at an optimal dose is key for maximum renal protection in hypertensive patients with diabetes and kidney disease, but opportunities are often limited due to hyperkalemia. Education on a low potassium diet is important and can address this problem. Also, with the availability of new safe daily oral potassium binders (patiromer, sodium zirconium cyclosilicate ZS-1) it may be possible to combine their use with ACE inhibitor/ARB therapy and reduce discontinuations due to hyperkalemia.

Angioedema is a rare but serious complication of ACE inhibitors, most often manifest as swelling of the lips or tongue, leading to airway obstruction in severe cases. This event occurs more often in Blacks, women, smokers, and nondiabetic patients. ACE inhibitors should be discontinued in patients with suspected ACE inhibitor associated angioedema, and this should be clearly documented in the allergy list to deter future prescription. Alternative treatment with an ARB may be initiated after a sufficient washout period of 2 to 3 months.

10. **As most patients will require more than one antihypertensive drug, is dual RAAS blockade (ACE inhibitor + ARB) a good option?**
Combining an ACE inhibitor with an ARB leads to modest additional SBP lowering of 2 to 4 mm Hg, but there are other adverse consequences. The Ongoing Telmisartan Alone and in Combination with Ramipril Global Endpoint Trial randomized 25,620 patients with CVD of which 9612 and 2781 had diabetes and microalbuminuria,

respectively, to ramipril, telmisartan, or the combination of both. Two thirds had a diagnosis of hypertension at baseline. The primary outcome was a cardiovascular composite, and there were no differences in the primary outcome between the groups despite greater BP reduction in the combination group. Although the combination group had lower proteinuria, it showed higher rates of hyperkalemia, renal impairment, need for dialysis, hypotension, syncope, and medication discontinuation rates due to poor tolerability. The VA-Nephron D trial specifically tested the safety and efficacy of a losartan-lisinopril combination in patients with T2DM with diabetic nephropathy (albuminuria of at least 300 mg/g creatinine). Due to safety concerns and the increased risk of hyperkalemia and acute kidney injury in the combination group, the trial was stopped early. Similarly, the ALTITUDE study failed to demonstrate a benefit when adding the direct renin inhibitor aliskiren to either an ACE inhibitor or an ARB in patients with diabetic nephropathy but showed increased adverse events largely due to increased stroke risk with the combination and was terminated early as well. In summary, there is likely no net benefit in dual RAAS blockade, and, given the increased risk of adverse events such as hyperkalemia and acute kidney injury, it is not generally recommended.

11. **What is the role of SGLT2 inhibitors in treating hypertension in patients with T2DM?**
Despite the demonstrated renoprotection of ARB therapy, many patients on RAAS blockade still ultimately progress to ESRD. Another pathologic mechanism in the diabetic nephron besides RAAS activation is SGLT2 upregulation. This luminal proximal tubular glucose-sodium cotransporter (SGLT2) is upregulated in the diabetic kidney in response to the hyperglycemic state with the aim of increasing the renal resorptive capacity and glucosuria threshold. This results in decreased sodium delivery to the macula densa and impaired tubuloglomerular feedback. The glomerular afferent arteriole remains vasodilated, promoting glomerular hyperperfusion, hyperfiltration, and hypertension. SGLT2 inhibitors (canagliflozin, empagliflozin, and dapagliflozin) were developed as antidiabetic drugs; however, in addition to causing glucosuria and lowering the HbA1c, they induce weight loss, are mildly diuretic, and cause a 3- to 4-mm Hg reduction in SBP. Cardiovascular safety trials were conducted with these glucose-lowering agents. The Empagliflozin, Cardiovascular Outcomes, and Mortality in Type 2 Diabetes trial (EMPA-Reg Outcome) demonstrated a significant reduction in major adverse cardiovascular events (nonfatal MI, stroke, or cardiovascular death) in patients with T2DM at increased cardiovascular risk ($>$90% on antihypertensive therapy) randomized to empagliflozin. SGLT2 inhibition was associated with a marked reduction in heart failure hospitalizations. Although not designed as a renal outcome trial, a prespecified renal outcome of incident nephropathy (worsening albuminuria, serum creatinine doubling, renal replacement therapy, renal death) was significantly lower with empagliflozin. The majority of patients ($>$80%) were already on RAAS blockade and had an eGFR greater than 60 mL/min/1.73 m^2 ($>$50%). Similarly, the Canagliflozin Cardiovascular Assessment Study (CANVAS), also a cardiovascular outcome trial, demonstrated significant cardiovascular benefits with canagliflozin. Secondary renal outcomes (40% reduction in composite of 40% eGFR reduction, renal replacement therapy, or renal death) were also lower with canagliflozin. These trials establish SGLT2 inhibitors as attractive add-on therapy for lowering blood sugar, BP, and reducing cardiovascular risk in patients with T2DM with hypertension who are at increased cardiovascular risk.

12. **Should SGLT2 inhibitors be used in hypertensive patients with T2DM with diabetic nephropathy?**
Kidney disease is a major comorbidity in hypertensive patients with T2DM, and the primary outcome in the EMPA-Reg and CANVAS trials was cardiovascular, which leaves the primary effect of SGLT2 inhibition on renal progression in these settings unanswered. Furthermore, the overall renal event rate and levels of proteinuria were low in these trials, thus capturing a lower renal risk population. The CREDENCE trial was a large randomized placebo-controlled trial using canagliflozin 100 mg daily on top the of maximum tolerated RAAS blockade in patients with T2DM with significant diabetic kidney disease (GFR of 30-90 mL/min/1.73m^2; mean eGFR 56 mL/min/1.73 m^2, and median albuminuria of 927 mg/g creatinine) and a primary renal composite of ESRD (dialysis, transplant, eGFR $<$15 mL/min/1.73 m^2), serum creatinine doubling, and renal or cardiovascular death. The prespecified efficacy criteria for early cessation of the trial were achieved with a reduction of the primary outcome in the canagliflozin group by 30% compared to placebo. Canagliflozin reduced SBP on average by 3.3 mm Hg compared to placebo, but the renoprotection was independent of the BP-lowering effect. This was the first renal-specific primary outcome trial for SGLT2 inhibition. In summary, SGLT2 inhibition (e.g., with canagliflozin 100 mg daily), in addition to reducing cardiovascular events in hypertensive patients with T2DM, also can be used as a renoprotective agent on top of RAAS blockade in those with significant diabetic kidney disease (eGFR as low as 30 mL/min/1.73 m^2 and albuminuria $>$300 mg/g). Given their established cardiovascular and renal protection, one may consider adding SGLT2 inhibitors as a second-line agent on top of RAAS blockade in all hypertensive patients with diabetes.

13. **What is the side effect profile of SGLT2 inhibitors?**
Likely due to increased glucosuria, SGLT2 inhibition is associated with more frequent genital mycotic infections (candida vaginitis in women and balanitis in men). However, most infections are mild and resolve with topical antifungals. The CREDENCE study did not find a difference in hyperkalemia and acute kidney injury risk between canagliflozin and placebo. A recent metaanalysis found a significant beneficial effect of SGLT2 inhibitors in

decreasing acute renal failure episodes. SGLT2 inhibitor use was not associated with increased hypoglycemic episodes. The CANVAS Program reported an increased amputation and fracture risk with canagliflozin in patients with known risk factors such as peripheral vascular disease or previous amputations, but this was not confirmed in CREDENCE or seen with SGLT2 inhibitors other than canagliflozin. Until more data emerges, the amputation risk remains controversial, but, generally, in the presence of risk factors (history of amputations, active foot ulcer) of SGLT2 inhibition, the risks versus the benefits of canagliflozin should be weighed.

KEY POINTS

1. There are conflicting guideline-based recommendations on BP targets in patients with diabetes, but currently the best available evidence supports an individualized approach with an SBP goal of at least 140 mm Hg or less.
2. First-line antihypertensive agents (thiazide, calcium channel blocker, ACE inhibitor, or ARB) are effective at reducing BP and reducing cardiovascular events in patients with T2DM.
3. Most patients will need a combination of two to three agents of different classes to reach goal BP.
4. Kidney disease (with or without albuminuria) is common in diabetic patients with hypertension, and RAAS activation is a key pathomechanism.
5. Given their effectiveness at preventing and delaying the progression of kidney disease in diabetes, RAAS inhibitors are preferred first-line treatment of hypertension in diabetes and also may be considered in the absence of hypertension.
6. In hypertensive patients with T2DM, SGLT2 inhibitors (canagliflozin, empagliflozin) are effective at reducing the cardiovascular risk and protecting the kidney in addition to inhibiting RAAS in those with significant kidney disease and may thus be considered second line after RAAS inhibitors in this setting.

BIBLIOGRAPHY

Brenner BM, Cooper ME, de Zeeuw D, et al. Effects of losartan on renal and cardiovascular outcomes in patients with type 2 diabetes and nephropathy. *N Engl J Med.* 2001;345(12):861–869.

Carey RM, Siragy HM. The intrarenal renin-angiotensin system and diabetic nephropathy. *Trends Endocrinol Metab.* 2003;14(6):274–281.

Climie RE, van Sloten TT, Bruno RM, et al. Macrovasculature and microvasculature at the crossroads between type 2 diabetes mellitus and hypertension. *Hypertension.* 2019;73(6):1138–1149.

de Boer IH, Bangalore S, Benetos A, et al. Diabetes and hypertension: a position statement by the American Diabetes Association. *Diabetes Care.* 2017;40(9):1273–1284.

Dwyer JP, Lewis JB. Nonproteinuric diabetic nephropathy: when diabetics don't read the textbook. *Med Clin North Am.* 2013;97(1):53–58.

Dwyer JP, Parving HH, Hunsicker LG, Ravid M, Remuzzi G, Lewis JB. Renal dysfunction in the presence of normoalbuminuria in type 2 diabetes: results from the DEMAND study. *Cardiorenal Med.* 2012;2(1):1–10.

Evans M, Palaka E, Furuland H, et al. The value of maintaining normokalaemia and enabling RAASi therapy in chronic kidney disease. *BMC Nephrol.* 2019;20(1):31.

Fried LF, Emanuele N, Zhang JH, et al. Combined angiotensin inhibition for the treatment of diabetic nephropathy. *N Engl J Med.* 2013;369(20):1892–1903.

Georgianos PI, Agarwal R. Revisiting RAAS blockade in CKD with newer potassium-binding drugs. *Kidney Int.* 2018;93(2):325–334.

Group AS, Cushman WC, Evans GW, et al. Effects of intensive blood-pressure control in type 2 diabetes mellitus. *N Engl J Med.* 2010;362(17):1575–1585.

Group SR, Wright Jr JT, Williamson JD, et al. A randomized trial of intensive versus standard blood-pressure control. *N Engl J Med.* 2015;373(22):2103–2116.

Haller H, Ito S, Izzo Jr JL, et al. Olmesartan for the delay or prevention of microalbuminuria in type 2 diabetes. *N Engl J Med.* 2011;364(10):907–917.

Heerspink HJL, Kosiborod M, Inzucchi SE, Cherney D.Z.I. Renoprotective effects of sodium-glucose cotransporter-2 inhibitors. *Kidney Int.* 2018;94(1):26–39.

Holman RR, Paul SK, Bethel MA, Neil HA, Matthews DR. Long-term follow-up after tight control of blood pressure in type 2 diabetes. *N Engl J Med.* 2008;359(15):1565–1576.

Investigators O, Yusuf S, Teo KK, et al. Telmisartan, ramipril, or both in patients at high risk for vascular events. *N Engl J Med.* 2008;358(15):1547–1559.

James PA, Oparil S, Carter BL, et al. 2014 evidence-based guideline for the management of high blood pressure in adults: report from the panel members appointed to the Eighth Joint National Committee (JNC 8). *JAMA.* 2014;311(5):507–520.

Lewis EJ, Hunsicker LG, Clarke WR, et al. Renoprotective effect of the angiotensin-receptor antagonist irbesartan in patients with nephropathy due to type 2 diabetes. *N Engl J Med.* 2001;345(12):851–860.

Maahs DM, Kinney GL, Wadwa P, et al. Hypertension prevalence, awareness, treatment, and control in an adult type 1 diabetes population and a comparable general population. *Diabetes Care.* 2005;28(2):301–306.

Menne J, Dumann E, Haller H, Schmidt BMW. Acute kidney injury and adverse renal events in patients receiving SGLT2-inhibitors: a systematic review and meta-analysis. *PLoS Med.* 2019;16(12):e1002983.

Neal B, Perkovic V, Mahaffey KW, et al. Canagliflozin and cardiovascular and renal events in type 2 diabetes. *N Engl J Med.* 2017;377(7):644–657.

Officers A. Coordinators for the ACRGTA, Lipid-Lowering Treatment to Prevent Heart Attack T. Major outcomes in high-risk hypertensive patients randomized to angiotensin-converting enzyme inhibitor or calcium channel blocker vs diuretic: The Antihypertensive and Lipid-Lowering Treatment to Prevent Heart Attack Trial (ALLHAT). *JAMA.* 2002;288(23):2981–2997.

Parving HH, Brenner BM, McMurray JJ, et al. Cardiorenal end points in a trial of aliskiren for type 2 diabetes. *N Engl J Med*. 2012;367(23):2204–2213.

Parving HH, Lehnert H, Brochner-Mortensen J, et al. The effect of irbesartan on the development of diabetic nephropathy in patients with type 2 diabetes. *N Engl J Med*. 2001;345(12):870–878.

Perkovic V, Jardine MJ, Neal B, et al. Canagliflozin and renal outcomes in type 2 diabetes and nephropathy. *N Engl J Med*. 2019;380(24):2295–2306.

Petrie JR, Guzik TJ, Touyz RM. Diabetes, hypertension, and cardiovascular disease: clinical insights and vascular mechanisms. *Can J Cardiol*. 2018;34(5):575–584.

Raebel MA. Hyperkalemia associated with use of angiotensin-converting enzyme inhibitors and angiotensin receptor blockers. *Cardiovasc Ther*. 2012;30(3):e156–166.

Ruggenenti P, Cravedi P, Remuzzi G. The RAAS in the pathogenesis and treatment of diabetic nephropathy. *Nat Rev Nephrol*. 2010;6(6):319–330.

Ruggenenti P, Fassi A, Ilieva AP, et al. Preventing microalbuminuria in type 2 diabetes. *N Engl J Med*. 2004;351(19):1941–1951.

Shen JI, Nicholas SB, Williams S, Norris KC. Evidence for and against ACC/AHA 2017 guideline for target systolic blood pressure of <130 mmHg in persons with type 2 diabetes. *Curr Cardiol Rep*. 2019;21(11):149.

UK Prospective Diabetes Study Group. Tight blood pressure control and risk of macrovascular and microvascular complications in type 2 diabetes: UKPDS 38. UK Prospective Diabetes Study Group. *BMJ*. 1998;317(7160):703–713.

Umanath K, Lewis JB. Update on diabetic nephropathy: core curriculum 2018. *Am J Kidney Dis*. 2018;71(6):884–895.

Wanner C, Inzucchi SE, Lachin JM, et al. Empagliflozin and progression of kidney disease in type 2 diabetes. *N Engl J Med*. 2016;375(4):323–334.

Weber MA, Bakris GL, Jamerson K, et al. Cardiovascular events during differing hypertension therapies in patients with diabetes. *J Am Coll Cardiol*. 2010;56(1):77–85.

Whelton PK, Carey RM, Aronow WS, et al. 2017 ACC/AHA/AAPA/ABC/ACPM/AGS/APhA/ASH/ASPC/NMA/PCNA Guideline for the prevention, detection, evaluation, and management of high blood pressure in adults: executive summary: a report of the American College of Cardiology/American Heart Association task force on clinical practice guidelines. *Hypertension*. 2018;71(6):1269–1324.

Wright Jr JT, Bakris G, Greene T, et al. Effect of blood pressure lowering and antihypertensive drug class on progression of hypertensive kidney disease: results from the AASK trial. *JAMA*. 2002;288(19):2421–2431.

Zinman B, Wanner C, Lachin JM, et al. Empagliflozin, cardiovascular outcomes, and mortality in type 2 diabetes. *N Engl J Med*. 2015;373(22):2117–2128.

Zoungas S, Chalmers J, Neal B, et al. Follow-up of blood-pressure lowering and glucose control in type 2 diabetes. *N Engl J Med*. 2014;371(15):1392–1406.

CHAPTER 19

HYPERTENSION AFTER TRANSPLANTATION

Saed Shawar, MD, and Beatrice P. Concepcion, MBBS

QUESTIONS

1. **What is the definition of hypertension in transplant recipients?**
   The definition of hypertension in transplant recipients follows that of the general population. Most guidelines for the general population define hypertension as a persistent systolic blood pressure on two separate days of 140 mm Hg or higher and/or diastolic blood pressure of 90 mm Hg or higher if age is 18 years or older. More recent hypertension guidelines have established a definition of 130/85 mm Hg, but the applicability to transplant patients is unclear.

2. **What is the incidence and prevalence of hypertension after transplantation?**
   The reported incidence of hypertension varies among different solid organ transplants. In kidney transplant recipients, it ranges from 50% to 80% in adult recipients and from 47% to 82% in pediatric recipients. According to the International Society of Heart and Lung Transplantation registry, among heart transplant survivors with a 10-year follow-up between April 1994 and June 2006, hypertension was present in 98% of patients. In liver transplant recipients, the range has been reported to be from 50% to almost 100% in some series.

3. **What is the clinical importance of hypertension in kidney transplant recipients?**
   Hypertension in kidney transplant recipients is associated with an increased risk of cardiovascular death (CVD), increased risk of allograft failure and mortality, and increased risk of hospitalization.
   - *Increased risk of cardiovascular disease*
     - Hypertension is a traditional risk factor for CVD, which is the leading cause of death in patients with a functional kidney transplant. The annual rate of fatal or nonfatal CVD events is 3.5% to 5.0% in kidney transplant recipients, 50-fold higher than in the general population. Uncontrolled systolic and diastolic blood pressures are associated with worsening left ventricular hypertrophy at 5 years posttransplant, which is also associated with increased CVD.
     - In addition, it has been reported that for every 20-mm Hg increase in systolic blood pressure, there is an associated 32% increase in the risk for cardiovascular events. Of note, each 10-mm Hg decrease in diastolic blood pressure below the 70-mm Hg level was found to be associated with a 31% increase in cardiovascular risk, but no such association emerged for diastolic blood pressure levels less than 70 mm Hg.
   - *Increased risk of allograft failure and mortality*
     - Hypertension is a potent nonimmunological risk factor and is independently associated with an increased risk of both allograft failure and mortality. The Collaborative Transplant Study, a large cohort study of nearly 30,000 kidney transplant recipients showed a graded association between both systolic and diastolic blood pressure and allograft failure. Moreover, increasing systolic pressure was associated with decreased graft survival at any level of diastolic blood pressure. In addition to decreased allograft survival, hypertension after transplant was associated with decreased patient survival. Each 10-mm Hg increase in systolic blood pressure above 140 mm Hg was associated with a hazard ratio (HR) of death of 1.18 (95% confidence interval [CI], 1.12–1.23). This risk persisted after adjusting for allograft function.
   - *Increased risk of hospitalization*
     - Among kidney transplant recipients, hypertension is the second most common cause of cardiovascular-related hospitalization in the first year after transplantation, accounting for approximately 13% of admissions after heart failure. It is the fourth leading cause of hospitalization (approximately 7%) in the second year after transplantation.

4. **What is the pathogenesis of hypertension after kidney transplantation?**
   The pathogenesis of hypertension after kidney transplantation is related to several factors which are discussed below and are summarized in Fig. 19.1.
   - *Endothelial dysfunction*
     Endothelial dysfunction is associated with hypertension, and it predicts atherosclerosis progression and cardiovascular events in the general population. This is related to one or more of the following factors:
     - The imbalance between vasoconstrictive molecules (endothelin, thromboxane, and prostaglandins) and vasodilatory nitric oxide. This can be caused by calcineurin inhibitors (CNIs).

Hypertension after transplantation				
Endothelial dysfunction	**Arterial stiffness**	**Renin-angiotensin-aldosterone system activation**	**Sympathetic nervous system activation**	**Sodium and water retention**
Injury due to rejection	Hypertensive	Ischemic native kidneys	Obesity	Reduced GFR
Calcineurin inhibitors	VSMC	Transplant renal artery	Obstructive	Calcineurin
↑ Vasoconstrictors:	hypertrophy	stenosis	sleep apnea	inhibitors
• Endothelin	Calcineurin	Calcineurin inhibitors	Calcineurin	RAAS
• Thromboxane	inhibitors	Obesity	inhibitors	activation
• Prostaglandins	Steroid	Obstructive sleep apnea		
↓ Vasodilators:	activation	Sympathetic stimulation		
• Nitric oxide	of vascular GR	Steroid activation of MR		

Fig. 19.1 **Hypertension after transplantation.** *GFR,* Glomerular filtration rate; *GR,* glucocorticoid receptor; *MR,* mineralocorticoid receptor; *RAAS,* renin-angiotensin-aldosterone system; *VSMC,* vascular smooth muscle cell.

- Increased generation of reactive oxygen species which can be seen in chronic inflammation, ischemia-reperfusion injury (which can manifest as delayed graft function after transplant), and increased angiotensin II (Ang II).
- Acute rejection episodes, whether T-cell or antibody-mediated, leading to endothelial injury. This can alter renal blood flow, impair kidney function, and increase the risk of fibrosis and loss of kidney function.

- *Arterial stiffness*
  Arterial stiffness is a manifestation of hypertension but may also represent a cause of hypertension. Some studies have shown that CNIs accelerate the arterial stiffness process, whereas belatacept-based regimens seem to offer better vascular protection compared with CNIs.
- *Renin-angiotensin-aldosterone system (RAAS) activation*
  Activation of the RAAS leads to the production of Ang II, and acting through angiotensin II type 1 (AT_1) receptors on cell membranes, leads to potent vasoconstriction of all blood vessels. It also causes the adrenal glands to release aldosterone, which increases reabsorption of salt and water, thereby leading to an increase in blood volume and elevated blood pressure. Increased activity of RAAS is seen in the presence of remaining ischemic native kidneys, transplant renal artery stenosis, increased sympathetic stimulation, and CNIs, among others.
- *Sodium and water retention*
  Sodium and water retention can be seen in those with low nephron mass and low glomerular filtration rate (GFR), due to the kidney's reduced capacity to excrete sodium. CNIs cause increased sodium reabsorption via the increased activity of the thiazide-sensitive sodium-chloride cotransporter (NCC) and Na-K-2Cl cotransporter (NKCC2). As mentioned previously, upregulation of RAAS increases Ang II, leading to stimulation of aldosterone release. This induces the upregulation of Na^+/K^+-ATPase and epithelial sodium channel (ENaC) in the distal convoluted tubule and collecting duct. Ang II also stimulates the production of arginine vasopressin (AVP), which also modulates NCC function.
- *Sympathetic nervous system activation*
  Increased sympathetic nervous system activity has been implicated in the initiation, maintenance, and progression of posttransplant hypertension. Several factors can increase the activity of the sympathetic nervous system such as conditions that increase Ang II, comorbidities such as obesity and obstructive sleep apnea, and drugs such as CNIs.

5. **What are the risk factors for hypertension after kidney transplantation?**
   Risk factors for hypertension after transplantation can be divided into recipient factors, transplant factors, and donor factors. These are summarized in Table 19.1.

6. **How do CNIs affect hypertension after transplantation?**
   Both cyclosporine and tacrolimus induce or exacerbate hypertension in transplant recipients. Cyclosporine has a more potent effect on hypertension than tacrolimus. Multiple mechanisms have been suggested, all of which cause potent vasoconstriction and systemic hypertension. These include the following:
   - Activation of the sympathetic nervous system
   - Upregulation of endothelin, mediated via an imbalance of Treg and Th17 cell
   - Increased thromboxane A2 production
   - Activation of the renal NCC (thiazide-sensitive cotransporter)
   - Decreased prostaglandin production
   - Decreased nitric oxide production

Table 19.1 Risk Factors for Hypertension after Transplantation

Recipient Factors
Older age
Black ethnicity
Male gender
Obesity
Smoking
Diabetes mellitus
Pretransplant chronic kidney disease
Presence of native kidneys
Pretransplant hypertension
Obstructive sleep apnea
Hypercalcemia
Transplant Factors
Volume overload
Delayed graft function
Acute rejection mainly with angiotensin II type 1 receptor agonist antibody
Poor allograft function for any reason
Immunosuppressive medications, in particular calcineurin inhibitors
Renal artery stenosis
Page kidney
Transplant obstruction: ureteral stenosis, lymphocele, large perinephric fluid collection
Hyperuricemia
Primary hyperaldosteronism
Donor Factors
Older age
Donor hypertension or a donor with a family history of hypertension
Baseline allograft vascular disease and fibrosis
Donor-recipient size discrepancy

7. How do steroids affect hypertension after transplantation?

   Corticosteroids are thought to mediate about 15% of hypertension after transplantation, with the effect highest in those with preexisting hypertension. Their hypertensive effect is dose-dependent and is particularly crucial in the early posttransplant period. Hypertension may be mediated in part by stimulation of mineralocorticoid receptors, promoting sodium and water retention. Glucocorticoid receptor activation in vascular smooth muscles may also promote increased vascular tone, increased responsiveness to vasoconstrictors, and decreased vasodilator production.

8. How does belatacept affect hypertension after transplantation?

   Belatacept-based immunosuppression is associated with a reduction of approximately 10 and 5 mm Hg in systolic and diastolic blood pressures, respectively, compared to CNI-based immunosuppression. In the Belatacept Evaluation of Nephroprotection and Efficacy as a First-line Immunosuppression Trial (BENEFIT), systolic and diastolic blood pressures were lower in kidney transplant recipients who received belatacept compared with those who received cyclosporine for immunosuppression even though both treatment groups had the same baseline level of blood pressure.

9. What is the goal of blood pressure after kidney transplantation?

   There are no randomized controlled trials (RCTs) to determine the optimal blood pressure in kidney transplant recipients. Expert recommendations include the following:
   - The Kidney Disease: Improving Global Outcomes (KDIGO) Guideline suggests a blood pressure of less than 130/80 mm Hg in kidney transplant recipients.

- The 2017 American College of Cardiology/American Heart Association Guideline suggests that blood pressure target should be similar to that of the general chronic kidney disease population, a blood pressure of less than 130/80 mm Hg.
- The European Best Practice Guidelines recommend a blood pressure goal of less than 125/75 mm Hg for proteinuric patients.

10. **What is the significance of low diastolic blood pressure on kidney transplant recipients?**
The FAVORIT trial showed that cardiovascular disease risk increased by 31% for each 10-mm Hg decrease in diastolic blood pressure less than 70 mm Hg. In the absence of aortic valve insufficiency, the pattern of high systolic blood pressure, low diastolic blood pressure, and increased pulse pressure is a marker of vascular stiffness.

11. **What approaches should be utilized for treatment of hypertension after kidney transplantation?**
- **Nonpharmacologic**
  - Avoid agents that can worsen hypertension, including nonsteroidal antiinflammatory drugs, decongestants, birth control pills, cocaine/amphetamine, and ergot-derived medicines.
  - Increase diet rich in vegetables, fruits, and whole grains such as the Dietary Approaches to Stop Hypertension (DASH) diet
  - Smoking cessation and limiting alcohol intake
  - Weight loss. Reduction in systolic blood pressure with a 10-kg weight loss is 5 to 10 mm Hg.
- **Pharmacologic**
  There are no RCTs that have investigated the optimal antihypertensive regimen in kidney transplant recipients. No single agent has been found to be more efficient than another. The choice of medications should be individualized and based on various comorbidities.

12. **How should calcium channel blockers be utilized in the treatment of hypertension after kidney transplantation?**
Dihydropyridine calcium channel blockers (CCBs) are considered first-line agents, particularly in the early transplant period. These agents counteract the vasoconstrictive effect of CNIs, possibly leading to improvements in GFR and graft survival.
- In a systematic review and metaanalysis by Pisano and colleagues, CCBs were found to decrease blood pressure, increase GFR, and reduce the risk for graft loss.
- A systematic review and metaanalysis by Cross and colleagues analyzed 60 RCTs with 3802 transplant patients. Twenty-nine trials compared CCBs with placebo or absence of treatment, 10 trials compared angiotensin-converting enzyme inhibitors (ACEIs) with a placebo or absence of treatment, and seven studies compared CCBs with ACEIs. The study found that CCBs improved GFR by a mean difference of +4.5 mL/min and reduced graft loss by 25%. The authors concluded that CCBs may be preferred as a first-line antihypertensive medication in adult kidney transplant recipients

  Nondihydropyridine CCBs such as verapamil and diltiazem are usually avoided due to their inhibition of cytochrome P450 which results in an increase in blood levels of CNIs and mTOR inhibitors. Alternatively, they may be useful in patients whose CNI levels remain subtherapeutic despite high doses of CNIs.

13. **How should diuretics be used in the treatment of hypertension after kidney transplantation?**
The use of loop and thiazide diuretics can help manage hypervolemia and hyperkalemia, which are seen frequently in transplant recipients. Moes and colleagues performed a randomized crossover trial comparing chlorthalidone with amlodipine in hypertensive kidney transplant recipients on tacrolimus immunosuppression. The study noted similar blood pressure control for chlorthalidone and amlodipine, with slightly lower estimated GFRs and less proteinuria with chlorthalidone and more lower extremity edema with amlodipine.

14. **How should ACEIs and Ang II receptor blockers be used in the treatment of hypertension after kidney transplantation?**
ACEIs and Ang II receptor blockers (ARBs) are usually avoided in the first 3 to 6 months after transplant due to concerns for worsening of anemia, hyperkalemia, and a possible decline in kidney function. In general, ACEIs and ARBs are usually used in kidney transplant recipients who have cardiovascular indications for RAAS inhibition, posttransplant erythrocytosis, or in patients with proteinuria. The KDIGO guideline has an ungraded recommendation of considering ACEIs or ARBs as first-line antihypertensive medications in transplant recipients with proteinuria. Although ACEIs and ARBs are effective in slowing the progression of chronic kidney disease in the nontransplant population, particularly those with proteinuria, there is no strong evidence that these medications confer a benefit on graft or patient survival in kidney transplant recipients.
- Ibrahim and colleagues conducted a double-blind, prospective randomized, placebo-controlled trial involving 155 patients comparing the effect of losartan versus placebo initiated within 3 months of transplantation and continued for 5 years. The study found no significant effect difference between the two groups on a composite outcome of doubling of the fraction of renal cortical volume occupied by interstitium from baseline to 5 years,

or end-stage renal disease (ESRD) from interstitial fibrosis/tubular atrophy. The study also found no significant effect of losartan on time to a composite of ESRD, death, or doubling of creatinine level.
- Knoll and colleagues conducted an RCT of ramipril versus placebo in kidney transplant recipients with proteinuria. The study enrolled 213 adult kidney transplant recipients who were at least 3 months from transplant with an estimated GFR of at least 20 mL/min/1.73m^2 and had proteinuria of at least 0.2 g/d. There was no significant difference between the ramipril and placebo groups in terms of the primary outcome, which was a composite of doubling of serum creatinine, ESRD, or death.
- Cheungpasitporn and colleagues performed a systematic review and metaanalysis of three RCTs and two cohort studies including 20,024 kidney transplant patients. This showed no significant reduction in the risk of allograft loss or mortality among kidney transplant recipients treated with ACEIs or ARBs.
- Hiremath and colleagues found similar results based on a systematic review and metaanalysis of eight RCTs with a total of 1502 participants. They found no significant difference in the risk of death in the group with renin-angiotensin system (RAS) blockade compared to the control group (risk ratio [RR], 0.96; 95% CI, 0.62–1.51), transplant failure (RR, 0.76; 95% CI, 0.49–1.18), or doubling of creatinine level (RR, 0.84; 95% CI, 0.51–1.39). There was a more than twofold greater risk of hyperkalemia with RAS blockade.

15. **Discuss the role of beta-blockers in the treatment of hypertension after kidney transplantation.**
- Beta-blockers are cardioprotective in patients with coronary artery disease and congestive heart failure, and so patients who are already on beta-blockers should continue to take them in the peritransplant period. Perioperative initiation of beta-blockers may be considered in kidney transplant candidates with established coronary artery disease or those who have two or more cardiovascular risk factors. However, caution must be taken in starting beta-blockers immediately prior to surgery as this has been associated with an increased risk of 30-day all-cause mortality and stroke in the nontransplant population.
- A retrospective study by Aftab and colleagues of 321 kidney transplant recipients followed for 10 years found that the use of beta-blockers was associated with reduced mortality (HR, 0.60; 95% CI, 0.36–0.98). This benefit was seen in all subgroups of patients with different comorbidities.

KEY POINTS

1. Hypertension in kidney transplant recipients is associated with an increased risk of CVD, increased risk of allograft failure and mortality, and increased risk of hospitalization.
2. Risk factors for hypertension after transplantation are due to a combination of recipient, transplant and donor factors.
3. Dihydropyridines CCBs are considered first-line agents, particularly in the early transplant period as they counteract the vasoconstrictive effect of CNIs.
4. ACEIs and ARBs are usually avoided in the first 3 to 6 months after transplant due to concerns for worsening anemia, hyperkalemia, and a possible decline in kidney function.

BIBLIOGRAPHY

Aftab W, Varadarajan P, Rasool S, Kore A, Pai RG. Beta and angiotensin blockades are associated with improved 10-year survival in renal transplant recipients. *J Am Heart Assoc.* 2013;2:e000091.

Aziz F, Clark D, Garg N, Mandelbrot D, Djamali A. Hypertension guidelines: how do they apply to kidney transplant recipients. *Transplant Rev.* 2018;32(4):225–233.

Brandes RP. Endothelial dysfunction and hypertension. *Hypertension.* 2014;64(5):924–928.

Calò LA, Ravarotto V, Simioni F, et al. Pathophysiology of post-transplant hypertension in kidney transplant: focus on calcineurin inhibitors induced oxidative stress and renal sodium retention and implications with RhoA/Rho kinase pathway. *Kidney Blood Press Res.* 2017;42:676–685.

Cardinal H, Dieude M, Hebert MJ. Endothelial dysfunction in kidney transplantation. *Front Immunol.* 2018;9:1130.

Carpenter M, John A, Weir M, et al. BP, cardiovascular disease, and death in the folic acid for vascular outcome reduction in transplantation trial. *J Am Soc Nephrol.* 2014;25(7):1554–1562.

Cheungpasitporn W, Thongprayoon C, Mao MA, Kittanamongkolchai W, Sathick IJ, Erickson SB. The effect of renin-angiotensin system inhibitors on kidney allograft survival: a systematic review and meta-analysis. *N Am J Med Sci.* 2016;8:291–296.

Cross N, Webster A, Masson P, O'Connell P, Craig J. Antihypertensive treatment for kidney transplant recipients. *Cochrane Database Syst Rev.* 2009;doi: 10.1002/14651858.cd003598.pub2.

Durlik M. Hypertension in solid organ transplant recipients. *Ann Transplant.* 2012;17(1):100–107.

European best practice guidelines for renal transplantation. Section IV: Long-term management of the transplant recipient. IV.5.2. Cardiovascular risks. Arterial hypertension. *Nephrol Dial Transplant.* 2002;17(Suppl 4):25.

Fisher J, Paton J. The sympathetic nervous system and blood pressure in humans: implications for hypertension. *J Hum Hypertens.* 2012;26:463–475.

Glicklich D, Lamba R, Pawar R. Hypertension in the kidney transplant recipient. *Cardiol in Rev.* 2017;25(3):102–109.

Heitzer T, Schlinzig T, Krohn K, et al. Endothelial dysfunction, oxidative stress, and risk of cardiovascular events in patients with coronary artery disease. *Circulation.* 2001;104:2673–2678.

Hiremath S, Fergusson DA, Fergusson N, Bennett A, Knoll GA. Renin angiotensin system blockade and long-term clinical outcomes in kidney transplant recipients: a meta-analysis of randomized controlled trials. *Am J Kidney Dis.* 2017;69:78–86.

Ibrahim HN, Jackson S, Connaire J, et al. Angiotensin II blockade in kidney transplant recipients. *J Am Soc Nephrol.* 2013;24:320.

Kidney Disease: Improving Global Outcomes (KDIGO) Transplant Work Group. KDIGO clinical practice guideline for the care of kidney transplant recipients. *Am J Transplant.* 2009;9(suppl 3):S1–S155.

Knoll GA, Blydt-Hansen TD, Campbell P, et al. Canadian Society of Transplantation and Canadian Society of Nephrology commentary on the 2009 KDIGO clinical practice guideline for the care of kidney transplant recipients. *Am J Kidney Dis.* 2010;56(2):219–246.

Knoll GA, Ferguson D, Chasse M, Herbert P, et al. Ramipril versus placebo in kidney transplant patients with proteinuria: a multicentre, double-blind, randomised controlled trial. *Lancet Diabetes Endocrinol.* 2016;4(4):318–326.

Kuźmiuk-Glembin I, Adrych D, Tylicki L, et al. Treatment of hypertension in renal transplant recipients in four independent cross-sectional analyses. *Kidney Blood Press Res.* 2018;43(1):45–54.

Lentine K, Costa SP, Weir MR, et al. Cardiac disease evaluation and management among kidney and liver transplantation candidates: a scientific statement from the American Heart Association and the American College of Cardiology Foundation. *J Am Coll Cardiol.* 2012;60(5):434–480.

Mangray M, Vella JP. Hypertension after kidney transplant. *Am J Kidney Dis.* 2011;57(2):331–341.

Masson P, Henderson L, Chapman J, Craig J, Webster A. Belatacept for kidney transplant recipients. *Cochrane Database Syst Rev.* 2014;doi: 10.1002/14651858.cd010699.pub2.

Melilli E, Manonelles A, Montero N, et al. Impact of immunosuppressive therapy on arterial stiffness in kidney transplantation: are all treatments the same?. *Clin Kidney J.* 2017;11(3):413–421.

Moes AD, Hesselink DA, van den Meiracker AH, Zietse R, Hoorn EJ. Chlorthalidone versus amlodipine for hypertension in kidney transplant recipients treated with tacrolimus: a randomized crossover trial. *Am J Kidney Dis.* 2017;69(6):796–804.

Opelz G, Dohler B. Improved long-term outcomes after renal transplantation associated with blood pressure control. *Am J Transplant.* 2005;5(11):2725–2731.

Opelz G, Wujciak T, Ritz E. for the Collaborative Transplant Study. Association of chronic kidney graft failure with recipient blood pressure. *Kidney Int.* 1998;53(1):217–222.

Pisano AB, Davide, Mallamaci F, et al. Comparative effectiveness of different anti-hypertensive agents in kidney transplantation: a systematic review and meta-analysis. Nephrol Dial Transplant 2020; 2019;35(5):878–887.

Rossi AP, Vella JP. Hypertension, living kidney donors, and transplantation: where are we today? *Adv Chron Kid Dis.* 2015;22(2):154–164. doi: 10.1053/j.ackd.2015.01.002.

Saran R, Robinson B, Abbott KC, et al. US Renal Data System 2019 Annual Data Report: epidemiology of kidney disease in the United States. *Am J Kidney Dis.* 2020;75(1)(suppl 1):Svi–Svii.

Soypacaci Z, Sengul S, Yıldız E, et al. Effect of daily sodium intake on post-transplant hypertension in kidney allograft recipients. *Transplant Proceed.* 2013;45(3):940–943.

Taler SJ, Agarwal R, Bakris GL, et al. KDOQI US Commentary on the 2012 KDIGO clinical practice guideline for management of blood pressure in CKD. *Am J Kidney Dis.* 2013;62(2):201–213.

Thomas B, Weir MR. The evaluation and therapeutic management of hypertension in the transplant patient. *Curr Cardiol Rep.* 2015;17(11):95. doi: 10.1007/s11886-015-0647-z.

United States Renal Data System. 2018 USRDS annual date report: epidemiology of kidney disease in the United States. National Institutes of Health, National Institute of Diabetes and Digestive and Kidney Diseases, Bethesda, MD, 2018. https://www.usrds.org/atlas10.aspx. Published 2020.

Weir M, Burgess E, Cooper J, et al. Assessment and management of hypertension in transplant patients. *J Am Soc Nephrol.* 2015;26(6):1248–1260.

Whelton PK, Carey RM, Aronow WS, Casey DE, et al. 2017 ACC/AHA/AAPA/ABC/ACPM/AGS/APhA/ASH/ASPC/NMA/PCNA Guideline for the Prevention, Detection, Evaluation, and Management of High Blood Pressure in Adults: A Report of the American College of Cardiology/American Heart Association Task Force on Clinical Practice Guidelines. *Circulation.* 2018;138(17):e484–e594.

CHAPTER 20

TREATMENT OF HYPERTENSION IN OBESITY

Carlos A. Schiavon, MD, and Luciano F. Drager, MD

QUESTIONS

1. **What is the epidemiology of obesity and hypertension?**

   Overweight and obesity are defined as abnormal or excessive fat accumulation that may impair health (World Health Organization). Body mass index (BMI) is the simplest way to classify overweight (BMI between 25 and 29.9 kg/m²) and obesity (BMI > 30 kg/m²) in adults.[1]

   Worldwide obesity has nearly tripled since 1975, and almost a third of the world's adult population are overweight and obese today. Unfortunately, children and adolescents aged 5 to 19 can also become overweight or obese. In 2016, 18% of this population was classified as being either overweight or obese.

   The prevalence of obesity is greater in women than men and increases with age.

   In the United States, 39.8% of the adult population are obese. Hispanics (47%) and non-Hispanic Blacks (46.8%) have the highest age-adjusted prevalence of obesity, followed by non-Hispanic Whites (37.9%) and non-Hispanic Asians (12.7%).

   Obesity is a risk factor for developing hypertension and cardiorenal and metabolic disorders.[2] The Framingham Heart Study suggests that 78% of primary hypertension in men and 65% in women can be attributed to excess weight gain. Central obesity is a better predictor than subcutaneous fat for the development of obesity, and duration of obesity also has a negative impact on blood pressure (BP) levels.

2. **How does obesity cause and/or aggravate hypertension?**

   The pathophysiological mechanisms involved in obesity-related hypertension are complex and have not been fully elucidated. Adipose tissue, particularly with excess visceral fat, serves as an endocrine organ producing multiple hormones and cytokines, which increase the risk of developing hypertension and cardiovascular disease.[2] Obesity is accompanied by increases in macrophages and other immune cells in adipose tissue, in part because of tissue remodeling in response to adipocyte apoptosis. These immune cells secrete proinflammatory cytokines, which contribute to insulin resistance, sympathetic activation, and vascular remodeling.

   Compression of the kidney by surrounding adipose tissue may also contribute to relative ischemia, renin-angiotensin activation, increased sodium reabsorption, and hypertension. Obesity also is often accompanied by an increase in pharyngeal soft tissues, which can contribute to the respiratory events observed in obstructive sleep apnea (OSA). Once present, this common sleep-disordered breathing (especially moderate and severe OSA) amplifies sympathetic activation, aldosterone production, inflammation, and oxidative stress observed in obesity.[3] These contributions provide additional indirect mechanisms by which obesity may promote hypertension.

3. **What is the impact of the nonpharmacologic (and nonsurgical) intervention to obesity treatment over hypertension?**

   Lifestyle modifications can significantly decrease BP in patients with hypertension. Proven nonpharmacologic interventions for obesity that also improve hypertension control include physical activity (especially aerobic exercises), which reduces BP by approximately 5 to 8 mm Hg. Weight loss strategies including caloric restriction may be expected to reduce BP by 1 mm Hg for every 1 kg reduction in body weight. Most evidence on weight loss is based on short-term follow-up, and a high rate of recidivism over a longer timeframe negatively impacts the effects of lifestyle modifications on hypertension control in clinical practice.[4–6]

4. **What are the effects of antiobesity drugs in hypertension?**

   Only a few specific drugs have been formally approved for obesity treatment by the Food and Drug Administration in the United States, with the most promising cardiovascular benefits associated with weight loss induced by glucagon-like peptide-1 (GLP-1) agonists.[7] Although not the primary intent of weight loss, investigations of these pharmacologic interventions measured BP as a secondary endpoint. In the SCALE trial, once daily subcutaneous GLP-1 agonist liraglutide (3.0 mg) promoted greater weight loss than placebo at 56 weeks (difference of −5.6 kg; 95% confidence interval [CI], −6.0 to −5.1; P < .001).[8] Liraglutide also significantly decreased systolic blood pressure (SBP) by 2.8 mm Hg (−3.56 to −2.09, P < .001). The long-acting GLP-1 agonist semaglutide (2.4 mg once weekly) similarly reduced body weight (difference of −12.7 mm Hg; 95% CI, −11.7 to −13.7;

$P < .001$) and SBP (difference of -5.10 mm Hg; 95% CI, -6.34 to -3.87; $P < .001$) to a greater extent than placebo at 65 weeks.[9] The variability in BP reduction was partially explained by degree of weight loss achieved during liraglutide treatment.

The effects of other antiobesity drugs on BP varies, and some concerns may exist according to their mechanism of action. The combination drug therapy of naltrexone/bupropion may slightly raise BP (both office and ambulatory BP monitoring [ABPM]) despite promoting weight loss, although this finding has been inconsistent. Phentermine-topiramate reduces weight and BP but increases heart rate slightly, likely due to sympathomimetic activity, and is not generally recommended in patients with cardiovascular disease or uncontrolled hypertension.[10] Some supplements for weight loss contain sympathomimetic agents associated with increased BP and cardiovascular events without appropriate labeling (e.g., ephedra, phentermine, sibutramine, etc.). Several of these agents have been removed from the market in the United States and are not generally recommended. In summary, GLP-1 agonists simultaneously reduce body weight and BP, but many weight-loss dietary supplements may contain drugs that exacerbate BP control or hypertension.

5. **What BP measurement technique should be used in patients with obesity?**

BP measurement techniques for patients with obesity should follow the same procedures for obtaining a reliable measurement. Attention should be devoted to use of an appropriately sized cuff, which requires appropriate measurement of arm circumference. BP monitoring during and after surgical procedures (including bariatric surgery) is also a concern.[11] With the rise in the incidence and severity of obesity, hospitals should supply a wide range of BP cuff sizes to adequately measure BP during surgical procedures and in the hospital. Conically shaped arms present a major challenge for appropriately fitting cuffs. Although innovative technology is in development, none have been validated for general use.

6. **What are the treatment options for overweight and obesity grade 1?**

Obesity is a complex multifactorial disease, and its treatment involves many interventions based on the severity of the disease and the presence of comorbidities.

As stated earlier (question 3), lifestyle intervention is mandatory for all patients who need to lose weight. It includes exercise, dietary therapy, and behavior modification.

Drug therapy is indicated for patients with BMI greater than 30 kg/m^2 and for those with BMI between 27 and 29.9 kg/m^2 with a comorbidity. Liraglutide, orlistat, and phentermine-topiramate are the most commonly used options that reduce body weight, although their long-term cardiovascular benefits remain to be proven.

The same indications to start a drug therapy apply to the indication of endoscopic devices. Intragastric balloons are approved in most countries as well as in the United States. The most common intragastric balloon is implanted with endoscopy and should be explanted after 6 months. Complications are rare. The procedure typically achieves short-term weight loss of approximately 10%, but the success rate decreases over time in most patients.

7. **Which is the best treatment option when the baseline BMI is greater than 35 kg/m^2?**

Although there are many controversies about the use of BMI, it is always present in any algorithm to treat obesity. The National Institutes of Health defined classic indications based on BMI for bariatric surgery in 1991, and these guidelines remain the standard of care today. Patients with a BMI between 35 and 39.9 kg/m^2 should be referred to surgery if significant comorbidities such as hypertension, type 2 diabetes, dyslipidemia, heart failure, atrial fibrillation, sleep apnea, or orthopedic problems are present. Patients with a BMI greater than 40 kg/m^2 should be referred for surgical evaluation regardless of the presence of comorbidities.

With appropriate patient selection and surgical expertise, bariatric surgery has low morbidity and mortality rates. The weight loss, metabolic improvements, and cardiovascular benefits are accompanied by some complications such as nutritional deficiencies, highlighting the need for appropriate follow-up.

8. **Does bariatric surgery reduce BP?**

BP control clearly improves after bariatric surgery. Compared to medically treated patients, the incidence of resistant hypertension (2.3% vs. 15.0%; $P < .07$) and the number of antihypertensive medications (1 [0–2] vs. 3 [2.8–4] classes; $P < .001$) improved markedly after Roux-en-Y gastric bypass (RYGB) and achieved similar BP between groups.[12,13] Notably, hypertension completely resolved (BP $<140/90$ mm Hg) in 35% of patients after RYGB, as verified by 24-hour ABPM with the patient off all medications.[12]

9. **How should hypertension be managed in the perioperative period of a bariatric surgery?**

Many patients undergoing bariatric surgery require multiple antihypertensive drugs to achieve adequate control of hypertension.[14] Rapid weight loss after bariatric surgery also may be accompanied by rapid reduction in BP. Therefore attention to BP and appropriate reduction of the number and doses of the medications should be a primary focus during postsurgical follow-up. These evaluations should balance the risks of hypotension with hypertension control. The GATEWAY Trial protocol modified antihypertensive medication according to the following protocols[12,13]:
- Discontinue or reduce medications for SBP less than 130 mm Hg or diastolic blood pressure (DBP) less than 80 mm Hg if symptoms of orthostatic hypotension are present.

- In patients with SBP less than 110 mm Hg and DBP less than 70 mm Hg, attempt to reduce antihypertensive medications even in the absence of orthostatic symptoms. Continue the reduced doses if SBP and DBP are sustained at less than 140/90 mm Hg or 130/80 mm Hg, depending on desired BP targets.
- For patients referred for bariatric surgery:
  - Monitor BP closely during the postoperative period while in the hospital.
  - If BP remains controlled (<140/90 mm Hg), do a trial without antihypertensive medications to avoid hypotension at home. Instruct patients to self-monitor home BP on a daily basis in the immediate postoperative period, in the first visit 1 week after the procedure, and in the remaining follow-up visits.
  - If BP is not controlled (>140/90 mm Hg) during the hospital stay, maintain at least one drug of the patient's regimen. An angiotensin-converting enzyme inhibitor or an angiotensin II receptor blocker are generally preferred. Generally, avoid the use of a diuretic because patients cannot drink a lot of liquids after bariatric surgery, and diuretics may increase the risk of volume depletion. Reintroduce or reduce medications as described.

Ideally ABPM can be utilized to verify BP control over 24 hours. Sometimes patients need to modify the doses and the time to take medications.

10. **Is there a better surgical technique for a patient with hypertension?**
The most frequently performed techniques are RYGB and sleeve gastrectomy (SG). Contemporary guidelines indicate that the choice of one technique should be based on therapeutic goals, expertise of the surgeon, patients' preferences, risk stratification, and cost-effectiveness. Preliminary evidence suggests that RYGB performs superiorly to SG for weight loss and resolution of comorbidities including hypertension and diabetes. STAMPEDE found a greater efficacy of RYGB in the resolution or improvement of type 2 diabetes mellitus.[15] Similar results from the SLEEVEPASS and SM-BOSS studies generally support the superiority of RYGB for diabetes, although results were not significant. A greater percentage of patients in the SLEEVPASS study were able to discontinue all antihypertensive agents after RYGB (51%) than the SG group (29%; *P* = .02 for difference).[16] Despite these data, there is currently no consensus whether a specific bariatric surgery technique is superior for patients with hypertension.

KEY POINTS

1. Obesity is a major risk factor for the development of hypertension.
2. Besides lifestyle intervention, the use of GLP-1 agonists showed significant weight loss and mild SBP reduction.
3. Patients with obesity grade 2 and 3 and hypertension should be referred for a bariatric surgery evaluation.
4. Bariatric surgery has the potential to reduce BP (with a significant rate of hypertension remission) and other cardiovascular risk factors. Morbidity and mortality attributed to bariatric surgery are very low, but nutritional follow-up is mandatory.

REFERENCES

1. Heymsfield SB, Wadden TA. Mechanisms, pathophysiology, and management of obesity. *N Engl J Med.* 2017;376:254–266.
2. Sun K, Kusminski CM, Scherer PE. Adipose tissue remodeling and obesity. *J Clin Invest.* 2011;121:2094–2101.
3. Drager LF, Bortolotto LA, Figueiredo AC, Silva BC, Krieger EM, Lorenzi-Filho G. Obstructive sleep apnea, hypertension, and their interaction on arterial stiffness and heart remodeling. *Chest.* 2007;131:1379–1386.
4. Brook RD, Appel LJ, Rubenfire M, et al. Beyond medications and diet: alternative approaches to lowering blood pressure: A scientific statement from the American Heart Association. *Hypertension.* 2013;61:1360–1383.
5. Rejeski WJ, Ip EH, Bertoni AG, et al. Lifestyle change and mobility in obese adults with type 2 diabetes. *N Engl J Med.* 2012;366:1209–1217.
6. Whelton PK, Carey RM, Aronow WS, et al. 2017 ACC/AHA/AAPA/ABC/ACPM/AGS/APHA/ASH/ASPC/NMA/PCNA guideline for the prevention, detection, evaluation, and management of high blood pressure in adults: a report of the American College of Cardiology/American Heart Association task force on clinical practice guidelines. *Hypertension.* 2018;71:e13–e115.
7. Cohen JB, Gadde KM. Weight loss medications in the treatment of obesity and hypertension. *Curr Hypertens Rep.* 2019;21:16.
8. Pi-Sunyer X, Astrup A, Fujioka K, et al. A randomized, controlled trial of 3.0 mg of liraglutide in weight management. *N Engl J Med.* 2015;373:11–22.
9. Wilding JPH, Batterham RL, Calanna S, et al. Once-weekly semaglutide in adults with overweight or obesity. *N Engl J Med.* 2021;384:989–1002.
10. Gadde KM, Allison DB, Ryan DH, et al. Effects of low-dose, controlled-release, phentermine plus topiramate combination on weight and associated comorbidities in overweight and obese adults (conquer): a randomised, placebo-controlled, phase 3 trial. *Lancet.* 2011;377:1341–1352.
11. Rogge DE, Nicklas JY, Schon G, et al. Continuous noninvasive arterial pressure monitoring in obese patients during bariatric surgery: an evaluation of the vascular unloading technique (clearsight system). *Anesth Analg.* 2019;128:477–483.
12. Schiavon CA, Bhatt DL, Ikeoka D, et al. Three-year outcomes of bariatric surgery in patients with obesity and hypertension: a randomized clinical trial. *Ann Intern Med.* 2020;173:685–693.
13. Schiavon CA, Ikeoka D, Santucci EV, et al. Effects of bariatric surgery versus medical therapy on the 24-hour ambulatory blood pressure and the prevalence of resistant hypertension. *Hypertension.* 2019;73:571–577.

14. Pareek M, Bhatt DL, Schiavon CA, Schauer PR. Metabolic surgery for hypertension in patients with obesity. *Circ Res.* 2019;124:1009–1024.
15. Schauer PR, Bhatt DL, Kirwan JP, et al. Bariatric surgery versus intensive medical therapy for diabetes—3-year outcomes. *N Engl J Med.* 2014;370:2002–2013.
16. Salminen P, Helmio M, Ovaska J, et al. Effect of laparoscopic sleeve gastrectomy vs laparoscopic Roux-en-Y gastric bypass on weight loss at 5 years among patients with morbid obesity: the SLEEVEPASS randomized clinical trial. *JAMA.* 2018;319:241–254.

CHAPTER 21

HYPERTENSION IN BLACKS

Akshan Puar, MD, and J. Howard Pratt, MD

QUESTIONS

1. **What is the prevalence of hypertension in Blacks in the United States?**
   According to (the National Health and Nutrition Examination Survey from 2017–18, the age-adjusted prevalence of hypertension in adults was noted to be higher in non-Hispanic Blacks (57.1%) as compared with non-Hispanic Whites (43.6%) and Hispanics (43.7%). When looking at men and women separately, the age-adjusted prevalence of hypertension was also found to be higher in non-Hispanic Blacks as compared with non-Hispanic Whites and Hispanics. The definition of hypertension used in this survey was a cut off of blood pressure (BP) of 130/80 mm Hg or greater or taking medication for hypertension. The previous guidelines used a definition of 140/90 mm Hg. Interestingly, with this new definition of BP goal of less than 130/80 mm Hg (according to the 2017 American Heart Association and American College of Cardiology guidelines), 3.5 million more Black men would fit the definition of having hypertension (Fig. 21.1).

2. **Does hypertension have an earlier age of onset in Blacks in comparison to Whites?**
   The number of children and adolescents with hypertension is relatively small, and to get meaningful comparative data is difficult. We do know that BPs are, on average, significantly higher in normotensive Black children than in normotensive White children.
   There is an increased number of Blacks who develop hypertension by middle age when compared with their White counterparts. According to the findings of the (Coronary Artery Risk Development in Young Adults study published in 2018, three in four Black men and women were likely to have hypertension by age 55 in contrast to 55% of White men and 40% of White women by the same age.

3. **How does the hypertension in Blacks compare with the hypertension in Whites?**
   Compared to all other population groups, for Blacks the risk for hypertension is greater, and the likelihood of developing serious complications such as stroke, heart failure, or end-stage renal disease is increased considerably.

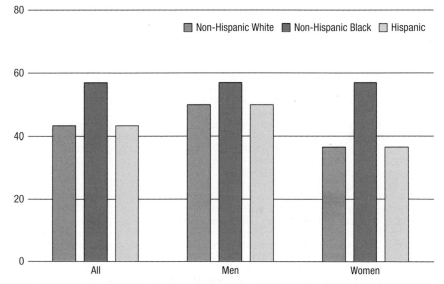

Fig. 21.1 Age-adjusted prevalence of hypertension among adults aged 18 and old by sex, race, and Hispanic origin, United States, 2017–18. Results are expressed as a percent. (From National Health and Nutrition Examination Survey, 2017–18.)

4. **Why is hypertension more prevalent and severe in Blacks compared with Whites?**
   There is no single correct answer. Hypertension, regardless of ethnicity, is complex and very multifactorial. Social issues, economic issues, and health care availability are all potential barriers that may or may not be surmountable. With that having been said, there appears to be underlying physiological mechanisms in Blacks resulting in a steady state of sodium retention. This is evidenced by the salt sensitivity of BP and the lower renin levels in many Black patients. In addition, there is aldosterone sensitivity where BP is proportional to the plasma aldosterone concentration. Aldosterone sensitivity has been described in Black children and Black young adults but is virtually absent in young White individuals. Blacks and Whites differ with respect to the intensity with which they reabsorb and accumulate sodium and water. There is a plasma volume expansion that creates an increase in arterial pressure, which, through pressor natriuresis, balances sodium excretion with sodium intake.

   What does not immediately fit with this schematic is that aldosterone secretion is lower in Blacks than in Whites by 30% to 40%. It can be proposed that the aldosterone sensitivity in Blacks fills in for the decrease in aldosterone secretion. This is indeed speculative, but we also know that spironolactone, which lowers BP in Blacks, does so by blocking the mineralocorticoid receptor (MR). It is a compelling explanation for the sodium retention that places Blacks at great risk for developing hypertension and its complications. Added to this mechanism is the relative nonsuppressibility of aldosterone secretion normally regulated by angiotensin II.

5. **What laboratory tests and results are helpful in directing treatment for Black patients?**
   In addition to the basic metabolic panel, which includes serum creatinine to assess kidney function, the next single most important test would be plasma renin activity.

6. **Should renin (or renin activity) be measured in all Blacks with hypertension?**
   Almost anyone with significant hypertension should probably have renin measured as it is an indicator of the extracellular fluid volume. Patients with low renin levels are more volume expanded and more likely to respond to a standard diuretic as well as the treatment proposed here of blocking the MR or directly inhibiting the epithelial sodium channel also known as ENaC, the principal target of aldosterone.

7. **Should aldosterone also be measured?**
   Knowing the plasma aldosterone concentration allows for consideration of primary aldosteronism. If the level of aldosterone is low and takes on features of a Liddle syndrome phenotype, these patients may respond better to amiloride or triamterene than to an MR blocker.

8. **Can a different approach to treating hypertension lead to better outcomes for Black patients?**
   When targeting an approach to treat hypertension in Blacks, lifestyle modifications and other nondrug interventions can play a role. Numerous community-based interventions, including recognizing and treating hypertension at barbershops and churches, have shown benefit. Of particular note is the (Dietary Approaches to Stop Hypertension study in which a reduction in sodium intake had a profound effect on BP in Blacks.

   Many Blacks with hypertension have low renin levels, are salt sensitive, and respond well to MR antagonists and ENaC inhibitors. By understanding these mechanisms, offering treatment with medications such as spironolactone can be valuable. This is a reasonable approach if there are no contraindications such as serum electrolyte abnormalities or elevated serum creatinine level. It could be helpful diagnostically as well.

9. **Spironolactone vs. eplerenone—which one is preferred?**
   More advantages seem to reside with spironolactone—it has twice the potency of eplerenone, needs to be given only once daily (eplerenone may be more effective if given twice daily), and it is inexpensive, whereas eplerenone is relatively expensive (both drugs are generic).

   In men, however, a disadvantage to using spironolactone is that it also binds to the androgen receptor, causing estrogenic influences that can lead to breast tenderness, gynecomastia, and loss of libido. However, at the dose of 25 mg/day, spironolactone produces these symptoms in only 10% of patients. Therefore the use of spironolactone should not necessarily be limited to female patients.

   Spironolactone should not be used in pregnancy.

   Spironolactone use has been associated with leg cramps.

10. **Why are drugs that reduce ENaC activity so underutilized?**
    Earlier studies often used much higher doses of spironolactone, as much as 400 mg/day. Side effects were the rule, and the drug's reputation was one that led to infrequent use in men. These drugs were also not included and thus not tested in several historically important clinical trials of antihypertensive drugs: Veterans Affairs studies of monotherapies from different population groups, ALLHAT (Antihypertensive and Lipid-Lowering Treatment to Prevent Heart Attack Trial), and AASK (African American Study of Kidney Disease and Hypertension). In addition, these drugs are no longer receiving patent protection, and therefore they may not be promoted as vigorously.

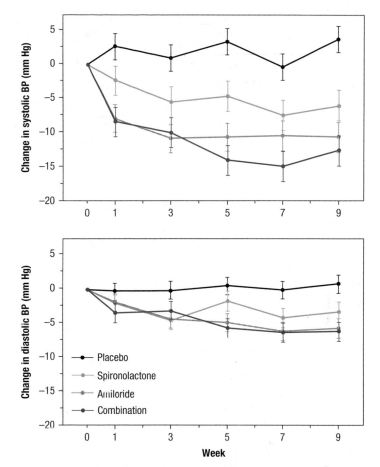

Fig. 21.2 Changes from baseline in systolic and diastolic blood pressure (BP). The decrease in systolic BP was significant in all treatment groups in comparison to placebo, $P < .001$ for amiloride, $P < .010$ for spironolactone, and $P < .001$ for the combination. Diastolic BP was significant for the amiloride-treated group ($P = .003$) and for the combination-treated group ($P = .002$). (From Saha C, Eckert GJ, Ambrosius WT, et al. Improvement in blood pressure with inhibition of the epithelial sodium channel in blacks with hypertension. *Hypertension* 2005;46:481–487.)

11. **Amiloride and triamterene are used mostly as potassium-sparing agents in patients. How effective are they as antihypertensive drugs?**
    Triamterene, as an ENaC inhibitor, is prescribed almost exclusively for its potassium-sparing properties when used in combination with diuretics such as hydrochlorothiazide. But triamterene alone lowers BP. In an observational study by Tu et al. of 17,291 hypertensive patients treated with hydrochlorothiazide (average dose 25 mg/day), ~60% of the patients were Black. Of the total number, 3131 were also given triamterene, 37.5 mg/day on average. The mean systolic BP was 3.8 mm Hg lower in those who also received triamterene ($P < .0001$).
    A second clinical trial is presented in Fig. 21.2. This was a 9-week, placebo-controlled, randomized, double-blind study by Saha et al. (with 2 × 2 factorial design). All the patients were Black with low renin levels. They compared the changes from baseline BP. There were four treatment groups: placebo, amiloride 10 mg/day, spironolactone 25 mg/day, and the combination of amiloride and spironolactone. Systolic BP was significantly reduced from baseline for all treatment groups. Amiloride lowered BP significantly more than did spironolactone.
    Black patients with hypertension benefit from both MR blockers and ENaC inhibitors—BP is lowered, and hypokalemia is avoided.

12. **To what extent are these drugs accepted by patients?**
    Patient satisfaction is typically very high. As the BP normalizes and fewer pills are required (the usual case), compliance with taking medications may improve.

KEY POINTS

1. Hypertension in Blacks is a major public health problem.
2. Most Blacks with hypertension have a suppressed renin-angiotensin system due to plasma volume expansion, a result of excessive sodium retention mediated, at least in part, by aldosterone.
3. Treatment of the hypertension with drugs that mitigate the activity of ENaC can be highly effective in lowering BP in Blacks.
4. Blacks and, to a much lesser extent, Whites demonstrate aldosterone sensitivity. For a given plasma level of aldosterone, there is a proportionately higher BP in Blacks than in Whites.
5. Blacks produce less aldosterone than Whites. This could result from a suppressed renin-angiotensin system or from the presence of greater aldosterone sensitivity in Blacks.
6. Management of hypertension in Blacks should focus more on aldosterone as an antihypertensive target.

BIBLIOGRAPHY

ALLHATCollaborative Research Group: Major outcomes in high-risk hypertensive patients randomized to angiotensin-converting enzyme inhibitor or calcium channel blocker vs diuretic: The Antihypertensive and Lipid-Lowering Treatment to Prevent Heart Attack Trial (ALLHAT). *JAMA.* 2002;288:2981–2997.

Carnethon MR, Pu J, Howard G, et al. Cardiovascular health in African Americans: a scientific statement from the American Heart Association. *Circulation.* 2017;136:e393–e423.

Flack JM, Hamaty M. Difficult-to-treat hypertensive populations: focus on African-Americans and people with type 2 diabetes. *Journal of Hypertension. Supplement: Official Journal of the International Society of Hypertension.* 1999;17(1):S19–24.

Liddle GW, Bledsoe T, Coppage Jr WS. A familial renal disorder simulating primary aldosteronism but with negligible aldosterone secretion. *Trans Assoc Am Physicians.* 1963;76:199–213.

Lifton RP. Molecular genetics of human blood pressure variation. *Science.* 1996;272:676–680.

Luft FC, Grim CE, Fineberg NS, Weinberger MH. Effects of volume expansion and contraction in normotensive Whites, Blacks, and subjects of different ages. *Circulation.* 1979;59:643–650.

Palacios C, Wigertz K, Martin BR, et al. Sodium retention in Black and White female adolescents in response to salt intake. *J Clin Endocrinol Metab.* 2004;89:1858–1863.

Pratt JH, Jones JJ, Miller JZ, Wagner MA, Fineberg NS. Racial differences in aldosterone excretion and plasma aldosterone concentrations in children. *N Engl J Med.* 1989;321:1152–1157.

Roush GC, Sica DA. Diuretics for hypertension: a review and update. *Am J Hypertens.* 2016;29:1130–1137.

Sacks FM, Svetkey LP, Vollmer WM, et al. Effects on blood pressure of reduced dietary sodium and the Dietary Approaches to Stop Hypertension (DASH) diet. DASH-Sodium Collaborative Research Group. *N Engl J Med.* 2001;344:3–10.

Saha C, Eckert GJ, Ambrosius WT, et al. Improvement in blood pressure with inhibition of the epithelial sodium channel in blacks with hypertension. *Hypertension.* 2005;46:481–487.

Sowers JR, Zemel MB, Zemel P, Beck FWJ, Walsh MF, Zawada ET. Salt sensitivity in Blacks. *Hypertension.* 1988;12:485–490.

Spence JD, Rayner BL. Hypertension in Blacks. *Hypertension.* 2018;72(2):263–269.

Thomas SJ, Booth JN, Dai C, et al. Cumulative incidence of hypertension by 55 years of age in Blacks and Whites: The CARDIA study. *J Am Heart Assoc.* 2018;7(14):e007988.

Tu W, Decker BS, He Z, et al. Triamterene enhances the blood pressure lowering effect of hydrochlorothiazide in patients with hypertension. *J Gen Intern Med.* 2016;31(1):30–36.

Tu W, Eckert GJ, Hannon TS, et al. Racial differences in sensitivity of blood pressure to aldosterone. *Hypertension.* 2014;63:1212–1218.

Tu W, Li R, Bhalla V, Eckert GJ, Pratt JH. Age-related blood pressure sensitivity to aldosterone in Blacks and Whites. *Hypertension.* 2018;72:247–252.

Wright JT, Bakris G, Aask G, et al. Effect of blood pressure lowering and antihypertensive class on progression of hypertensive kidney disease: results from the AASK trial. *JAMA.* 2002;288:2421–2431.

CHAPTER 22

HYPERTENSION IN THE ELDERLY

Christine Dillingham, MD, and Aldo J. Peixoto, MD

QUESTIONS

1. **What is the epidemiology of hypertension in the elderly?**

   In this chapter, we will refer to the "elderly" as those individuals aged 65 years or older, as this is the definition used by the United Nations in its reports on aging. This rapidly growing segment of the population accounts for 9% of individuals globally and 16.5% in the United States and is expected to reach 22% by 2050.

   Hypertension prevalence increases with age, with a sharp rise in people older than age 55 years. In the elderly, hypertension is the rule, afflicting more than two-thirds of individuals. Data from the National Health and Nutrition Examination Surveys (NHANES) show that 64% of men and 69% of women between ages 64 and 74 years have hypertension, which is defined as blood pressure (BP) of 140/90 mm Hg or higher or antihypertensive therapy. Hypertension affects 67% of men and 79% of women aged 75 years or older.

   In 2017 the American College of Cardiology and the American Heart Association (ACC/AHA) updated their hypertension guidelines and redefined hypertension as BP of 130/80 mm Hg or higher. Using these new thresholds, the estimated prevalence of hypertension increased to 77% among patients aged 65 years or older.

   In recent years, the rate of BP control to levels under 140/90 mm Hg has increased among the elderly. Current NHANES estimates indicate that approximately 49% of elderly hypertensives have controlled BP with similar numbers among men and women.

2. **What are some issues of specific importance when evaluating elderly hypertensive patients?**
   - **BP Measurement – Evaluation of Both Arms.** Significant inter-arm BP differences (>10 mm Hg) are observed in ~11% of all hypertensive patients. Inter-arm differences are associated with underlying peripheral arterial disease and are more common among older men than other groups. Because of the impact such differences can have on treatment decisions, it is recommended that all patients be screened by simultaneous BP measurements (or in rapid sequence). If a disparity is noted, the higher level is always used. Even though not formally recommended by guidelines, it is reasonable to rescreen elderly patients for inter-arm differences periodically.
   - **BP Measurement – Pseudohypertension.** Older patients often have arterial calcification that may lead to limited compressibility of the brachial **artery** resulting in falsely high BP readings. This should be considered in patients with very high BP levels and no evidence of target organ damage or in those with hypotensive symptoms despite high measured BP. In the past, the Osler sign (the brachial and radial artery remain palpable distal to a maximally inflated BP cuff) was thought to be diagnostic, but it has limited diagnostic reliability. Therefore if pseudohypertension is suspected, intra arterial measurements are necessary to settle the issue.
   - **BP Measurement – Orthostatic Vital Signs.** Orthostatic hypotension, often asymptomatic, occurs in up to a third of older patients with hypertension. It is defined as a BP fall greater than 20/10 mm Hg with standing. Some guidelines have recommended checking orthostatic vital signs in the elderly as well as in patients with chronic kidney disease and diabetes. Although it is best to perform orthostatic testing after at least 5 minutes of supine rest followed by 3 minutes of standing, we recognize the difficulties of doing this in a busy clinical practice. A reasonable compromise is to measure BP in the seated position followed by BP after 1 minute standing. Because this technique is less sensitive, the proposed threshold to diagnose orthostatic hypotension using this abbreviated method is a BP drop greater than 15/7 mm Hg with standing.
   - **Out-of-Office BP Assessment.** Out-of-office BP monitoring with 24-hour ambulatory BP or home BP monitoring is now uniformly recommended for the diagnosis of hypertension, and the 2017 ACC/AHA guidelines also endorse its use to guide therapy. Despite these recommendations, the uptake by physicians at large is still suboptimal. This is problematic in the elderly because both white coat hypertension (elevated office BP with normal ambulatory BP) and masked hypertension (normal office BP with high ambulatory BP) are more common with aging, thus demanding the use of out-of-office BP monitoring to avoid both over- and undertreatment. White coat hypertension was observed in 3.2% of those younger than age 60 years and 29% of those 60 years or older. Likewise, NHANES estimated the prevalence of masked hypertension to increase significantly with aging, from 8% in adults younger than 44 years, to 17% in those 45 to 64 years, to 28% in those 65 years

or older. These data support a recommendation for routine out-of-office BP measurement for evaluation and management of elderly hypertensive patients.

3. What is the distribution of hypertensive subtypes in elderly patients?
Both systolic blood pressure (SBP) and diastolic blood pressure (DBP) increase with age up to the sixth decade of life. After that, DBP starts to decline, resulting in increased pulse pressure (PP). Consequently, isolated diastolic and systo-diastolic hypertension are the predominant subtypes in younger patients. In the elderly, data from NHANES indicate that isolated systolic hypertension (ISH, defined as SBP ≥ 140 mm Hg with DBP < 90 mm Hg) is the predominant subtype, representing 80% to 90% of cases.

4. What is the major mechanism of ISH in the elderly?
The major pathogenic factor in ISH is increased arterial stiffness. Aging results in elastin fragmentation and degradation followed by collagen deposition in place of elastin fibers in the large elastic arteries, rendering them stiffer. Multiple mechanisms underlie this process including excessive activity of several matrix metalloproteinases, collagen cross-linking by advanced glycation end-products, vascular smooth cell proliferation and stiffening, calcification of the vascular media, endothelial dysfunction, and vascular wall inflammation and fibrosis. Other common prohypertensive factors are often increased in elderly patients such as salt sensitivity, increased sympathetic tone, and relative increase in activity of the renin-angiotensin system. Finally, arterial stiffening is accelerated by many common age-associated disorders such as atherosclerosis, diabetes mellitus, the metabolic syndrome, chronic kidney disease, and hypertension itself (i.e., high BP is both result and cause of arterial injury and stiffening).

Under normal conditions, an incident pulse wave generated during systole travels to the periphery and is reflected back, returning to the aortic root in diastole and augmenting diastolic pressure. Arterial stiffening, however, increases pulse wave velocity, thus making the incident forward wave travel faster to the periphery and the reflected wave return faster to the central circulation. Because of faster travel, the reflected wave reaches the aortic root while systole is still occurring. This results in increased SBP and greater decay of the DBP curve (thus lower diastolic DBP), resulting in widening of the PP. Although arterial stiffness can be measured using a variety of clinical tools, high brachial SBP with low DBP and increased PP are the "poor man's" clinical hallmarks of arterial stiffness.

Increased left ventricular pressure during systole results in pressure-induced left ventricular hypertrophy. Systolic stress also leads to increased cardiomyocyte energy consumption leading to relative ischemia, particularly given the associated impairment in diastolic coronary perfusion produced by the decrease in DBP. These mechanisms are important mediators of the increased incidence of cardiovascular events and death in patients with ISH.

5. What is the role of salt sensitivity in the elderly?
Salt sensitivity is a physiological trait characterized by sustained BP increase with increased salt intake and significant BP fall with salt depletion. Salt sensitivity is normally distributed and cannot yet be effectively predicted using current biomarkers—only formal testing of the BP responses to variable sodium intake can identify it. Salt sensitivity increases with age. Average reductions in BP with sodium depletion in hypertensive patients are significantly greater in patients over the age of 60 years (16 mm Hg) compared with younger patients (6 mm Hg for patients age 31–40, 10 mm Hg for patients age 41–60). Although this varies from person to person and many will not be salt-sensitive at all, it is worth recognizing that salt sensitivity is more common in the elderly to remind us of the importance of advice on sodium restriction and the use of diuretics for treatment.

6. Are there differences in benefit from treatment of hypertension in the elderly compared to younger patients?
A metaanalysis comparing the observed risk reduction associated with the treatment of hypertension in patients above or below 65 years of age did not detect any significant differences. Patients in both age groups had similar benefits as summarized in Table 22.1. In this study similar numerical risk reductions occurred in patients older than 80 years, with statistically significant reductions in the risk of stroke (-32%) and heart failure (-62%).

7. What should the BP treatment targets be for elderly patients?
Evidence supporting hypertension treatment in the elderly, especially systolic hypertension, is a relatively recent achievement. The European Working Party on High Blood Pressure in the Elderly Trial in 1985 enrolled 840 patients with BP levels of 160 to 239/90 to 119 mm Hg (average 183/101 mm Hg) randomized to a thiazide-based therapy or placebo. Reduced BP in the treated group at 1 year (151/88 vs. 172/95 mm Hg) and throughout the study resulted in 27% reduction in cardiovascular mortality ($P = .03$) and a nonsignificant 9% reduction in total mortality after 4.6 years of follow-up. In 1991 the treatment of ISH in the elderly was reshaped by the results of the Systolic Hypertension in the Elderly Program (SHEP). In SHEP, the goal BP depended on a participant's baseline BP. Individuals with SBP over 180 mm Hg had a reduction goal to under 160 mm Hg. For individuals with SBP between 160 and 179, goal was a reduction of at least 20 mm Hg. Achieved SBP in the active treatment group was 144 mm Hg (~ 26 mm Hg lower than baseline) compared to 155 mm Hg in the control group (~ 9 mm Hg

Table 22.1 Comparison of Treatment-Induced Event Rate Reduction in Hypertensive Patients According to Age

	AGE ≥65	AGE <65
Blood pressure change with treatment	−6.7/− 3.2 mm Hg	−6.9/− 3.8 mm Hg
Stroke ↓	33%	29%
Coronary disease ↓	22%	6%
Heart failure ↓	40%	53%
Cardiovascular death ↓	24%	15%
All-cause death ↓	9%	13%

lower than baseline). Over the 4.5 years of follow up, this favorable BP difference resulted in reductions of 36% in stroke, 32% in cardiovascular events, and 13% in all-cause death. Since then, many studies in different populations have replicated these results.

Treatment of very elderly patients (aged 80 years or older) received additional attention because some subanalyses suggested increased all-cause mortality with aggressive hypertension treatment. This uncertainty led to the Hypertension in the Very Elderly Trial, which enrolled patients aged 80 years or older with baseline BP 160 to 199/90 to 109 mm Hg (average 173/91 mm Hg). After 2 years of follow-up, BP in the treatment group was 15/6 mm Hg lower than the placebo group (143/78 vs. 158/84 mm Hg), resulting in a reduction of 30% for strokes, 34% for any cardiovascular event, and 21% in all-cause death.

The results consolidated the importance of decreasing SBP to the 140-mm Hg range in all elderly patients. To evaluate the question of "how low to go," the Systolic Blood Pressure Intervention Trial (SPRINT) evaluated the effect of intensive (SBP <120 mm Hg) compared with standard (SBP <140 mm Hg) antihypertensive treatment on cardiovascular disease outcomes and all-cause mortality in patients at high cardiovascular risk. SPRINT-Senior was the portion of the SPRINT trial enriched by patients aged 75 years or older. In SPRINT-Senior, both intensive and standard treatment groups had a baseline seated SBP of 142 mm Hg and, after treatment, the achieved SBP was 123 mm Hg and 135 mm Hg in the intensive and standard groups, respectively. After a follow up of 3.1 years, patients randomized to intensive BP reduction experienced a reduction in the primary endpoint of incident cardiovascular disease by 34% (2.6% vs. 3.9% per year, number needed to treat 27), 38% reduction in heart failure (0.9% vs. 1.4% per year), and 33% reduction in all-cause mortality (1.8% vs. 2.6% per year).

The results from SPRINT-Senior fueled a push for more intensive treatment of older adults. The 2017 ACC/AHA guidelines recommended an SBP goal of under 130/80 mm Hg for ambulatory, noninstitutionalized patients aged 65 years or older. However, there are certain caveats that must be discussed. In contrast, the 2018 European Society of Hypertension and European Society of Cardiology (ESH/ESC) guidelines were a bit more conservative in the elderly and recommended an SBP goal of less than 140/80 mm Hg but not less than 130 mm Hg.

Most patients studied in clinical trials are typically active and independent. Institutionalized patients and those heavily dependent on others for their activities of daily living have not been studied. This needs to be taken into account when choosing BP targets (see question 9).

8. How does low DBP affect the treatment decisions in ISH?

Low DBP (<70 mm Hg, and especially <60 mm Hg) is associated with increased rates of de novo and recurrent cardiovascular events in older hypertensive patients. In ISH, treatment targeting SBP usually also lowers DBP (see question #11), thus raising concerns about coronary risk. In SPRINT, low DBP was associated with worse cardiovascular outcomes. However, intensive therapy resulted in better outcomes than the standard target regardless of DBP category at baseline. Given the uncertainty in the literature, we take a conservative approach. We tolerate DBP levels above 55 to 60 mm Hg. If DBP is under 55 to 60 mm Hg, we review risks with the patient to make a joint decision about treatment escalation to address persistently elevated SBP levels.

9. Does frailty modify BP goals?

Frailty is an aging-related state of poor response to stressor events leading to progressive physiological and cognitive decline, loss of autonomy, and decreased survival. Clinically, it can be observed by slowing of mobility and gait speed, need for help with instrumental activities of daily living, often progressing to complete dependence, and requirement for full-time care either at home or in a nursing home.

Stratified analysis of the SPRINT-Senior trial, according to gait speed and a frailty index score, showed similar outcomes across all strata of frailty. Whereas SPRINT-Senior did have 33% of patients qualify as "frail" based on their frailty index and 28% had a gait speed slower than 0.8 m/s, study subjects were not institutionalized and had to have enough independence to participate in the trial, thus limiting the generalizability of these results to severely frail patients. Furthermore, multiple observational studies have determined that hypertensive patients with advanced frailty have worse outcomes when SBP falls below 130 mm Hg. The ACC/AHA guidelines provide expert opinion on the subject: for elderly patients with a high burden of comorbidity and limited life expectancy, the use of "clinical judgment, patient preference, and a team-based approach to assess risk/benefit" is indicated. We typically settle for a target SBP under 150 mm Hg for these severely frail patients.

10. **Is the approach to antihypertensive drug therapy different for older patients?**
    The overall treatment approach proposed by both the ACC/AHA and the ESH/ESC guidelines is similar across the age spectrum, with a few caveats:
    - Polypharmacy is common: ~50% of community elderly adults are prescribed five or more medications, and ~20% receive more than 10 concomitant prescription drugs! Given age-associated changes in pharmacokinetics and pharmacodynamics, polypharmacy increases the risk of drug-related adverse events and is associated with worse outcomes in the elderly, including decreased adherence to treatment, increased hospitalizations, poorer physical and cognitive performance, and possibly increased mortality. Therefore choosing to add multiple medications to achieve BP goals needs to be a balanced decision that must include an assessment of overall expected benefit from the treatment of hypertension and the competing interests related to the treatment of other comorbidities. The clinician and patient need to decide together how to prioritize based on specific risk profile and patient preferences. There are tools to help guide the use of medications in vulnerable elderly patients such as the Beers Criteria of the American Geriatrics Society, which can be found for use in pocket cards and on a mobile app.
    - Although guidelines favor the use of combination therapy to maximize adherence and efficacy, older patients (particularly those >80 years old) may be more safely managed with monotherapy to avoid undue side effects.
    - Initial doses are often lower, particularly in frail patients to minimize unexpectedly excessive BP reductions and/or orthostatic hypotension.
    - It is reasonable to escalate therapy at a slower pace in frail elderly patients. In a study evaluating treatment escalation every 2 weeks compared to every 6 weeks, the overall rate of adverse events was similar, but the occurrence of severe adverse events was twice as common in the group undergoing fast treatment titration. Although this study was not restricted to elderly patients, clinical experience indicates that slower titration (every 4–6 weeks) is often better tolerated by older individuals.
    - Beta-blockers underperform in comparison to the other major drug classes used to treat hypertension (calcium channel blockers [CCBs], angiotensin-converting enzyme inhibitors (ACEis), angiotensin receptor blockers, thiazide-type diuretics). A metaanalysis showed that, when used alone as backbone of therapy, beta-blockers are associated with significantly higher rates of strokes (risk ratio 1.26 [1.15–1.38]) and all-cause death (risk ratio 1.08 [10.02–1.14]) compared with other antihypertensive treatment. Patients in included trials were often in the elderly range, and efficacy was low in two trials restricted to the elderly. Therefore the ACC/AHA guidelines recommend against the use of beta-blockers as part of the initial regimen to treat hypertension in all ages, particularly in the elderly.

11. **Are there drugs that specifically target ISH?**
    Most traditional antihypertensive drug classes have similar effects on SBP and PP. A few agents, however, appear to have a more significant effect on SBP, thus lowering PP. Sacubitril-valsartan, approved for the treatment of heart failure with reduced ejection fraction but not for hypertension, is a very effective antihypertensive agent. In a study of patients with hypertension without heart failure, it reduced ambulatory PP significantly more than valsartan alone (4.8 vs. 0.8 mm Hg at peak doses). Similar results were observed with omapatrilat (a "vasopeptidase inhibitor," a class that combines an ACEi with the neutral endopeptidase inhibitor neprilysin, which blocks the degradation of natriuretic peptides), thus suggesting that the enhancement of natriuretic factors by neprilysin, in combination with blockade of the renin-angiotensin system, may have a favorable effect on SBP without further reduction in DBP, thus lowering PP. The underlying mechanisms of this effect are not understood but likely involve improvements in aortic stiffness.

    Several studies have shown that nitrates (isosorbide dinitrate and mononitrate) and the phosphodiesterase-5 inhibitor sildenafil (a nitrate donor) are effective in lowering SBP and improving wave reflection patterns in ISH. Interestingly, contrary to the antianginal effect, there is no apparent tolerance to the BP-lowering effect despite continuous use. The presumed mechanism is its vasodilatory effects that lead to a decrease in the magnitude of the reflected pulse wave.

    Most large clinical trials of ISH have used either thiazide-type diuretics or dihydropyridine CCBs, making some lean toward the use of these classes in ISH. However, the Avoiding Cardiovascular Events through Combination Therapy in Patients Living with Systolic Hypertension (ACCOMPLISH) trial compared two combination treatments using an ACEi backbone (benazepril/hydrochlorothiazide vs. benazepril/amlodipine) in elderly patients with ISH. In this study the ACEi/CCB combination resulted in better outcomes than the ACEi/diuretic combination (20% fewer fatal and nonfatal cardiovascular events, $P < .001$) despite equivalent BP reduction. Therefore the combination of an ACEi with a nondihydropyridine CCB is a useful and well-tested approach to ISH.

12. **What impact does hypertension treatment have on cognition?**

Progressive cognitive impairment is a common and dreaded complication of aging. The prevalence of mild cognitive impairment (MCI) and dementia in the elderly in the United States is estimated to be ~15% to 20% and ~10%, respectively. Hypertension in mid-life is associated with increased risk of dementia in later life. Studies on the ability of antihypertensive treatment to improve cognition had been inconclusive. However, a metaanalysis including 12 studies published through 2019 demonstrated that BP lowering with antihypertensive drugs was associated with a statistically significant but numerically small reduction in incident dementia or MCI over a mean follow-up of 4.1 years (7.0% vs. 7%, odds ratio 0.93). However, studies that prospectively evaluated cognition scores did not reveal an association between drug treatment and improved cognitive scores.

A substudy of SPRINT (SPRINT-MIND) showed a 17% reduction in incident dementia (7.2 vs. 8.6 cases per 1000 person-years, $P = .10$) and a 19% reduction in MCI (14.6 vs. 18.3 cases per 1000 person-years, $P = .007$). In addition, brain magnetic resonance imaging in the SPRINT-MIND cohort showed that the rate of increase of white matter hyperintensities (a marker of microvascular disease) was slower in those in the intensive treatment group (change in lesion volume 0.92 cm^3 vs. 1.45 cm^3, $P < .001$). Similar results were observed in the Intensive Versus Standard Ambulatory Blood Pressure Lowering to Prevent Functional Decline In the Elderly (INFINITY) trial, which randomized patients aged 75 years or older to a target 24-hour SBP of 130 mm Hg or lower vs. 145 mm Hg or lower (0.29% vs. 0.48% increase in lesion volume, $P = .03$). However, there were no differences in cognitive outcomes in INFINITY.

Overall, these data indicate a modest effect of BP reduction on the incidence or progression of cognitive impairment and dementia in elderly hypertensive patients. On the other hand, these results are reassuring to practicing clinicians as they quell previous concerns that BP lowering could worsen cognition due to sustained cerebral hypoperfusion. No such effect was observed in the intensive arms of SPRINT-MIND and INFINITY.

13. **Are there concerns about increased adverse effects from antihypertensive drugs in elderly patients?**

Elderly patients, particularly those subject to polypharmacy (see earlier), are more susceptible to adverse drug reactions. In the setting of hypertension, the main concerns are related to excessive BP reduction and its complications (falls, syncope), electrolyte disorders (hypokalemia, hyperkalemia, hyponatremia), and acute renal failure, usually due to hypoperfusion often amplified by intrarenal hemodynamic effects from ACEis or angiotensin receptor blockers. Alpha-blockers are associated with an additional increased risk of orthostatic hypotension and falls in the elderly and should be used with caution.

In SPRINT, a study marked by aggressive BP targets, the rates of significant adverse events "of interest" (hypotension, syncope, bradycardia, electrolyte abnormalities, acute renal failure) were 19% to 39% higher in elderly patients (i.e., the SPRINT-Senior cohort) than in patients younger than 65 years. However, the overall rates of events were surprisingly low and often not significantly different between intensive and standard treatment groups. Only hypotension (3.3% intensive vs. 2.0% standard, $P = .04$) reached statistical significance, although relevant trends were observed for electrolyte abnormalities (4.6% intensive vs. 3.3% standard, $P = .07$) and acute renal failure (5.5% intensive vs. 4.2% standard, $P = .07$). Interestingly, injurious falls were more common in the standard group (11.6% intensive vs. 14.1% standard, $P = .04$). It has been speculated that better BP control leads to better gait stability, although this hypothesis could not be confirmed in the INFINITY trial, which specifically tested gait performance.

Within SPRINT-Senior, adverse events increased with increasing levels of frailty and slower gait speed. For example, overall event rate for all events "of interest" combined was 14% among fit elderly compared to 22% in those classified as "less fit" and 30% in those in the frail category.

The risk of hyponatremia and hypokalemia with thiazide-type diuretics increases with age. Likewise, the risk of significant declines in renal function and hyperkalemia are more common in elderly patients receiving ACEis, angiotensin receptor blockers, mineralocorticoid antagonists, and aliskiren. Consequently, monitoring of renal function and electrolytes is necessary for 1 to 2 weeks after treatment initiation and following dose titrations, in addition to periodic longitudinal monitoring.

KEY POINTS

1. Hypertension prevalence increases with age. Using the 2017 ACC/AHA threshold of 130/80 mm Hg to define hypertension, it affects 77% of individuals aged 65 years or older.
2. White coat hypertension and masked hypertension are more common in older patients. Integration of out-of-office BP monitoring is important.
3. ISH is the most common BP subtype in the elderly. Increased arterial stiffness is the major underlying factor.
4. Ambulatory, noninstitutionalized, elderly patients should be treated to a target BP below 130 to 140/80 mm Hg to optimize cardiovascular and cognitive outcomes.
5. Antihypertensive drug choices for the elderly are similar to those for younger hypertensive patients.

BIBLIOGRAPHY

American Geriatrics Society Beers Criteria Update Expert Panel. American Geriatrics Society 2019 updated AGS Beers Criteria(R) for potentially inappropriate medication use in older adults. *J Am Geriatr Soc.* 2019;(4):674–694. doi: 10.1111/jgs.15767.

Amery A, Birkenhager W, Brixko P, et al. Mortality and morbidity results from the European Working Party on High Blood Pressure in the Elderly trial. *Lancet.* 1985;1(8442):1349–1354. doi: 10.1016/s0140-6736(85)91783-0.

Bavishi C, Bangalore S, Messerli FH. Outcomes of intensive blood pressure lowering in older hypertensive patients. *J Am Coll Cardiol.* 2017;69(5):486–493. doi: 10.1016/j.jacc.2016.10.077.

Bavishi C, Goel S, Messerli FH. Isolated systolic hypertension: an update after SPRINT. *Am J Med.* 2016;129(12):1251–1258. doi: 10.1016/j.amjmed.2016.08.032.

Benetos A, Bulpitt CJ, Petrovic M, et al. An expert opinion from the European Society of Hypertension-European Union Geriatric Medicine Society Working Group on the management of hypertension in very old, frail subjects. *Hypertension.* 2016;67(5):820–825. doi: 10.1161/HYPERTENSIONAHA.115.07020.

Benetos A, Petrovic M, Strandberg T. Hypertension management in older and frail older patients. *Circ Res.* 2019;124(7):1045–1060. doi: 10.1161/CIRCRESAHA.118.313236.

Butt DA, Harvey PJ. Benefits and risks of antihypertensive medications in the elderly. *J Intern Med.* 2015;278(6):599–626. doi: 10.1111/joim.12446.

Chirinos JA, Segers P, Hughes T, Townsend R. Large-artery stiffness in health and disease: JACC state-of-the-art review. *J Am Coll Cardiol.* 2019;74(9):1237–1263. doi: 10.1016/j.jacc.2019.07.012.

Clark CE, Taylor RS, Shore AC, Campbell JL. Prevalence of systolic inter-arm differences in blood pressure for different primary care populations: systematic review and meta-analysis. *Br J Gen Pract.* 2016;66(652):e838–e847. doi: 10.3399/bjgp16X687553.

Duchier J, Iannascoli F, Safar M. Antihypertensive effect of sustained-release isosorbide dinitrate for isolated systolic systemic hypertension in the elderly. *Am J Cardiol.* 1987;60(1):99–102. doi: 10.1016/0002-9149(87)90993-3.

Elijovich F, Weinberger MH, Anderson CA, et al. Salt sensitivity of blood pressure: a scientific statement from the American Heart Association. *Hypertension.* 2016;68(3):e7–e46. doi: 10.1161/HYP.0000000000000047.

Ernst ME, MacLaughlin EJ. From clinical trials to bedside: the use of antihypertensives in aged individuals. Part 2: approach to treatment. *Curr Hypertens Rep.* 2019;21(11):83. doi: 10.1007/s11906-019-0988-x.

Flack JM, Yunis C, Preisser J, et al. The rapidity of drug dose escalation influences blood pressure response and adverse effects burden in patients with hypertension: the Quinapril Titration Interval Management Evaluation (ATIME) Study. ATIME Research Group. *Arch Intern Med.* 2000;160(12):1842–1847. doi: 10.1001/archinte.160.12.1842.

Franklin SS, Gokhale SS, Chow VH, et al. Does low diastolic blood pressure contribute to the risk of recurrent hypertensive cardiovascular disease events? The Framingham Heart Study. *Hypertension.* 2015;65(2):299–305. doi: 10.1161/HYPERTENSIONAHA.114.04581.

Franklin SS, Jacobs MJ, Wong ND, L'Italien GJ, Lapuerta P. Predominance of isolated systolic hypertension among middle-aged and elderly US hypertensives: analysis based on National Health and Nutrition Examination Survey (NHANES) III. *Hypertension.* 2001;37(3):869–874. doi: 10.1161/01.hyp.37.3.869.

Franklin SS, Thijs L, Hansen TW, et al. Significance of white-coat hypertension in older persons with isolated systolic hypertension: a meta-analysis using the International Database on Ambulatory Blood Pressure Monitoring in Relation to Cardiovascular Outcomes population. *Hypertension.* 2012;59(3):564–571. doi: 10.1161/HYPERTENSIONAHA.111.180653.

Hughes D, Judge C, Murphy R, et al. Association of blood pressure lowering with incident dementia or cognitive impairment: a systematic review and meta-analysis. *JAMA.* 2020;323(19):1934–1944. doi: 10.1001/jama.2020.4249.

Lindholm LH, Carlberg B, Samuelsson O. Should beta blockers remain first choice in the treatment of primary hypertension? A meta-analysis. *Lancet.* 2005;366(9496):1545–1553. doi: 10.1016/S0140-6736(05)67573-3.

MacLaughlin EJ, Ernst ME. From clinical trials to bedside: the use of antihypertensives in aged individuals. Part 1: evaluation and evidence of treatment benefit. *Curr Hypertens Rep.* 2019;21(11):82. doi: 10.1007/s11906-019-0987-y.

Muntner P, Hardy ST, Fine LJ, et al. Trends in blood pressure control among US adults with hypertension, 1999-2000 to 2017-2018. *JAMA.* 2020;324(12):1190–1200. doi: 10.1001/jama.2020.14545.

Oliver JJ, Hughes VE, Dear JW, Webb DJ. Clinical potential of combined organic nitrate and phosphodiesterase type 5 inhibitor in treatment-resistant hypertension. *Hypertension.* 2010;56(1):62–67. doi: 10.1161/HYPERTENSIONAHA.109.147686.

Ritchey MD, Gillespie C, Wozniak G, et al. Potential need for expanded pharmacologic treatment and lifestyle modification services under the 2017 ACC/AHA hypertension guideline. *J Clin Hypertens (Greenwich).* 2018;20(10):1377–1391. doi: 10.1111/jch.13364.

Ruilope LM, Dukat A, Bohm M, Lacourciere Y, Gong J, Lefkowitz MP. Blood-pressure reduction with LCZ696, a novel dual-acting inhibitor of the angiotensin II receptor and neprilysin: a randomised, double-blind, placebo-controlled, active comparator study. *Lancet.* 2010;375(9722):1255–1266. doi: 10.1016/S0140-6736(09)61966-8.

SHEP Investigators. Prevention of stroke by antihypertensive drug treatment in older persons with isolated systolic hypertension. Final results of the Systolic Hypertension in the Elderly Program (SHEP). SHEP Cooperative Research Group. *JAMA.* 1991;265(24):3255–3264.

Sobieraj P, Lewandowski J, Sinski M. Low on-treatment diastolic blood pressure is not independently associated with increased cardiovascular risk: an analysis of the SPRINT trial. *Eur Heart J.* 2019;40(25):2094–2095. doi: 10.1093/eurheartj/ehz225.

Sprint Mind Investigators for the SPRINT Research Group, Nasrallah IM, Pajewski NM, et al. Association of intensive vs standard blood pressure control with cerebral white matter lesions. *JAMA.* 2019;322(6):524–534. doi: 10.1001/jama.2019.10551.

Sprint Mind Investigators for the SPRINT Research Group, Williamson JD, Pajewski NM, et al. Effect of intensive vs standard blood pressure control on probable dementia: a randomized clinical trial. *JAMA.* 2019;321(6):553–561. doi: 10.1001/jama.2018.21442.

Staessen JA, Fagard R, Thijs L, et al. Randomised double-blind comparison of placebo and active treatment for older patients with isolated systolic hypertension. The Systolic Hypertension in Europe (Syst-Eur) Trial Investigators. *Lancet.* 1997;350(9080):757–764. doi: 10.1016/s0140-6736(97)05381-6.

Stokes GS, Bune AJ, Huon N, Barin ES. Long-term effectiveness of extended-release nitrate for the treatment of systolic hypertension. *Hypertension.* 2005;45(3):380–384. doi: 10.1161/01.HYP.0000156746.25300.1c.

Thomopoulos C, Parati G, Zanchetti A. Effects of blood pressure-lowering treatment on cardiovascular outcomes and mortality: 13 - benefits and adverse events in older and younger patients with hypertension: overview, meta-analyses and meta-regression analyses of randomized trials. *J Hypertens.* 2018;36(8):1622–1636. doi: 10.1097/HJH.0000000000001787.

Wang YC, Shimbo D, Muntner P, Moran AE, Krakoff LR, Schwartz JE. Prevalence of masked hypertension among US adults with nonelevated clinic blood pressure. *Am J Epidemiol*. 2017;185(3):194–202. doi: 10.1093/aje/kww237.

Whelton PK, Carey RM, Aronow WS, et al. 2017 ACC/AHA/AAPA/ABC/ACPM/AGS/APhA/ASH/ASPC/NMA/PCNA Guideline for the prevention, detection, evaluation, and management of high blood pressure in adults: executive summary: a report of the American College of Cardiology/American Heart Association task force on clinical practice guidelines. *Hypertension*. 2018;71(6):1269–1324. doi: 10.1161/HYP.0000000000000066.

White WB, Wakefield DB, Moscufo N, et al. Effects of intensive versus standard ambulatory blood pressure control on cerebrovascular outcomes in older people (INFINITY). *Circulation*. 2019;140(20):1626–1635. doi: 10.1161/CIRCULATIONAHA.119.041603.

Williams B, Cockcroft JR, Kario K, et al. Effects of Sacubitril/valsartan versus olmesartan on central hemodynamics in the elderly with systolic hypertension: the PARAMETER study. *Hypertension*. 2017;69(3):411–420. doi: 10.1161/HYPERTENSIONAHA.116.08556.

Williams B, Mancia G, Spiering W, et al. 2018 ESC/ESH guidelines for the management of arterial hypertension. *Eur Heart J*. 2018;39(33):3021–3104. doi: 10.1093/eurheartj/ehy339.

Williamson JD, Supiano MA, Applegate WB, et al. Intensive vs standard blood pressure control and cardiovascular disease outcomes in adults aged >/ = 75 years: a randomized clinical trial. *JAMA*. 2016;315(24):2673–2682. doi: 10.1001/jama.2016.7050.

Wimmer BC, Cross AJ, Jokanovic N, et al. Clinical outcomes associated with medication regimen complexity in older people: a systematic review. *J Am Geriatr Soc*. 2017;65(4):747–753. doi: 10.1111/jgs.14682.

CHAPTER 23

HYPERTENSION IN PREGNANCY

Cassandra Kovach, MD, and Anna Burgner, MD

QUESTIONS

1. **How does pregnancy normally affect blood pressure?**
   Renin, angiotensin, and aldosterone are all increased in normal pregnancy so you might predict blood pressure (BP) would increase. However, systolic blood pressure (SBP) and diastolic blood pressure (DBP) are both significantly lower as early as 6 to 7 weeks from the last menstrual period, suggesting that these hormonal changes are secondary. Arterial pressure usually declines until 24 to 26 weeks, gestation and then slowly increases, returning to prepregnancy levels postpartum. Venous pressures do not change during pregnancy. Supine hypotension occurs in about 10% of pregnant women due to compression of the great vessels by the uterus in the supine position.

   Renin is produced by the woman's kidneys and by the placenta. Angiotensinogen is produced by the maternal liver in larger amounts during pregnancy due to estrogen production, and the fetal liver also produces angiotensinogen. However, pregnant women become refractory to angiotensin II due to increased progesterone, and this effect is lost within 15 to 30 minutes after placenta delivery.

2. **Describe the classification of hypertension disorders that occur in pregnancy.**
   Table 23.1 defines the blood pressure disorders in pregnancy.

Table 23.1 Hypertension disorders in pregnancy.

Disorder	Definition
Preeclampsia-eclampsia	Preeclampsia—new onset of hypertension (SBP $\geq$140 or DBP $\geq$90 mm Hg) and proteinuria or end-organ dysfunction with onset after 20 weeks' gestation. Eclampsia—preeclampsia with superimposed seizures.
Chronic (preexisting) hypertension	Hypertension that is present before pregnancy, before the 20th week of pregnancy, or persists longer than 12 weeks' postpartum.
Preeclampsia-eclampsia superimposed upon chronic hypertension	Chronic hypertension that worsens during pregnancy and is associated with proteinuria or other end-organ damage.
Gestational hypertension	New onset of hypertension (SBP $\geq$140 or DBP $\geq$90) on two occasions at least 4 hours apart) detected after 20 weeks' gestation in the absence of other features of preeclampsia and resolves by 12 weeks' postpartum.

3. **When should secondary causes of hypertension be considered as the cause of hypertension in pregnancy?**
   Secondary causes of hypertension should be considered in pregnancy when the woman has difficulty to control BP requiring three or more medications, hypertension diagnosed at a younger age, sudden onset hypertension, hypokalemia, an abdominal bruit, symptoms of obstructive sleep apnea, substance use, clinical features of hypercortisolism, or a lack of lifestyle factors that put them at risk for high BP (obesity, high sodium diet, or decreased physical activity). The main secondary causes of hypertension are primary hyperaldosteronism, pheochromocytoma, renal artery stenosis (primarily from fibromuscular dysplasia in this group of patients), Cushing syndrome, and obstructive sleep apnea. Women with secondary causes of hypertension are at higher risks for adverse outcomes in pregnancy.

4. **How do you diagnose preeclampsia?**
   Preeclampsia carries an increased risk of maternal and neonatal morbidity and mortality, so proper diagnosis and expert care is of utmost importance for the health of both the mother and infant. The diagnosis of preeclampsia requires the following criteria (ACOG, 2020):

Blood Pressure as Defined by:

- SBP of 140 mm Hg or more OR DBP of 90 mm Hg or more on two occasions at least 4 hours apart after 20 weeks' gestation in a woman with previously normal BP
- SBP of 160 mm Hg or more OR DBP of 110 mm Hg or more on two occasions within minutes

AND Either Proteinuria as Defined as One of the Following:

- 300 mg or more per 24-hour urine collection
- Protein/creatinine ratio of 0.3 or more
- Dipstick reading of 2+ (used only if other quantitative methods not available)

OR Evidence of End-Organ Damage as Defined by One of the Following:

- Platelets $<100 \times 10^9$/L
- Serum creatinine >1.1 mg/dL or a double of the serum creatinine in the absence of other kidney disease
- Liver transaminases $2\times$ the upper limit of normal (aspartate aminotransferase [AST] is increased more than alanine aminotransferase [ALT])
- Pulmonary edema
- Cerebral or visual symptoms (new onset headache unresponsive to medication and not accounted for by alternative diagnoses, blurred vision, flashing lights)

Adapted from American College of Obstetricians and Gynecologists (ACOG). Practice Bulletin No. 222: Gestational hypertension and preeclampsia. *Obstet Gynecol.* 2020; 135(6): e237-e260.

Severe features of preeclampsia include:
- SBP over 160 mm Hg OR DBP over 110 mm Hg on two occasions at least 4 hours apart
- Platelets less than 100×10^9/L
- Transaminases greater than $2\times$ the upper limit of normal and severe persistent right upper quadrant or epigastric pain unresponsive to medication and not accounted for by alternative diagnosis
- Serum creatinine greater than 1.1 mg/dL or doubling of serum creatinine in the absence of other kidney disease
- Pulmonary edema
- New-onset headache unresponsive to medication and not accounted for by alternative diagnoses
- Visual disturbances

Eclampsia is preeclampsia plus seizures.

Other serious disorders can present similarly to preeclampsia and need to be considered before diagnosing preeclampsia, including thrombotic thrombocytopenic purpura, hemolytic-uremic syndrome, molar pregnancy, underlying kidney disease, or autoimmune disease. If the clinical features are present before 20 weeks' gestation or if atypical features are present, one of these other causes should be considered.

Importantly, preeclampsia can also be diagnosed postpartum. Most cases of postpartum preeclampsia develop within 48 hours of delivery, but it can develop as late as 6 weeks after childbirth.

5. **What is HELLP syndrome?**

HELLP stands for Hemolysis, Elevated Liver enzymes, and Low Platelet count. HELLP syndrome is probably a severe form of preeclampsia, although the relationship is controversial. It is associated with increased rates of morbidity and mortality. The following criteria make the diagnosis:
- Lactate dehydrogenase of 600 IU/L or greater
- AST and ALT elevated greater than $2\times$ the upper limit of normal
- Platelets less than 100×10^9/L

HELLP syndrome usually occurs in the third trimester, but it can also occur postpartum. The typical presenting symptoms include right upper quadrant pain, generalized malaise, and nausea and vomiting. In about 15% of the cases, either hypertension or proteinuria is not present.

6. **What are risk factors for developing preeclampsia?**

High-Risk Factors for Preeclampsia	Moderate-Risk Factors for Preeclampsia
Previous pregnancy with preeclampsia	First pregnancy
Multifetal gestation	Maternal age of 35 years or older
Chronic kidney disease	Body mass index more than 30
Autoimmune disease	Family history of preeclampsia
Type 1 or type 2 diabetes mellitus	
Chronic hypertension	

7. What is currently known about the pathogenesis of preeclampsia?

Preeclampsia develops because of maternal and fetal/placental factors. Placental vasculature appears to develop abnormally early in pregnancy, which leads to placental ischemia. Placental ischemia then causes the release of antiangiogenic factors into the maternal circulation, which affects maternal endothelial function. Although the exact causes and mechanisms of these events is unknown, preeclampsia is characterized by consistent pathologic and laboratory abnormalities.

Abnormal spiral artery remodeling and trophoblast invasion are characteristic findings in hypertension disorders of pregnancy. Normally, spiral artery remodeling is completed by 20 weeks' gestation and results in the spiral arteries being large capacitance vessels with low resistance, which facilitates blood flow to the placenta. In preeclampsia, this spiral artery remodeling is abnormal; the vessels remain small and narrow, and placental ischemia occurs.

A normal placenta produces a balance between proangiogenic (VEGF, PIGF) and antiangiogenic (sFlt-1, soluble endoglin) factors. In preeclampsia, systemic levels of sFlt-1 and endoglin are increased. In animal studies, an increase in sFlt-1 causes endothelial damage, vascular oxidative stress, vasoconstriction, and increased sensitivity to angiotensin II, and endoglin overexpression leads to increased vascular permeability and modest hypertension without proteinuria. Overexpression of sFlt-1 and endoglin causes severe vascular damage, nephrotic-range proteinuria, severe hypertension, HELLP syndrome, and fetal growth restriction in pregnant rats.

Immunologic factors, genetic factors, environmental factors (low calcium intake and obesity), inflammation, increased sensitivity to angiotensin II, and complement activation also are felt to potentially play a role.

8. What can be done to prevent preeclampsia?

Low-dose aspirin in women at moderate or high risk for preeclampsia has been shown to decrease the frequency of preeclampsia and its gestational complications. Therefore women with at least one high-risk factor for preeclampsia or women with at least two of the moderate-risk factors for preeclampsia should start low-dose (81 mg/day) aspirin for preeclampsia prophylaxis between 12 and 28 weeks' gestation (ideally before 16 weeks' gestation), and it should be continued until delivery. Although low-dose aspirin is safe, high-dose aspirin or other nonsteroidal antiinflammatory agents (e.g., ibuprofen, naproxen) should be avoided in pregnancy due to the risk of premature closure of the ductus arteriosus.

9. What can be done to treat preeclampsia?

The definitive treatment of preeclampsia is delivery. Treatment of severe hypertension can reduce the typical cardiovascular complications of hypertension but does not address the underlying pathophysiology of preeclampsia and does not prevent progression of disease. The decision of whether to deliver or do expectant management is dependent on gestational age, severity of preeclampsia, and maternal and fetal condition.

For women at term (37+0 weeks' gestation), the treatment is delivery. Preeclampsia alone is not an indication for cesarean delivery, and these patients can deliver vaginally unless they have the usual obstetric indications for cesarean section.

For women who are late preterm (34+0–36+6 weeks' gestation), expectant management is recommended unless they have features of severe preeclampsia or standard obstetric indications for earlier delivery. Delivery is recommended once they reach 37+0 weeks' gestation.

For women who are early preterm (<34 weeks' gestation), expectant management is generally recommended unless they have features of severe preeclampsia or standard obstetric indications for earlier delivery. However, some data suggests that even those with severe features can be treated expectantly as long as maternal and fetal conditions are stable. Delivery is recommended once they reach 37+0 weeks' gestation.

Expectant management includes laboratory monitoring (platelet count, liver function tests, kidney function tests), BP monitoring, assessment of maternal symptoms, and evaluation of fetal growth and well-being.

Antihypertensive medications are given for persistently elevated SBP of 160 mm Hg or higher or DBP of 110 mm Hg or higher to prevent stroke. Treating hypertension does not prevent eclampsia. Giving antihypertensives for SBP less than 160 mm Hg and DBP less than 110 mm Hg does not decrease morbidity or mortality.

Seizure prophylaxis is recommended for women with severe preeclampsia intrapartum and postpartum, and is frequently done for those without severe features despite no clear consensus. The first-line treatment for seizure prophylaxis is magnesium.

Women with preeclampsia are at risk for serious complications following delivery. There is no standardized approach to postpartum maternal monitoring and follow up, but it is generally recommended that these women have close monitoring of BP for at least 72 hours after delivery, often as an inpatient. Persistent, severe hypertension should be treated, and patients may require antihypertensives after discharge.

10. What are potential complications of preeclampsia?

Sixteen percent of maternal deaths can be attributed to hypertensive disorders. The mortality rate for women with preeclampsia or eclampsia is estimated to be up to 1.8% in developed countries, and the fetal death rate in developed countries has been reported to be as high as 11.8%.

In the long-term, women with preeclampsia are at risk for recurrent preeclampsia with future pregnancies, development of chronic kidney disease (including an increased risk for development of end-stage renal disease), chronic hypertension, and ischemic heart disease.

11. **What is the target BP in pregnant patients?**
    There is no high-quality clinical evidence to guide us in target BP in pregnant patients. The American College of Obstetricians and Gynecologists (ACOG) guidelines recommend the initiation of antihypertensive medications for chronic hypertension, gestational hypertension, or preeclampsia when SBP is 160 mm Hg or higher and/or DBP is 110 mm Hg or higher. Tight BP control does not reduce the risk of pregnancy loss, high-level neonatal care, or overall maternal complications. Less-tight control is associated with a significantly higher frequency of severe maternal hypertension.

    If there is evidence of end-organ damage, antihypertensive treatment is recommended at lower thresholds, usually SBP less than 150 mm Hg and DBP less than 100 mm Hg, to reduce the risk of further end-organ damage or hemorrhagic stroke.

    There is no data regarding the decision to continue or discontinue therapy for women with chronic hypertension with SBP less than 160 mm Hg or DBP less than 110 mm Hg who were receiving antihypertensive medications prior to pregnancy.

12. **Which antihypertensive agents have acceptable safety profiles to be used in pregnancy?**
    All antihypertensive agents cross the placenta, and there is not adequate data to recommend one antihypertensive over another. The most commonly used antihypertensive agents that are considered to have acceptable safety profiles in pregnancy include methyldopa, labetalol, and nifedipine. Other agents that are used less frequently because of their side effects but are generally considered safe in pregnancy include hydralazine, thiazide diuretics, and clonidine.

    Methyldopa takes 3 to 6 hours to work so it should not be used to lower BP acutely, and often it is dose limited due to its sedative side effects at higher doses.

    There has been conflicting data as to whether beta-blockers are associated with congenital birth defects; however, a recent international metaanalysis is reassuring. Labetalol's onset of action is typically less than 2 hours and can be used to acutely lower BP. It has been associated with maternal hepatotoxicity, which is typically reversible. Metoprolol and pindolol are also considered acceptable alternatives; however, nonselective beta-adrenergic blockers (propranolol) are typically avoided as well as beta-adrenergic blockers that lack alpha-blocking properties (atenolol).

    Extended-release nifedipine is considered to be safe in pregnancy. Immediate-release nifedipine, which typically has an onset of action within 10 minutes as opposed to an hour with the extended-release, is endorsed by ACOG for emergent treatment of severe hypertension. However, tachycardia and headache are common and the duration of action is short. There is less data to support the use of amlodipine or the nondihydropyridine calcium antagonists during pregnancy, although it is generally thought that their use is safe.

    Hydralazine is often used in acute hypertension in pregnancy; however, because it can cause reflex tachycardia and fluid retention, it is less useful chronically.

    Thiazide diuretic use during pregnancy is controversial; there is a theoretic risk of intravascular volume depletion from diuretics leading to fetal growth restriction or oligohydramnios, although this has not been born out in study. Thiazides can be continued in those who were taking it prior to pregnancy.

    Clonidine works similarly to methyldopa and is considered safe in pregnancy; however, given the rebound hypertension that can develop if it is stopped suddenly, its use is typically limited.

13. **Which antihypertensive agents should be avoided in pregnancy?**
    Angiotensin-converting enzyme (ACE) inhibitors, angiotensin II receptor blockers (ARBs), direct renin inhibitors (DRIs), mineralocorticoid receptor antagonists, and nitroprusside should be avoided in pregnancy.

    ACE inhibitors, ARBs, and DRIs, when given in the first trimester, are associated with an increase in congenital malformations, particularly of congenital heart disease and central nervous system malformations. When given in the second and third trimester, these agents can cause kidney failure, kidney dysplasia, hypotension, oligohydramnios, fetal growth restriction, pulmonary hypoplasia, stillbirth, and neonatal death.

    Spironolactone is a concern due to its antiandrogen activity, and there has been a case report of ambiguous genitalia in the newborn of a mother treated with spironolactone. Eplerenone has not been studied enough to draw a conclusion on its safety. Nitroprusside is the last resort for management of refractory severe hypertension and should only be used in emergencies because of its risk of fetal cyanide poisoning.

14. **What considerations to type of antihypertensive agents should be made in breastfeeding women?**
    Beta-adrenergic blockers and calcium channel blockers enter breast milk but appear to be safe during lactation. There is a concern that diuretics may decrease milk production. Table 23.2 lists common agents and their effects on infants receiving breastmilk.

Table 23.2 Antihypertensive Medications in Breastfeeding Women

No Known Adverse Effects on Infants Receiving Breastmilk:

Atenolol
Captopril
Enalapril
Hydrochlorothiazide
Labetalol
Metoprolol
Nifedipine
Spironolactone

Insufficient Safety Evidence to Recommend Use in Breastfeeding Mothers:

Angiotensin receptor blockers
Amlodipine
Angiotensin converting enzyme inhibitors other than enalapril and captopril
Chlorthalidone
Clonidine
Doxazosin
Eplerenone
Indapamide

Not Recommended:

Methyldopa—considered safe for newborns, but, given its association with maternal depression, its use is not typically recommended for postpartum women

KEY POINTS

1. During normal pregnancy both the SBP and DBP are significantly lower than baseline.
2. Low-dose daily aspirin is the only thing that has been shown to reduce the likelihood of the development of preeclampsia.
3. Preeclampsia leads to increased morbidity and mortality both in the short and long term.
4. ACE inhibitors, ARBs, and DRIs should be avoided during pregnancy.

BIBLIOGRAPHY

Abalos E, Duley L, Steyn DW. Antihypertensive drug therapy for mild to moderate hypertension during pregnancy. *Cochrane Database Syst Rev.* 2014;(2):CD002252.

American College of Obstetricians and Gynecologists. Emergent therapy for acute-onset, severe hypertension during pregnancy and the postpartum period. ACOG committee opinion No. 767. *Obstet Gynecol.* 2019.

American College of Obstetricians and Gynecologists (ACOG). Practice Bulletin No. 222: gestational hypertension and preeclampsia. *Obstet Gynecol.* 2020;135(6):e237–e260.

American College of Obstetricians and Gynecologists (ACOG). Practice Bulletin No. 203: chronic hypertension in pregnancy. *Obstet Gynecol.* 2019;133:e26–e50.

Beardmore KS, Morris JM, Gallery ED. Excretion of antihypertensive medications into human breast milk: a systematic review. *Hypertens Pregnancy.* 2002;21(1):85.

Douglas KA, Redman CWG. Eclampsia in the United Kingdom. *BMJ.* 1994;309:1395.

Fitton CA, et al. In-utero exposure to antihypertensive medication and neonatal and child health outcomes: a systematic review. *J Hypertens.* 2017 Nov;35(11):2123–2137.

Kattah AG, Garovic VD. The management of hypertension in pregnancy. *Adv Chronic Kidney Dis.* 2013;20(3):229–239.

Khan KS, Wojdyla D, Say L, Gulmezoglu AM, Van Look PFA. WHO analysis of causes of maternal death: a systematic review. *Lancet.* 2006;367:1066–1074.

Maternal physiology. In: Cunningham F, Leveno KJ, Bloom SL, et al., eds. *Williams Obstetrics.* 25th ed. New York, NY: McGraw-Hill; 2018. http://accessmedicine.mhmedical.com/content.aspx?bookid=1918&sectionid=144754618. Accessed February 23, 2020.

Roberge S, Nicolaides K, Demers S, Hyett J, Chaillet N, Bujold E. The role of aspirin dose on the prevention of preeclampsia and fetal growth restriction: systematic review and meta-analysis. *Am J Obstet Gynecol.* 2017;216:110–20e6.

Smith M, Waugh J, Nelson-Piercy C. Management of postpartum hypertension. *Obstet Gynaecol.* 2013;15:45–50.

CHAPTER 24

HYPERTENSION IN HEART DISEASE

Simon W. Rabkin, MD, FRCPC, FESC, FACC

QUESTIONS

TREATMENT OF HYPERTENSION IN PATIENTS WITH CORONARY ARTERY DISEASE AND STABLE ANGINA PECTORIS

1. **How does hypertension and its management contribute to coronary artery disease?**
   There is overwhelming evidence that hypertension plays a role in the development of coronary atherosclerosis. Furthermore, there is abundant evidence that the treatment of hypertension reduces the development of the adverse consequences of coronary artery disease (CAD) including myocardial infarction and heart failure.

   There are data from 22,672 patients with stable CAD who were enrolled in the ProspeCtive observational LongitudinAl Reglstry oF patients with stable coronary arterY disease (CLARIFY) registry that included patients from 45 countries who were treated for hypertension. The primary outcome was the composite of cardiovascular death, myocardial infarction, or stroke. Increased systolic blood pressure (SBP) of 140 mm Hg or more and diastolic blood pressure (DBP) of 80 mm Hg or more were each associated with increased risk of cardiovascular events. Blood pressure (BP) targeted to less than 140 mm Hg systolic and less than or equal to 80 mm Hg diastolic is suggested.

2. **What drugs are recommended for the treatment of hypertension in patients with CAD?**
   The principle of utilizing a single drug that would address hypertension and angina pectoris has led to guideline recommendations for the use of beta-blockers or calcium channel blockers (CCBs). Some recommendations prefer beta-blockers as the first choice based on the greater amount of data on cardio protection for beta-blockers that arises from the use of beta-blockers in myocardial infarction. The use of either agent as first-line therapy has also gained credibility because of the lower antihypertensive efficacy of beta-blockers in older individuals who are usually in the age group with a greater prevalence of patients with CAD. Other antihypertensive agents can be utilized for hypertension management except for hydralazine, which has the potential to produce a reflex tachycardia and potentially precipitate myocardial ischemia.

3. **What are the determinants of coronary artery blood flow, and how would this impact your management of patients with hypertension and CAD?**
   Coronary (artery) blood flow (CBF) usually occurs during diastole and is dependent on or determined by myocardial perfusion pressure (MPP), which is a function of (1) DBP, (2) the degree of coronary stenosis, which determines MPP distal to the stenosis, and (3) the resistive properties of the coronary vascular bed. The myocardium exerts an extravascular pressure on the intramural coronary vasculature to reduce CBF. Coronary artery resistance is affected by circulating neurohumoral factors and the autonomic nervous system, as well as factors released by circulating elements such as platelets.

   The presence of CAD leading to coronary artery narrowing or stenosis reduces CBF significantly after the degree of stenosis exceeds 80%. Myocardial (oxygen) demands influence symptoms so that increased physical exercise will increase myocardial oxygen requirements in excess of the ability of the stenotic artery to increase myocardial blood flow, producing myocardial ischemia or angina pectoris.

4. **How would consideration of the determinants of CBF impact your management of patients with hypertension and CAD?**
   Patients with hypertension and CAD have a range of degrees of coronary artery stenosis that is often not known at the time of treatment. Specifically, does the patient have a 70%, 80%, or 90% stenosis in one or several coronary arteries? In a patient group with moderate coronary artery stenosis, a direct measurement of MPP, the coronary artery pressure distal to the stenosis, was used to estimate CBF at different potential levels of DBP. DBP of 60 mm Hg or less was associated with unacceptably low MPPs and CBF. As the degree of coronary stenosis is unknown in most patients with hypertension and CAD, clinicians should be cautioned about the potential for myocardial ischemia at low DBP.

5. **Does the data on low DBP extend to clinical trial data?**
   In a post hoc analysis of a large clinical trial treating 22,576 patients with hypertension and CAD (INternational VErapamil SR Trandolapril STudy, INVEST), the relationship between BP and the primary outcome, all-cause death, and total myocardial infarction (MI) was J-shaped, particularly for diastolic pressure, with a nadir at

119/84 mm Hg. There were substantially more myocardial infarctions than strokes with low BPs. Their data suggest that it is due to the severity of CAD because low DBP was associated with relatively less risk for adverse outcomes in patients who have had revascularization compared to those without revascularization.

6. **What is the impact of left ventricular hypertrophy on CBF in hypertension?**
   In a metaanalysis of studies that directly measured CBF in patients with hypertension and left ventricular hypertrophy (LVH), there was a significant and 2.9-fold higher CBF in hypertension. The increase in CBF was due to the increase in left ventricular (LV) mass because metaanalysis showed a significant decrease in CBF per gram of LV mass in hypertension. There was a significant inverse correlation between LV mass and CBF per gram of LV mass. In contrast to pathological LVH produced by hypertension, physiological LVH produced by exercise training is associated with a greater CBF per gram of LV mass. These data suggest that patients with hypertension are at greater risk for myocardial ischemia should they develop other factors that limit CBF or myocardial oxygen delivery such as coronary disease.

   LVH in the setting of isolated systolic hypertension is characterized by an increased pulse pressure caused by reduced aortic compliance; the accompanying reduction in diastolic pressure will result in a lower coronary flow reserve, as myocardial perfusion occurs primarily in diastole. One can develop an approach to treatment of patients with hypertension and CAD considering the presence of LVH.

7. **Why are patients with aortic regurgitation and accompanied increase in SBP and markedly reduced DBP not experiencing major myocardial ischemia?**
   Aortic regurgitation (AR) is associated with a significant increase in the amount of stroke volume or forward blood flow, which includes CBF that occurs during systole and a decrease in the amount of blood flow that occurrs in diastole. The ratio of systolic/diastolic myocardial blood flow is increased. The increase in systolic systemic arterial blood flow in AR is responsible for the increase in systolic CBF. CBF is reduced in diastole because of lowered DBP, but this is compensated for by the increase in CBF during systole. Increased systolic CBF is the mechanism whereby CBF is maintained in severe AR. (This explanation is valid when there is no associated severe CAD.)

HYPERTENSION IN PATIENTS WITH ACUTE CORONARY SYNDROMES

8. **What is the impact of hypertension on the prognosis of patients with acute myocardial infarction, and does antihypertensive drug treatment alter the prognosis?**
   Hypertension is an indicator of an adverse prognosis for patients with acute myocardial infarction. Antihypertensive drug treatment reduces the risk of cardiac complications. The choice of agents involved are beta-blockers and angiotensin-converting enzyme (ACE) inhibitors (ACEis). If the patient is hemodynamically stable, the recommendations are:
   - a short-acting β1-selective beta-blocker without intrinsic sympathomimetic activity, such as metoprolol tartrate,
   - an ACEi, especially in a patient with an anterior myocardial infarction with LV dysfunction,
   - a diuretic, especially if there is pulmonary venous congestion,
   - nitroglycerin, especially if there is ongoing chest pain.

   The data are convincing. Placebo control trials permit an examination of the effect of hypertension in the absence of treatment during myocardial infarction. For example, in the placebo-controlled trial of ramipril following acute myocardial infarction, Acute Infarction Ramipril Efficacy (AIRE), antecedent hypertension was a significant indicator of adverse prognosis in the placebo-treated patients (hazard ratio 1.49). In contrast, ramipril-treated patients did not have a significant increase in overall adverse outcomes. A similar pattern was observed for the risks of sudden death and severe/resistant heart failure. These data are consistent with a retrospective analysis of data from the Trandolapril Cardiac Event (TRACE) study, that randomized patients with acute myocardial infarction and heart failure (ejection fraction $\leq$35%) to trandolapril or placebo 3 to 7 days after the infarction. Treatment with trandolapril resulted in a relative risk of death from any cause for the hypertensive patients of 0.59 (compared to 0.85 in normotensive patients).

   Microvascular changes induced by hypertension may play a role in the adverse effect of hypertension in acute myocardial infarction. A history of hypertension in patients with acute ST-elevation myocardial infarction (STEMI) is independently associated with less improvement in LV systolic function (especially in women), a propensity to heart failure, and an increased risk of all-cause events. Hypertensive-induced vascular disease, which leads to an increase in myocardial hemorrhage reflecting severe microvascular injury, was postulated as an explanation for the adverse effect of hypertension.

TREATMENT OF HYPERTENSION IN PATIENTS WITH HEART FAILURE

9. **What is the main current way to categorize heart failure?**
   Heart failure is categorized as heart failure with a:
   - reduced ejection fraction (HFrEF; i.e., LV ejection fraction of 40% or less),
   - preserved ejection fraction (HFpEF) normal ejection fraction, (i.e., LV ejection fraction of 50% or greater),
   - mid-ranged reduction in LV ejection fraction (HFmEF; i.e., LV ejection fraction of 41% to 49%).

This categorization is useful when considering the clinical trials data on drugs that have been shown to be effective in management of heart failure. There is, however, controversy whether HFmEF is simply a transition state to HFrEF.

10. **Which drugs are useful in lowering BP and reducing cardiovascular mortality in patients with hypertension and heart failure, and which drugs are not?**

A. **Heart failure with reduced ejection fraction**

Hypertension is a major factor responsible for heart failure. Most clinical trials of drugs in the management of heart failure have a high proportion of individuals with hypertension. Most agents that are useful in heart failure are the agents that lower BP. Thus it is usually agreed that these agents should be used in patients with hypertension and heart failure. It is not simply BP reduction that is useful in chronic heart failure as there are some antihypertensive agents that do not lower mortality in patients with heart failure so that the general recommendation has been to use agents with demonstrated efficacy to reduce cardiovascular (all-cause preferably) mortality as well as the morbidity of hospital readmissions. Treating physicians need to be aware of antihypertensive drugs and their effect not only on BP but also on morbidity and mortality in selecting medications and to utilize.

1. Agents that effectively lower both BP and mortality in heart failure:
   - ACEis or angiotensin-receptor blockers (ARBs).
   - Beta-blockers. The effectiveness of beta-blockers to lower BP in heart failure is not high but their effect to lower mortality has been consistently demonstrated.
   - Mineralocorticoid receptor antagonists (MRAs), especially in combination with ACEis, have been demonstrated to improve outcome and reduce heart failure, as well as lower BP.
   - Angiotensin receptor plus neprilysin inhibitor (ARNI).
   - Sodium-glucose cotransporter-2 (SGLT2) inhibitors have recently been demonstrated to produce a small reduction in BP and improve cardiovascular outcomes in patients with heart failure, whether or not they have diabetes mellitus.

2. Agents that lower BP and marginally improve prognosis in the absence of ACEis/ARBs:
   - Hydralazine plus transdermal nitrates (mainly in individuals of African heritage).

3. Agents that lower BP and may not improve but do not worsen prognosis:
   - Dihydropyridine CCBs such as amlodipine.

4. Agents that lower BP and do not improve mortality or may exacerbate heart failure:
   - Nondihydropyridine CCBs such as diltiazem.
   - Alpha-blockers—prazosin, doxazosin.

5. Agents that lower BP and increase mortality (contraindicated):
   - Central sympathetic inhibition agents. Moxonidine is representative of the class of central sympathetic inhibitors and was found to increase mortality in patients with HFrEF.

A metaanalysis suggests that renin-angiotensin-aldosterone system (RAAS) inhibitors (ACEis or ARBs) achieve greater BP reduction than beta-blockers in patients with heart failure so that these agents should be used first in patients with hypertension and heart failure. The next lines of therapy are MRAs (spironolactone or eplerenone). If the patient is still in heart failure, the next step is angiotensin receptor plus ARNI, which currently is treatment with the combination of the neprilysin inhibitor sacubitril plus the ARB valsartan. This combination produced a 20% reduction in cardiovascular death and a 21% lower rehospitalization rate for patients with heart failure compared to ACE inhibition, which was usually associated with beta-blocker and MRA treatment. ARB plus ARNI treatment is associated with a higher proportion of patients with hypotension and nonserious angioedema but lower proportions with renal impairment or hyperkalemia compared with ACEi treatment.

If the patient is still hypertensive and has HFrEF, the next step involves administering agents with antihypertensive efficacy but with less or no beneficial effect on heart failure mortality, respectively hydralazine plus nitrates or the dihydropyridine CCB amlodipine. These agents are also of value in patients who have contraindications to ACEis, ARBs, MRAs, and beta-blockers.

B. **Heart failure with preserved ejection fraction**

No agent has been found to improve mortality in HFpEF yet. Sodium-glucose cotransporter-2 (SGLT2) inhibitors have recently been demonstrated to produce a small reduction in BP and improve cardiovascular outcomes in patients with HFrEF, whether or not they have diabetes mellitus, in a single trial. Other trials are soon expected to confirm these promising results. Diuretics are useful for symptomatic relief and can assist in BP reduction. Other antihypertensive agents are encouraged to be utilized in order to reduce BP and reduce the progression of HFpEF.

11. **What is the target BP for patients with heart failure and hypertension, and what is the evidence for it?**

The target BP in patients with hypertension and HFrEF has not been studied in clinical trials that treated patients to specific BP targets. Thus guidelines often encourage titrating heart failure drugs according to tolerance irrespective of achieved BP.

12. **Does the level of initial BP influence treatment with BP-lowering drugs in HFrEF?**
    This question addresses whether individuals with minimal BP elevation do not need or should not be treated with the agents in the classes listed previously. Usually this question is circumvented by the need to treat patients with HFrEF with agents that will reduce mortality and heart failure severity. However, the data suggest that the benefits of antihypertensive agents is consistent across levels of baseline of BP (i.e., patients with small BP elevations benefit from antihypertensive drug therapy).

KEY POINTS

1. The principle of utilizing a single drug that would address hypertension and angina pectoris has led to guideline recommendations for the use of beta-blockers or CCB in patients with CAD.
2. Because the degree of coronary stenosis is unknown in most patients with hypertension and CAD, clinicians should be cautioned about the potential for myocardial ischemia at low DBP.
3. It is not simply BP reduction that is useful in chronic heart failure as there are some antihypertensive agents that do not lower mortality in patients with heart failure. Thus the general recommendation has been to use agents with demonstrated efficacy to reduce cardiovascular mortality as well as the morbidity of hospital readmissions.
4. In HFrEF, guidelines often encourage titrating heart failure drugs according to tolerance, irrespective of achieved BP.

BIBLIOGRAPHY

Carrick D. Hypertension, microvascular pathology, and prognosis after an acute myocardial infarction. *Hypertension.* 2018;72(3):720–730.

Duncker DJ, Koller A, Merkus D, Canty JM. Regulation of coronary blood flow in health and ischemic heart disease. *Prog Cardiovasc Dis.* 2015;57:409–422.

Gustafsson F, Torp-Pedersen C, Kober L, Hildebrandt P. on behalf of the TRACE study group. Effect of angiotensin converting enzyme inhibition after acute myocardial infarction in patients with arterial hypertension. *J Hypertens.* 1997;15(7):793–798.

Kario K, Ferdinand KC, O'Keefe JH. Control of 24-hour blood pressure with SGLT2 inhibitors to prevent cardiovascular disease. *Prog Cardiovasc Dis.* 2020;63:249–262.

Lewington S, Clarke R, Qizilbash N, et al. Age-specific relevance of usual blood pressure to vascular mortality: a meta-analysis of individual data for one million adults in 61 prospective studies. [Erratum appears in Lancet. 2003; 361(9362):1060]. *Lancet.* 2002;360(9349):1903–1913.

McMurray JJV, Packer M, Desai AS, et al. Angiotensin–neprilysin inhibition versus enalapril in heart failure. *New Engl J Med.* 2014;371:993–1004.

Messerli FH, Mancia G, Conti CR, et al. Dogma disputed: can aggressively lowering blood pressure in hypertensive patients with coronary artery disease be dangerous? *Ann Intern Med.* 2006;144(12):884–893.

Pinho-Gomes AC, Azevedo L, Bidel Z, et al. Effects of blood pressure-lowering drugs in heart failure: a systematic review and meta-analysis of randomized controlled trials. *J Hypertens.* 2019;37(9):1757–1767.

Rabkin SW. Differences in coronary blood flow in aortic regurgitation and systemic arterial hypertension have implications for diastolic blood pressure targets: a systematic review and meta-analysis. *Clin Cardiol.* 2013;36(12):728–736.

Rabkin SW. Considerations in understanding the coronary blood flow-left ventricular mass relationship in patients with hypertension. *Curr Cardiol Rev.* 2017;13(1):75–83.

Rabkin SW, Waheed A, Poulter RS, Wood D. Myocardial perfusion pressure in patients with hypertension and coronary artery disease: implications for DBP targets in hypertension management. *J Hypertens.* 2013;31(5):975–982.

Spargias K, Ball S, Hall A. The prognostic significance of a history of systemic hypertension in patients randomised to either placebo or ramipril following acute myocardial infarction: evidence from the AIRE study. Acute Infarction Ramipril Efficacy. *J Hum Hypertens.* 1999;13(8):511–516.

Vidal-Petiot E, Ford I, Greenlaw N, et al. CLARIFY Investigators. Cardiovascular event rates and mortality according to achieved systolic and diastolic blood pressure in patients with stable coronary artery disease: an international cohort study. *Lancet.* 2016;388(10056):2142–2152.

CHAPTER 25

HYPERTENSION IN STROKE

James M. Luther, MD, MSCI, Michel Shamy, MD, MA, FRCPC, and Swapnil Hiremath, MD

QUESTIONS

1. **What is the epidemiology of stroke?**
A stroke refers to the development of focal neurological symptoms such as the sudden loss of movement, sensation, or coordination that arises due to impaired blood flow to the brain or spinal cord. A transient ischemic attack (TIA) is a temporary period of symptoms similar to those of a stroke that resolves spontaneously. A TIA usually lasts only a few minutes and does not cause permanent damage. A TIA is often a warning sign of impending stroke.

   Globally, stroke is the second largest cause of death (5·5 million deaths in 2016) after ischemic heart disease, and also the second most common cause of disability. There were 14 million incident and 80 million prevalent cases of stroke globally in 2016. There is significant geographical variation, with east Asia, followed by Eastern Europe having the highest incidence. Even in United States, the incidence of stroke is highest in the southeastern region, often referred to as the "stroke belt." There is an increasing risk of stroke with increasing age, and a slightly higher risk for men compared to women, which equalizes approximately after the age of 80 years. In less developed regions, the average age of stroke is younger, likely due to the different population age structure and competing causes of death.[1]

2. **What are the major classifications of stroke and which types are associated with hypertension?**
Strokes are broadly classified as ischemic (88%) or hemorrhagic (12%). In ischemic stroke, an intracranial artery becomes blocked; in hemorrhagic stroke, it ruptures. The proportion of hemorrhagic strokes is higher in Asia, at about 20% to 30%.[1,2] Common causes of ischemic stroke include small vessel disease, cardio emboli, and large artery atherosclerotic plaque rupture. About 20% of strokes are cryptogenic, in that a clear cause cannot be identified despite thorough investigations. An independent phenomenon that may present in a similar fashion is subarachnoid hemorrhage due to rupture of an intracranial aneurysm.

   Hypertension is the primary cause of intracerebral hemorrhage, accounting for a population attributable risk of about 60%.[1] Hypertension is also the primary cause of lacunar infarcts. The risk of stroke rises steadily as blood pressure level rises and doubles for every 7.5 mm Hg increment in diastolic blood pressure, with no lower threshold.

3. **What are the risk factors for stroke?**
Risk factors for ischemic and hemorrhagic stroke are shown in Table 25.1.[3] Metabolic risk factors (high systolic blood pressure [BP], high body-mass index, high fasting plasma glucose, high total cholesterol, and low glomerular filtration rate) account for the major proportion of the attributable risk, followed by behavioral factors (smoking, poor diet, and low physical activity), and environmental risks (e.g., air pollution and lead exposure).[1]

   The relationship of stroke mortality to usual BP is strong and direct at all ages, with no good evidence of a threshold at any age in the range of usual systolic BP (SBP) above 115 mm Hg or of usual diastolic BP (DBP) above 75 mm Hg. At ages 40 to 69 years, each difference of 20 mm Hg usual SBP (or ~ 10 mm Hg usual DBP) is associated with more than a twofold difference in the stroke death rate.[4] See Fig. 25.1 for a representation of this risk from a systematic review of multiple cohorts including about one million individuals.

4. **What is the "acute hypertensive response in stroke?"**
The classic response is called "Cushing's response" after Harvey Cushing who described it over a century ago. In response to raised intracranial pressure, the SBP rises, in combination with bradycardia and irregular respiration due to autonomic activation. This triad signifies impending brain herniation and hence is a poor prognostic sign. A specific equation relates intracranial pressure (ICP), mean arterial pressure (MAP), and cerebral perfusion pressure (CPP) (CPP = MAP − ICP). In this setting hypertension is thought to be a homeostatic mechanism to maximize cerebral perfusion pressure in the setting of raised intracranial pressure. It can be seen with any cause of raised intracranial pressure.

Table 25.1 Stroke Risk Factors

	ISCHEMIC CVA	CARDIOEMBOLIC CVA	HEMORRHAGIC CVA
Traditional risk factors	Hypertension Smoking Obesity ↑LDL cholesterol ↓HDL cholesterol Diabetes		Hypertension Intracranial aneurysm Arteriovenous malformation (AVM)
Comorbid conditions	Diabetes Peripheral arterial disease	Atrial fibrillation Valvular heart disease Patent foramen ovale Endocarditis	
Unusual causes	Carotid or vertebrobasilar dissection Aortic dissection Fibromuscular dysplasia Vasculitis		

CVA, Cerebrovascular accidents; *HDL,* high-density lipoprotein; *LDL,* low-density lipoprotein.

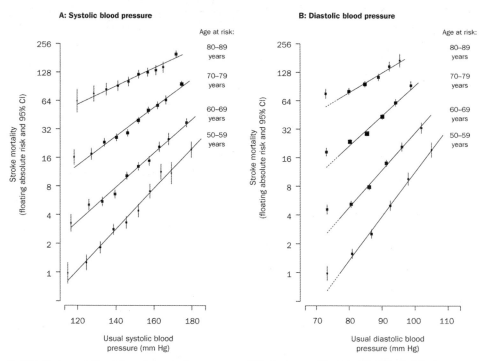

Fig. 25.1 Stroke mortality rate in each decade of age versus usual blood pressure at the start of that decade. Rates for stroke mortality increased exponentially (demonstrated as a linear relationship on a logarithmic y-axis) with increasing systolic (A) and diastolic (B) blood pressure within each age strata. (From Lewington S, Clarke R, Qizilbash N, et al. Age-specific relevance of unusual blood pressure to vascular mortality: a meta-analysis of individual data for one million adults in 61 prospective studies. *Lancet* 2002;360(9349):1903-1913.)

5. How should hypertension be managed in the setting of an acute stroke?
   In acute stroke, 75% of patients have high BP and 50% of those have a prior history of hypertension. A U-shaped relationship between baseline SBP and stroke outcome has been described, in that both high and low SBP are associated with early as well as late mortality and disability. Normal cerebral autoregulation is impaired in acute

stroke, and the relationship between BP and cerebral perfusion becomes linear, and thus a rapid BP reduction could theoretically reduce cerebral blood flow and extend the infarction zone. Thus, decision-making regarding BP management involves considerations of timing of BP lowering, threshold of BP lowering, choice of BP lowering agents, and whether the setting is an ischemic or hemorrhagic stroke.[5,6]

Hemorrhagic Stroke:

On the basis of randomized controlled trials (RCTs) (primarily Antihypertensive Treatment of Acute Cerebral Hemorrhage [ATACH] and Intensive Blood Pressure Reduction in Acute Cerebral Haemorrhage Trial [INTERACT2]), intensive BP lowering in acute hemorrhagic stroke has been shown to be safe, with a signal for improved functional outcome, thought to be mediated by attenuation of hematoma expansion.[7,8] Hence the American Heart Association guidelines recommendations are to reduce SBP to 140 mm Hg or less in this setting within 6 hours of onset.

Ischemic Stroke:

The concerns about decreasing cerebral perfusion by rapid decrease in BP are important in this setting. Hence, for patients not eligible for thrombolytic therapy or mechanical thrombectomy, treatment of hypertension is not routinely indicated, unless it is elevated to extreme levels. Extreme BP elevation (e.g., SBP greater than 220 mm Hg or DBP greater than 120 mm Hg) should be treated to reduce the blood pressure by approximately 15%, and not more than 25%, over the first 24 hours. Subsequent to the first 24 to 48 hours, BP can be gradually reduced with pharmacotherapy for secondary prevention. It should be noted that initiating or reinitiating BP lowering therapy in the first 48 to 72 hours has been reported to be safe, but this strategy is not associated with improved mortality or functional outcomes.[9]

6. **Does hypertension affect decision making for acute thrombolysis in acute stroke?**

In the setting of thrombolysis, the risk of elevated BP is the occurrence of a hemorrhagic transformation of the ischemic stroke. There is indirect evidence from thrombolysis trials that this risk is higher when BP is greater than 185/110 mm Hg.[10] Hence BP higher than 185/110 mm Hg should be treated when thrombolysis is planned to reduce the risk of hemorrhagic transformation. It is standard care to lower BP below 185/110 mm Hg *prior* to thrombolytic therapy and to below 180/105 mm Hg for the next 24 hours. Labetalol (10–20 mg intravenously [IV] over 1–2 minutes, may repeat one time) and/or nicardipine (IV, at 5 mg/h, titrated up by 2.5 mg/h up to a maximum of 15 mg/h) are useful in these settings, with hydralazine and enalaprilat as other alternatives. If BP is not controlled despite this, or with DBP greater than 140 mm Hg, sodium nitroprusside could be considered.[5,6]

Similar considerations apply in the setting of mechanical thrombectomy, with indirect evidence only available as most RCTs have BP greater than 185/110 mm Hg as exclusion for eligibility. Additionally, care should be taken to avoid relative hypotension during the procedure, especially when general anesthesia is used. Lastly, SBP greater than 140 mm Hg is generally targeted during the procedure as a lower limit, as BP below this threshold has been shown to be independently predictive of poor neurologic outcomes after endovascular treatment.[11]

7. **Does hypertension treatment prevent first and recurrent stroke?**

Cardiovascular mortality has markedly decreased over the last 50 years, in part due to decreased risk of death from heart attack and stroke. Improved BP control is associated with this risk reduction, and the risk of hemorrhagic stroke (which is largely attributable to hypertension) has markedly decreased with the improved hypertension treatment rates over this period.

In addition to the epidemiologic data, multiple randomized clinical trials demonstrate that lowering BP reduces subsequent stroke risk. The BP Lowering Treatment Trialists Collaboration provides a summary effect of lowering SBP by 10 mm Hg, which lowers the risk of subsequent stroke by about 27%, irrespective of the initial SBP (Fig. 25.2).[12] From the same metaanalysis, beta-blockers were inferior, but all other first line BP lowering drugs were effective in reducing this risk of stroke.

For secondary prevention, strong consideration should be given to the initiation of antihypertensive therapy after the acute phase of the stroke. There are no RCT data to guide on the optimal timing on when to initiate BP lowering therapy, but it is reasonable that BP lowering therapy be initiated or modified before discharge from hospital, especially among those with BP more than 140/90 mm Hg. For long-term prevention, a goal of BP less than 130/80 mm Hg may be reasonable in these patients. In those previously untreated for hypertension who experience stroke and have a BP less than 140/90 mm Hg, the usefulness of initiating BP lowering therapy is unclear. RCTs of renin-angiotensin system (RAS) blockade and thiazide diuretics have demonstrated a clinical benefit in this population.

8. **What is the role of hypertension in cerebral aneurysm development and rupture?**

Hypertension, smoking, alcohol abuse, and sympathomimetic drug use are modifiable epidemiologic risk factors for the development and rupture of intracranial aneurysms.[13] Genetic risk factors associated with intracranial aneurysms (e.g., autosomal dominant polycystic kidney disease) and multiple genetic loci identified by GWAS are also associated with hypertension.[14] In animal models of intracranial aneurysmal rupture, blood pressure reduction with hydralazine reduces the risk of rupture in a dose-dependent manner and angiotensin converting enzyme (ACE) inhibition or mineralocorticoid receptor blockade reduced the risk of rupture at a dose that did not alter SBP.[15]

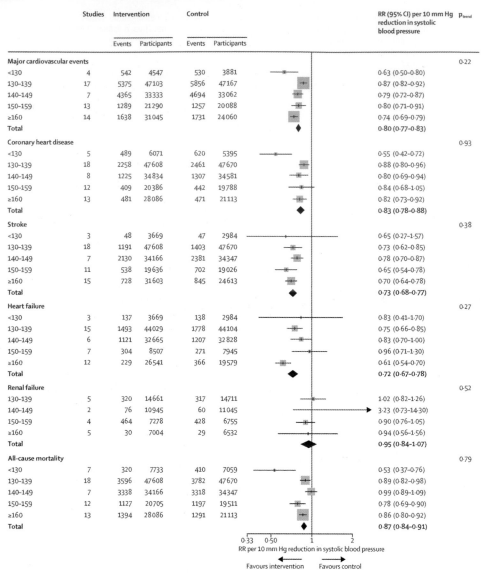

	Studies	Intervention		Control		RR (95% CI) per 10 mm Hg reduction in systolic blood pressure	p_trend
		Events	Participants	Events	Participants		
Major cardiovascular events							0·22
<130	4	542	4547	530	3881	0·63 (0·50–0·80)	
130–139	17	5375	47103	5856	47167	0·87 (0·82–0·92)	
140–149	7	4365	33333	4694	33062	0·79 (0·72–0·87)	
150–159	13	1289	21290	1257	20088	0·80 (0·71–0·91)	
≥160	14	1638	31045	1731	24060	0·74 (0·69–0·79)	
Total						0·80 (0·77–0·83)	
Coronary heart disease							0·93
<130	5	489	6071	620	5395	0·55 (0·42–0·72)	
130–139	18	2258	47608	2461	47670	0·88 (0·80–0·96)	
140–149	8	1225	34834	1307	34581	0·80 (0·69–0·94)	
150–159	12	409	20386	442	19788	0·84 (0·68–1·05)	
≥160	13	481	28086	471	21113	0·82 (0·73–0·92)	
Total						0·83 (0·78–0·88)	
Stroke							0·38
<130	3	48	3669	47	2984	0·65 (0·27–1·57)	
130–139	18	1191	47608	1403	47670	0·73 (0·62–0·85)	
140–149	7	2130	34166	2381	34347	0·78 (0·70–0·87)	
150–159	11	538	19636	702	19026	0·65 (0·54–0·78)	
≥160	15	728	31603	845	24613	0·70 (0·64–0·78)	
Total						0·73 (0·68–0·77)	
Heart failure							0·27
<130	3	137	3669	138	2984	0·83 (0·41–1·70)	
130–139	15	1493	44029	1778	44104	0·75 (0·66–0·85)	
140–149	6	1121	32665	1207	32828	0·83 (0·70–1·00)	
150–159	7	304	8507	271	7945	0·96 (0·71–1·30)	
≥160	12	229	26541	366	19579	0·61 (0·54–0·70)	
Total						0·72 (0·67–0·78)	
Renal failure							0·52
130–139	5	320	14661	317	14711	1·02 (0·82–1·26)	
140–149	2	76	10945	60	11045	3·23 (0·73–14·30)	
150–159	4	464	7278	428	6755	0·90 (0·76–1·05)	
≥160	5	30	7004	29	6532	0·94 (0·56–1·56)	
Total						0·95 (0·84–1·07)	
All-cause mortality							0·79
<130	7	320	7733	410	7059	0·53 (0·37–0·76)	
130–139	18	3596	47608	3782	47670	0·89 (0·82–0·98)	
140–149	7	3338	34166	3318	34347	0·99 (0·89–1·09)	
150–159	12	1127	20705	1197	19511	0·78 (0·69–0·90)	
≥160	13	1394	28086	1291	21113	0·86 (0·80–0·92)	
Total						0·87 (0·84–0·91)	

0·33   0·50   1   2
RR per 10 mm Hg reduction in systolic blood pressure

Favours intervention   Favours control

Fig. 25.2 Standardized effects of a 10 mm Hg reduction in systolic blood pressure stratified by blood pressure. *CI*, Confidence interval; *RR*, relative risk. (From Ettehad D, Emdin CA, Kiran A, et al. Blood pressure lowering for prevention of cardiovascular disease and death: a systematic review and meta-analysis. *Lancet* 2016;387(10022)957-967.)

In the setting of subarachnoid hemorrhage due to aneurysmal rupture, the risk of rebleeding is associated with prior sentinel headache, initial loss of consciousness, larger aneurysm size, and SBP greater than 160 mm Hg.[13] Because the risk of rapidly reducing BP can also decrease cerebral perfusion and increase the risk of delayed cerebral ischemia (DCI), a titratable agent such as intravenous nicardipine is preferred to decrease SBP to less than 160 mm Hg with avoidance of hypotension in the acute setting.

Patients with subarachnoid hemorrhage due to aneurysmal rupture are at risk of DCI, i.e., ischemic stroke nearby to the ruptured aneurysm. DCI is related to cerebral vasospasm, though the pathophysiology of this process remains poorly understood. Arterial vasospasm and typically DCI occur 7 to 10 days after aneurysm rupture. The treatment of DCI includes hemodynamic augmentation by acutely raising arterial blood pressure with intravenous fluids and vasopressor agents.[13] Treatment includes the use of the oral calcium channel blocker nimodipine within 48 hours of the event and continued for 21 days, although evidence of efficacy is of poor quality.[16]

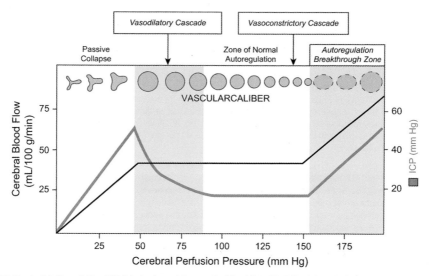

Fig. 25.3 Cerebral Autoregulation. With intact autoregulation, cerebral blood flow *(black line, left y-axis)* is maintained constant within the typical normal cerebral perfusion pressure range of 50 to 150 mm Hg *(x-axis)*. This is achieved in part by the vascular myogenic reflex which alters the vascular caliber in direct response to pressure. This autoregulatory mechanism fails at pressures above or below the normal range and is shifted rightward in the setting of chronic hypertension. *ICP,* Intracranial pressure (grey line, right y-axis). (From Wartenberg KE, Schmidt JM, Mayer SA. Multimodality monitoring in neurocritical care. *Crit Care Clin* 2007;23:507-538.)

After recovery, blood pressure should be targeted to a goal consistent with relevant comorbidities. The incidence of aneurysmal subarachnoid hemorrhage has not decreased over time despite more intensive cardiovascular therapy, but improved treatment has decreased mortality from subarachnoid hemorrhage.[17]

9. **Which antihypertensive agents should be preferred or avoided in intracerebral hemorrhage?**
   The general principles are to use drugs with a rapid onset of action when quick BP reduction is necessary, as summarized previously. In the specific setting of subarachnoid hemorrhage, the calcium channel blocker nimodipine is standard, as it may have a specific effect on calcium influx at the neuronal level. Multiple trials and a systematic review support the benefit of nimodipine at this time to improve neurological outcomes.[18] The effect of other calcium channel blockers in this setting is uncertain.

10. **How should blood pressure be managed differently in the setting of severe intracranial atherosclerosis?**
    Patients with severe and inoperable **intracranial atherosclerotic disease** (ICAD) pose a unique issue due to concerns for decreased perfusion when blood pressure is reduced below a certain threshold. Although the optimal target blood pressure has not been firmly established in ICAD, stroke rates are lowest in participants of intensive medical therapy studies who achieved SBP less than 140 mm Hg.[19,20] These patients also have a high risk of future stroke and death and warrant intensive cardiovascular risk modification with aspirin and statin treatment, smoking cessation, diabetes optimization, and blood pressure control. Patients with ICAD who present with TIA have a 14% risk of stroke or death at 1 year, and that risk is 23% among those presenting with stroke.[21–23] Aggressive medical treatment is preferable as a first line treatment, with endovascular approaches such as intracranial stenting considered only when medical therapy has failed.[22,23]

11. **Which antihypertensive agents should be preferred or avoided in ischemic stroke?**
    On the basis of RCTs of BP lowering, calcium channel blockers, thiazide and thiazide-like diuretics, and RAS blockers have been demonstrated to lower the risk of subsequent stroke, with beta-adrenergic antagonists being the notable exception.[12] Though specific comparative RCTs between different classes of BP lowering drugs post-stroke to prevent risk of secondary stroke are not available, existing RCTs support a benefit of angiotensin converting enzyme inhibitors and thiazide diuretics in this setting.[24]

12. What is PRES and how should it be treated?

Posterior reversible leukoencephalopathy syndrome (PRES) is a radiological phenomenon that was initially described in patients presenting with posterior-predominant white matter hyperintensities on MRI in the setting of clinical syndromes including severe hypertension, headache, mental status changes, seizures, and vision disturbance.[25] We now understand these radiological features to be the imaging correlate of a spectrum of presentations including hypertensive encephalopathy and preeclampsia. Moreover, we now appreciate that the "posterior" pattern is not universal and the complications are not always reversible.

The occurrence of PRES should prompt a thorough search for a secondary cause of hypertension including severe renal artery stenosis, cyclosporine immunosuppressant use, or kidney disease. Cerebral edema may be contributed to by failure of cerebrovascular autoregulation (Fig. 25.3), volume overload, endothelial dysfunction, and other factors. Treatment includes acute reduction in blood pressure and proper identification and treatment of the underlying cause.[26]

KEY POINTS

1. Hypertension is the most important factor for both ischemic and hemorrhagic stroke, with an exponential relationship between increasing blood pressure and stroke risk, and stroke mortality.
2. Reduction of systolic blood pressure by 10 mm Hg is associated with a subsequent lowering of stroke by about 25%–35%.
3. In the setting of acute hemorrhagic stroke, systolic blood pressure should be reduced to less than 140 mm Hg within 6 hours of onset.
4. In the setting of an ischemic stroke, consideration of thrombolysis drive decisions about the speed of blood pressure lowering. When thrombolysis is planned, blood pressure should be reduced to 180/105 mm Hg at least. When thrombolysis is not planned, blood pressure reduction should be more gradual.
5. Controlling blood pressure is the most important intervention to prevent recurrent stroke.

REFERENCES

1. Johnson CO, Nguyen M, Roth GA, et al. Global, regional, and national burden of stroke, 1990-2016: a systematic analysis for the global burden of disease study 2016. *Lancet Neurol.* 2019;18:439–458.
2. Kleindorfer DO, Towfighi A, Chaturvedi S, et al. 2021 guideline for the prevention of stroke in patients with stroke and transient ischemic attack: a guideline from the American Heart Association/American Stroke Association. *Stroke.* 2021;52:e364–e467.
3. Boehme AK, Esenwa C, Elkind MS. Stroke risk factors, genetics, and prevention. *Circ. Res.* 2017;120:472–495.
4. Lewington S, Clarke R, Qizilbash N, et al. Age-specific relevance of usual blood pressure to vascular mortality: a meta-analysis of individual data for one million adults in 61 prospective studies. *The Lancet.* 2002;360:1903–1913.
5. Powers WJ, Rabinstein AA, Ackerson T, et al. Guidelines for the early management of patients with acute ischemic stroke: 2019 update to the 2018 guidelines for the early management of acute ischemic stroke: A guideline for healthcare professionals from the American Heart Association/American Stroke Association. *Stroke.* 2019;50:e344–e418.
6. Boulanger JM, Lindsay MP, Gubitz G, et al. Canadian stroke best practice recommendations for acute stroke management: prehospital, emergency department, and acute inpatient stroke care, 6th edition, update 2018. *Int. J. Stroke.* 2018;13:949–984.
7. Antihypertensive Treatment of Acute Cerebral Hemorrhage i.Antihypertensive treatment of acute cerebral hemorrhage. *Crit. Care Med.* 2010;38:637–648.
8. Anderson CS, Heeley E, Huang Y, et al. Rapid blood-pressure lowering in patients with acute intracerebral hemorrhage. *N. Engl. J. Med.* 2013;368:2355–2365.
9. Lee M, Ovbiagele B, Hong KS, et al. Effect of blood pressure lowering in early ischemic stroke: Meta-analysis. *Stroke.* 2015;46: 1883–1889.
10. Ahmed N, Wahlgren N, Brainin M, et al. Relationship of blood pressure, antihypertensive therapy, and outcome in ischemic stroke treated with intravenous thrombolysis: retrospective analysis from Safe Implementation of Thrombolysis in Stroke-International Stroke Thrombolysis Register (SITS-ISTR). *Stroke.* 2009;40:2442–2449.
11. Davis MJ, Menon BK, Baghirzada LB, et al. Anesthetic management and outcome in patients during endovascular therapy for acute stroke. *Anesthesiology.* 2012;116:396–405.
12. Ettehad D, Emdin CA, Kiran A, et al. Blood pressure lowering for prevention of cardiovascular disease and death: A systematic review and meta-analysis. *Lancet.* 2016;387:957–967.
13. Connolly Jr ES, Rabinstein AA, Carhuapoma JR, et al. Guidelines for the management of aneurysmal subarachnoid hemorrhage: a guideline for healthcare professionals from the American Heart Association/American Stroke Association. *Stroke.* 2012;43: 1711–1737.
14. Bakker MK, van der Spek RAA, van Rheenen W, et al. Genome-wide association study of intracranial aneurysms identifies 17 risk loci and genetic overlap with clinical risk factors. *Nat. Genet.* 2020;52:1303–1313.
15. Tada Y, Wada K, Shimada K, et al. Roles of hypertension in the rupture of intracranial aneurysms. *Stroke.* 2014;45:579–586.
16. Barker 2nd FG, Ogilvy CS. Efficacy of prophylactic nimodipine for delayed ischemic deficit after subarachnoid hemorrhage: a metaanalysis. *J. Neurosurg.* 1996;84:405–414.
17. Mackey J, Khoury JC, Alwell K, et al. Stable incidence but declining case-fatality rates of subarachnoid hemorrhage in a population. *Neurology.* 2016;87:2192–2197.
18. Dorhout Mees SM, Rinkel GJ, Feigin VL, et al. Calcium antagonists for aneurysmal subarachnoid haemorrhage. *The Cochrane database of systematic reviews.* 2007;:CD000277.

19. Turan TN, Cotsonis G, Lynn MJ, Chaturvedi S, Chimowitz M, Warfarin-Aspirin Symptomatic Intracranial Disease Trial I. Relationship between blood pressure and stroke recurrence in patients with intracranial arterial stenosis. *Circulation.* 2007;115:2969–2975.

20. Banerjee C, Chimowitz MI. Stroke caused by atherosclerosis of the major intracranial arteries. *Circ. Res.* 2017;120:502–513.

21. Barnard ZR, Alexander MJ. Update in the treatment of intracranial atherosclerotic disease. *Stroke and vascular neurology.* 2020;5: 59–64.

22. Zaidat OO, Fitzsimmons BF, Woodward BK, et al. Effect of a balloon-expandable intracranial stent vs medical therapy on risk of stroke in patients with symptomatic intracranial stenosis: The VISSIT randomized clinical trial. *JAMA.* 2015;313:1240–1248.

23. Zaidat OO, Castonguay AC, Fitzsimmons BF, et al. Design of the VITESSE intracranial stent study for ischemic therapy (VISSIT) trial in symptomatic intracranial stenosis. *J. Stroke Cerebrovasc. Dis.* 2013;22:1131–1139.

24. Group PC. Randomised trial of a perindopril-based blood-pressure-lowering regimen among 6,105 individuals with previous stroke or transient ischaemic attack. *Lancet.* 2001;358:1033–1041.

25. Hinchey J, Chaves C, Appignani B, et al. A reversible posterior leukoencephalopathy syndrome. *N. Engl. J. Med.* 1996;334:494–500.

26. Fugate JE, Claassen DO, Cloft HJ, Kallmes DF, Kozak OS, Rabinstein AA. Posterior reversible encephalopathy syndrome: associated clinical and radiologic findings. *Mayo Clin. Proc.* 2010;85:427–432.

CHAPTER 26

HYPERTENSION IN THE PATIENT WITH AORTIC DISSECTION

Tara A. Holder, MD J. Matt Luther, MD MSCI, and Joshua A. Beckman, MD MS

QUESTIONS

1. **What are the acute aortic syndromes?**

   Acute aortic syndromes (AAS) are a group of emergent aortic pathologies with similar clinical characteristics. AAS occur when blood penetrates the medial layer of the aorta either from a tear or ulceration of the intima or rupture of the vessels within the media. These syndromes include aortic dissection (AoD), penetrating atherosclerotic ulcer (PAU), and intramural hematoma (IMH). AoD is a tear within the ascending or descending aorta that allows blood to separate the medial layer from either the intima or external layers, creating a false lumen within the aortic wall. PAU is the erosion of the wall of the intima causing bleeding into the media and aneurysm formation. IMH occurs when there is bleeding in the aortic wall due to rupture of the vessels within the media (vasa vasorum) or via an undetectable intimal tear. In contrast to AoD, a false lumen is not created in PAU and IMH. In both PAU and IMH, bleeding can extend within the media and lead to AoD or aortic free-wall rupture.

2. **What are the risk factors for AAS?**

   Risk factors for AAS include aortic abnormalities (e.g., aneurysm) and increased aortic wall stress, most commonly secondary to trauma or hypertension. Other acquired causes of AAS are pregnancy, inflammatory aortitis, and cocaine or other stimulant use. Aortic and valvular pathology related to congenital abnormalities and genetic diseases (syndromic and nonsyndromic) are more commonly seen in younger patients under 40 years old and are associated with increased risk of AoD or rupture (Table 26.1). Patients of 40 years or older are more likely to have hypertension as the primary risk factor for AAS. Atherosclerosis does not appear to be an independent risk factor for AoD.

3. **What are typical presenting symptoms for the patient with an acute AoD?**

   AAS typically cause acute, severe chest and/or back pain generally localized to the location of aortic injury. Radiating or changing pain may indicate progression to other areas of the aorta. AAS are potentially fatal and should be considered in the initial evaluation of chest pain in addition to acute coronary syndrome, pulmonary embolism, pneumothorax, and esophageal perforation.

4. **How should blood pressure be assessed in the patient with an AAS?**

   A thorough vascular examination may detect absent or diminished pulses, which can indicate a severely affected artery. Blood pressure (BP) should be measured in all extremities to determine highest central BP, which should then be used to target therapy. Pulse pressure on presentation has prognostic value. In patients with Type A AoD, a narrow pulse pressure (<40 mm Hg) indicates increased risk of intrathoracic complications, such as periaortic hematoma and cardiac tamponade, whereas elevated pulse pressure (>75 mm Hg) is associated with extension into the abdominal aorta.

5. **What are unique causes of hypertension in AAS?**

   Cocaine or methamphetamine-induced hypertension is a significant risk factor for AoD. Young smokers with underlying hypertension have the greatest risk of AoD in the setting of cocaine use. Similarly, chronic amphetamine abuse/dependence is associated with increased risk of thoracoabdominal AoD in adults 18 to 49 years. Cocaine and methamphetamine abuse causes catecholamine-induced tachycardia and hypertension, augmenting shear force on the aorta. Repeated episodes of hypertension cause oxidant stress and endothelial dysfunction, weaken the aortic wall, and predispose to AoD.

6. **Do all patients with AAS need aggressive treatment of hypertension?**

   Hypertension is more common at the onset of type B versus type A aortic pathology, in part, due to an initial catecholamine surge. Severe complications that produce hypotension occur more frequently in patients with type A AoD, such as cardiac tamponade, myocardial infarction, aortic insufficiency, and aortic rupture. Initial management for all AAS includes surgical consultation, invasive hemodynamic monitoring, BP, and pain control. The goal of medical therapy should be to decrease shear stress on the aorta by reducing heart rate, which reduces velocity of ventricular contraction (dP/dt) and BP. In AoD, goal BP is less than 100–120/60–70 mm Hg with heart rates less than 60 bpm. In patients with BP at goal, antihypertensives should be avoided to decrease the risk of malperfusion.

Table 26.1   Risk Factors for Developing Acute Aortic Syndromes

Acquired
Hypertension
Trauma
Pregnancy
Inflammatory aortitis
Cocaine or methamphetamine use
Genetic Diseases
Bicuspid aortic valve
Marfan syndrome
Turner syndrome
Ehlers-Danlos syndrome
Loeys-Dietz syndrome
Familial thoracic aortic aneurysm and dissection syndrome
Other mutations in genes (e.g., fibrillin, tumor growth factor-beta receptor, SMAD3, myosin heavy chain)

Modified from Hiratzka LF, Bakris GL, Beckman JA, et al. 2010 ACCF/AHA/AATS/ACR/ASA/SCA/SCAI/SIR/STS/SVM guidelines for the diagnosis and management of patients with thoracic aortic disease: a report of the American College of Cardiology Foundation/ American Heart Association Task Force on Practice Guidelines, American Association for Thoracic Surgery, American College of Radiology, American Stroke Association, Society of Cardiovascular Anesthesiologists, Society for Cardiovascular Angiography and Interventions, Society of Interventional Radiology, Society of Thoracic Surgeons, and Society for Vascular Medicine. *Circulation.* 2010;121(13):e266-369.

7. **What medications are recommended for hypertension control in acute AoD?**
   Intravenous beta-blockers, including metoprolol, esmolol, labetalol, or propranolol, are first-line therapy for AoD due to their ability to decrease heart rate and shear stress on the aorta.[1] If heart rate is not adequately controlled with beta-blockers, additional sympathetic blockade with a centrally acting agent (e.g., clonidine, guanfacine, or methyldopa), verapamil, or diltiazem is often required. In patients with contraindications to beta-blockers, verapamil and diltiazem may be considered to achieve heart rate control.[1]

   If goal BP is not attained with initial antihypertensive drugs, angiotensin-converting enzyme/angiotensin II receptor blockers (ACE/ARBs) are useful as initial vasodilatory agents that do not cause reflex tachycardia. Short-acting vasodilators (e.g., nicardipine, clevidipine, sodium nitroprusside, and nitroglycerine) should not be used as a first-line agent or in the absence of adequate heart rate control because they routinely cause reflex tachycardia, increased left ventricular (LV) contractility, and increased shear stress.[1]

   Multiple antihypertensives are typically required to achieve goal BP in AoD. Sodium nitroprusside is the first choice in hypertension refractory to initial beta-blocker therapy due to rapid onset and effect on both arterial and venous vasodilation. Alternatively, nicardipine or clevidipine may be considered as an initial agent for additional BP control refractory to beta blockade alone, but vasodilator treatment should only be initiated once adequate heart rate control is obtained. Nifedipine and clevidipine are both dihydropyridine calcium channel antagonists with rapid-onset and selective arterial vasodilation (Table 26.2).

   In addition to antihypertensive treatment, opioid analgesics are recommended to reduce pain and decrease the sympathetic release of catecholamines driving tachycardia and hypertension.[1] Central alpha-2 agonists (e.g., guanfacine, clonidine, and methyldopa) are also helpful to reduce sympathetic activity and also may have additional analgesic effects.

8. **What are the goals of hypertension control prior to repair?**
   - **Type A AoD:** Prior to emergent surgical repair of type A AoD, the goal of BP management should be to minimize dissection extension to prevent aortic rupture, coronary ischemia, aortic insufficiency, or tamponade.
   - **Type B AoD:** The majority of type B AoDs do not result in life-threatening complications, and medical management is the standard of care. The goal of BP management is to limit propagation of the false lumen, thereby preventing end-organ ischemia and infarction. End-organ ischemia may occur by three mechanisms: (1) propagation of dissection flap into branch vessels resulting in vascular obstruction; (2) vessel inlet obstruction caused by mobile true lumen bulging into branch vessels; (3) compression of branch vessels by false lumen thrombus or hematoma.

Table 26.2 Intravenous Antihypertensives for the Management of Acute Aortic Syndromes

THERAPY	DOSE
Beta-Blocker	
Metoprolol	5-mg bolus, repeat every 5 min for 3 doses; additional doses of 5–10 mg every 4–6 h as needed
Esmolol	500–1000-μg/kg/min bolus, then 50-μg/kg/min infusion; maximum dose 200 μg/kg/min
Labetalol	0.3–1.0-mg/kg bolus (maximum 20 mg) repeat every 10 min as needed, or 0.4–1.0-mg/kg/h IV infusion up to 3 mg/kg/h. Maximum dose 300 mg. This can be repeated every 4–6 h
Propranolol	0.05–0.15 mg/kg every 4–6 h as needed
Calcium Channel Blocker	
Verapamil	0.075–0.15 mg/kg over 2 min, can give an additional 10-mg bolus after 15–30 min; initial infusion rate 5 mg/h
Diltiazem	0.25-mg/kg bolus over 5 min, infusion rate 5–15 mg/h
Short-Acting Vasodilators	
Nicardipine	5 mg/h increasing every 5 min by 2.5 mg/h; maximum 15 mg/h
Clevidipine	1–2 mg/h, double dose every 90 sec, maximum dose 32 mg/h
Sodium nitroprusside	0.3 μg/kg/min infusion, maximum infusion rate 2 μg/kg/min
Nitroglycerine	5 μg/min; increase every 5 min by 5 μg/min; maximum dose 20 μg/min
ACE (Enalaprilat)	1.25 mg over 5 min every 6 h; maximum 5 mg per dose every 6 h

ACE, Angiotensin-converting enzyme.
Data from Whelton PK, Carey RM, Aronow WS, et al. 2017 ACC/AHA/AAPA/ABC/ACPM/AGS/APhA/ASH/ASPC/NMA/PCNA Guideline for the prevention, detection, evaluation, and management of high blood pressure in adults: a report of the American College of Cardiology/ American Heart Association Task Force on Clinical Practice Guidelines. *Hypertension.* 2018;71(6):e13-e115.

9. **What are the goals of BP management in acute AoD?**
   Tight BP control is essential for acute management of both type A and type B AoD. Systolic BP should be reduced to less than 140 mm Hg within the first hour and then to less than 120 mm Hg.[2] After surgical repair or prevention of end-organ complications with BP control, patients should be carefully transitioned to an oral antihypertensive regimen to avoid rebound hypertension. Posthospitalization systolic BP goal is less than 120 mm Hg. Patients should have close follow-up to assess for over- or under treatment and to reinforce the importance of long-term control.

10. **What is the mechanism by which AAS cause complications?**
    - **Acute (first day):** In the acute phase of AoD, hypertension may cause dissection propagation. Retrograde propagation can lead to aortic insufficiency, tamponade, and myocardial ischemia. Dissection extension into branch arteries can compromise brachiocephalic, carotid, spinal, mesenteric, renal, or iliac artery circulation. Uncontrolled to hypertension can cause aortic rupture, leading to tamponade in type A AoD or to hemothorax in type B AoD.
    - **Subacute (first week to month):** In the subacute phase, partial thrombosis of the false lumen can occur. Partial thrombosis of the false lumen in the setting of hypertension may lead to extrinsic compression of the true lumen and impaired blood flow.[3]
    - **Chronic (after first month):** In the chronic phase, aortic dilation occurs predominantly in the upper descending aorta. The rate of aortic enlargement is based on the patency of the false lumen, the saccular type aneurysm formation, the number of entry tears, and the localization of false lumen. Increased mortality is seen in partial thrombosis of the false lumen where there is an increase in wall tension and localized wall weakening. Over time, the dissection flap stiffens and stabilizes, decreasing motion into the true lumen, which may affect the success of stent graft interventions.[4]

11. **What happens to the aorta over time in patients with AoD?**
    Medically managed AoDs can increase in diameter over time despite appropriate BP control. The false lumen can remain patent, partially thrombosed, or completely thrombosed. During chronic management, increased aortic diameter is seen in all patients. Partially thrombosed false lumen has a higher annual aortic diameter growth rate when compared with patent or completely thrombosed false lumen. Patients with partially thrombosed false

lumen are at the greatest risk of aneurysm formation, late rupture requiring operative management, and mortality, requiring close clinical monitoring and potentially earlier intervention.[3]

12. **What happens to the aorta over time in patients with IMH and PAU?**
    IMH has a variable natural history. The hematoma can completely resolve (~10%), convert to a dissection, enlarge, or rupture. Similar to AoDs, IMHs are categorized by type A (proximal aorta) and type B (distal aorta). In type A IMH, aortic diameter greater than 4.8 cm or IMH thickness greater than 11 mm are independent risk factors for surgery and mortality. Fortunately, the majority of cases are type B and medical management is the standard of care. However, type B IMH with an aortic diameter of 4 cm or greater or IMH thickness greater than 10 mm are at increased risk of aortic disease progression.

    PAU can cause medial hematoma, false aneurysm, dissection, or transmural rupture. Compared with AoD, the risk of rupture in PAU is considerably higher at ~40%. Follow-up for these patients should therefore be tailored to each individual with concurrent aggressive management of coexisting comorbidities.

13. **What medications are recommended in patients with AAS in the chronic setting?**
    Beta-blockers (e.g., metoprolol, carvedilol, bisoprolol, and atenolol) are associated with improved long-term survival and remain the cornerstone of hypertension management, decreasing the rate of aneurysm dilation and risk for operative repair in AAS.[5]

    Most patients need an additional antihypertensive medication to obtain target BP. ACE/ARBs are typically second-line therapy in the management of aortic syndromes, although data is limited in supporting their use to prevent disease progression and increase survival. An ACE inhibitor or an ARB remains the second-line therapy in patients with AoD for their potent antihypertensive effect.[5]

    Calcium channel blockers are reserved for third-line therapy and confer improved survival in patients with type B AoD but appear to be associated with worse long-term survival in patients with postsurgical type A AoD.[5]

14. **Does hypertension predict dissection recurrence and aneurysm formation?**
    Uncontrolled hypertension is a risk factor for AoD and aortic aneurysm formation. In patients with chronically managed AoD, hypertension does not appear to be an independent predictor of recurrent dissection or aortic aneurysm expansion.

KEY POINTS

1. Beta-blockers are the first-line treatment for inpatient and outpatient management of hypertension in AAS, with target systolic BP of 120 mm Hg.
2. Short-acting vasodilators should not be used as first-line therapy for acute AAS in the absence of adequate heart rate control because they routinely cause reflex tachycardia, increased LV contractility, and increased shear stress.
3. An ACE inhibitor or an ARB is the second-line therapy for management of hypertension due to their potent antihypertensive effect.

REFERENCES

1. Hiratzka LF, Bakris GL, Beckman JA, et al. 2010 ACCF/AHA/AATS/ACR/ASA/SCA/SCAI/SIR/STS/SVM guidelines for the diagnosis and management of patients with thoracic aortic disease: a report of the American College of Cardiology Foundation/American Heart Association Task Force on Practice Guidelines, American Association for Thoracic Surgery, American College of Radiology, American Stroke Association, Society of Cardiovascular Anesthesiologists, Society for Cardiovascular Angiography and Interventions, Society of Interventional Radiology, Society of Thoracic Surgeons, and Society for Vascular Medicine. *Circulation.* 2010;121(13):e266–369.
2. Whelton PK, Carey RM, Aronow WS, et al. 2017 ACC/AHA/AAPA/ABC/ACPM/AGS/APhA/ASH/ASPC/NMA/PCNA Guideline for the prevention, detection, evaluation, and management of high blood pressure in adults: a report of the American College of Cardiology/American Heart Association Task Force on Clinical Practice Guidelines. *Hypertension.* 2018;71(6):e13–e115.
3. Tsai TT, Evangelista A, Nienaber CA, et al. Partial thrombosis of the false lumen in patients with acute type B aortic dissection. *N Engl J Med.* 2007;357(4):349–359.
4. Yang CJ, Tsai SH, Wang JC, et al. Association between acute aortic dissection and the distribution of aortic calcification. *PLoS One.* 2019;14(7):e0219461.
5. Suzuki T, Isselbacher EM, Nienaber CA, et al. Type-selective benefits of medications in treatment of acute aortic dissection (from the International Registry of Acute Aortic Dissection [IRAD]). *Am J Cardiol.* 2012;109(1):122–127.

CHAPTER 27

RESISTANT AND PSEUDORESISTANT HYPERTENSION

Karen C. Tran, MD, FRCPC

QUESTIONS

1. **What is the prevalence of resistant hypertension?**

   Resistant hypertension (RH) is an emerging clinical and public health problem with increasing incidence because of increasing life expectancy and the growing global epidemic of obesity, diabetes mellitus, and obstructive sleep apnea. Likewise, the excessive dietary salt ingestion reported globally in most countries can contribute substantially to the risk of RH. RH carries a considerable public health problem due to increased treatment cost associated with disability and premature deaths. From the metaanalysis by Noubiap et al. of 3.2 million patients, 10.3% (95% confidence interval [CI]: 7.6% to 13.2%) have true RH. Similarly, the prevalence of apparent treatment-resistant and pseudoresistant hypertension (pseudo-RH) were 14.7% (95% CI: 13.1% to 16.3%) and 10.3% (95% CI: 6.0% to 15.5%), respectively. Specifically, the burden of RH is highest in patients with chronic kidney disease or renal transplant and in elderly patients.

2. **What is the definition of RH?**

   RH is defined as high blood pressure (BP) in a hypertensive patient that remains above goal despite concomitant use of three antihypertensive drugs of different classes usually including a long-acting calcium channel blocker (CCB), a blocker of the renin-angiotensin system (angiotensin-converting enzyme inhibitor [ACEi] or angiotensin receptor blocker [ARB]), and a diuretic. All antihypertensive medications should be administered at optimal or maximally tolerated doses and at the appropriate dosing frequency. Controlled RH is defined as BP that is controlled on four or less antihypertensive medications. The diagnosis of RH requires exclusion of common causes of pseudoresistance, which includes improper BP measurement technique, white coat hypertension (WCH), medication noncompliance, and treatment inertia.

   This definition of RH is based on BP response to standard therapy and identifies a group of high-risk patients who may benefit from specialist care and secondary work up of hypertension. Large epidemiological studies have shown that using the above definition of RH is associated with a higher risk of adverse cardiovascular (CV) outcomes. For example, in a cohort study of 205,750 patients with incident hypertension, it was reported that the risk of CV outcomes was higher in patients with RH with a hazard ratio of 1.47 (95% CI: 1.33 to 1.62).

   International hypertension guidelines have different targets for BP control for RH (e.g., the American College of Cardiology/American Heart Association [ACC/AHA] with a target of 130/80 mm Hg and the International Society of Hypertension and the European Society of Hypertension with a target of 140/90 mm Hg). For Hypertension Canada, the target for BP varies based on associated comorbid conditions (e.g., BP less than 140/90 mm Hg for those with no compelling indications, less than 130/80 mm Hg in those with diabetes, and systolic blood pressure [SBP] less than 120 mm Hg for those at high CV risk), and hence the diagnosis of RH takes this into account. See Table 27.1 for more details on the differences.

3. **What is the definition of pseudo-RH?**

   Most uncontrolled hypertension is not truly resistant to medical treatment, but results from other factors that lead to sustained elevated BP readings; this is termed *pseudo-RH*, or apparent treatment RH. Almost 1 in 10 individuals with hypertension have pseudo-RH, which highlights the high number of patients with hypertension wrongly classified as having RH. Identification of factors that contributes to pseudo-RH is important in preventing costly and potential invasive diagnostic tests or avoiding inappropriate intensification of treatment when unnecessary.

   Pseudo-RH is largely explained by nonadherence or poor adherence to treatment, improper BP measurement technique, suboptimal antihypertensive regimen, clinical inertia, and whitecoat effect (Table 27.2). Nonadherence or poor adherence to hypertensive medication has been incriminated as playing a major role in pseudo-RH as it is very common among patients with hypertension, reaching rates of 50% or more in some studies. To improve medication adherence, simplifying antihypertensive regiment with single-pill combination, patient education in self-management, and improved access to affordable medications are starting points. Assessment of medication adherence can be accomplished either through indirect measures of pill counting or pharmacy

Table 27.1 Definition and Diagnosis of Resistant Hypertension According to Different Professional Societies

GUIDELINE	ESH 2018(6)	ACC/AHA 2018(5)	HYPERTENSION CANADA 2020	ISH 2020
BP Threshold	SBP >140 and/or DBP >90	SBP >130 and/or DBP >80	Above target	BP >140/90
Number of anti-hypertensive medications	≥3 optimally tolerated or best tolerated	≥3 maximum or maximally tolerated, appropriate dosing intervals	≥3 drugs from different classes, at optimally tolerated dosages, used simultaneously	>3 drugs at optimal (or maximally tolerated) doses including a diuretic
Class of anti-hypertensive medications	ACEi/ARB, CCB, diuretic	3 different classes, commonly ACEi/ARB, CCB, diuretic	3 or more drugs of different classes, preferably including a diuretic	3 or more drugs of different classes, including a diuretic
Method of BP measurement	Confirmed with ABPM or HBPM	Consider ABPM or HBPM	Confirm with ABPM	Seated office BP; exclude white coat effect
Adherence	Confirm adherence	Assess for adherence	Assess for adherence	Exclude non-adherence

ABPM, Ambulatory blood pressure monitoring; *ACEi,* angiotensin-converting enzyme inhibitor; *ACC/AHA,* American College of Cardiology/American Heart Association; *ARB,* angiotensin receptor blocker; *BP,* blood pressure; *CCB,* calcium channel blocker; *DBP,* diastolic blood pressure; *ESH,* European Society of Hypertension; *HBPM,* home blood pressure monitoring; *ISH,* International Society of Hypertension; *SBP,* systolic blood pressure.

Table 27.2 Factors Contributing to Pseudoresistant Hypertension

FACTOR	HOW TO RULE OUT
Poor BP measurement technique	Automated office BP
White coat hypertension	24-h ABPM or home BP monitoring
Medication adherence	Pill counts, pharmacy refills, patient engagement
Treatment inertia	Follow A-C-D antihypertensive strategy; pay attention to drug doses (maximize) and duration (prefer long-acting)

ABPM, Ambulatory blood pressure monitoring; *A-C-D,* angiotensin-converting enzyme inhibitors or angiotensin receptor blockers (A) in combination with calcium channel blocker (C) and diuretic (D); *BP,* blood pressure.

refill data; however, these may not present a full picture and may be prone to overestimating adherence. More sophisticated techniques with direct measures, such as therapeutic drug monitoring or direct observed testing, provide a better assessment of medication adherence, but currently are research tools and not readily available for clinical use.

Improper BP measurement techniques can misclassify patients with RH 33% of the time, especially when using nonresting BP versus automated office BP devices. It is important that patients are rested, are in the seated position, have their back and arm supported, and are not talking during the time of BP measurement. Therefore most professional societies either support or require use of automated office BP for accurate measurement.

Furthermore, the presence of WCH (elevated office BP but normal out-of-office BP) can account for 37.5% of patients being misclassified as RH. Therefore it is important that patients with RH be preferably confirmed with 24-hour ambulatory blood pressure monitor (ABPM). If patients are unable to perform 24-hour ABPM, home BP monitoring may be an alternative.

Clinical or therapeutic inertia and improper drug choice or dosage may also contribute to pseudo-RH. Treatment inertia is the failure to escalate treatment to achieve target BP. The first-line drugs recommended for management of hypertension are renin-angiotensin system blockade (ACEi or ARB), CCB, and thiazide-like diuretics (i.e., indapamide or chlorthalidone). Choice of these three so-called A-C-D combination drug classes is commonly, though not exclusively, used as an inclusion criterion for randomized controlled trials (RCTs) in RH populations. Prior to diagnosing an individual with RH, it is pertinent that individuals are maximized on these classes of antihypertensive medications at the optimal and maximally tolerable doses.

4. What is the CV risk associated with RH?

RH is associated with an adverse prognosis. The presence of RH is an important predictor of CV risk beyond the level of BP alone. As compared with those with controlled BP, patients with RH have a higher risk of target end organ damage, including increased carotid intima-media thickness, retinopathy, and left ventricular hypertrophy. Similarly, patients with RH have up to 50% increased risk of CV events, 46% increased risk of heart failure, 24% increased risk of ischemic cardiac events, 32% increased risk of end-stage renal disease, 14% increased risk of stroke, and 6% increased risk of premature death.

It is unclear whether the increased CV risk in RH is related to the long duration of uncontrolled BP or whether specific pathophysiological factors are involved. Patients with RH do have a higher prevalence of comorbid conditions, including diabetes, obstructive sleep apnea, chronic kidney disease, ischemic heart disease, and stroke, which can themselves also greatly increase CV morbidity and mortality.

Additionally, the pathophysiology of RH resulting from the interplay of increase renin-angiotensin-aldosterone system (RAAS), sympathetic nervous system (SNS), hyperaldosteronism, and arterial stiffness can contribute to the high burden of CV disease in those with RH.

5. What is the pathophysiology of RH?

RH is a complex pathophysiological state with contributions from sodium retention, aldosterone excess, low renin states, and activation of the RAAS. Sodium retention can be mediated by increased sodium sensitivity, excessive salt intake, and renal dysfunction. Aldosterone excess is related to being overweight or obese, as adipocytes can directly secrete aldosterone or indirectly stimulate the release of aldosterone secretagogues. Aldosterone excess can lead to further sodium and fluid retention. Low renin causes involve distal nephron handling of sodium either through dysfunction of mineralocorticoid receptor or direct tubular pathology. Greater than two-thirds of patients with RH have a suppressed plasma renin activity despite using ACEi/ARB and diuretics. Cross talk with RAAS and mineralocorticoid receptor can cause further vasoconstriction of vascular smooth muscle cells, leading to worsening hypertension.

In contrast, refractory hypertension is defined as uncontrolled BP on greater than five antihypertensive medications, including diuretics, in particular a mineralocorticoid antagonist. The definition suggests that the mechanism here is unlikely to be due to sodium retention but is more likely neurogenic in pathogenesis and attributable to heightened sympathetic outflow. Studies show these individuals have persistent higher heart rates, greater arterial stiffness, and greater 24-hour urine excretion of norepinephrine. In this patient population, agents that block sympathetic drive, (i.e., beta-blockers, alpha-1 blockers, or alpha-2 agonists) may be more beneficial at reducing BP.

6. What is the work-up for RH?

In patients with suspected RH, confirmation of RH first needs to be made with thorough medication review to assess adherence, accurate in-office BP measurement with an automated office BP machine, out-of-office BP monitoring with 24-hour ABPM, and home BP monitoring to rule out WCH. Given the strong association with sleep apnea, an overnight oximetry should be done to assess for sleep apnea. Secondary causes of hypertension should be considered depending on the clinical scenario and whether the patient has signs or symptoms (Table 27.3). Specifically, patients should be worked up for primary aldosteronism with upright plasma aldosterone/renin ratio and confirmatory testing as indicated, for thyroid disease with thyroid stimulating hormone, and for parathyroid disease with serum calcium. Patients should be assed for pheochromocytoma and Cushing syndrome if they are symptomatic. Furthermore, renal causes of RH should be assessed with baseline creatinine, estimated glomerular

Table 27.3 Work-Up of Secondary Hypertension

SECONDARY HYPERTENSION	INVESTIGATIONS REQUIRED
Obstructive sleep apnea	Overnight oximetry
Endocrine	
Primary aldosteronism	Upright plasma aldosterone/renin ratio
Pheochromocytoma	24-h urine metanephrines and fractionated catecholamines
Cushing syndrome	24-h urine cortisol, dexamethasone suppression test, or midnight salivary cortisol
Thyroid disease	Thyroid-stimulating hormone (TSH)
Parathyroid disease	Calcium
Renal	
Chronic kidney disease	Creatinine, estimated glomerular filtration rate, urine for albuminuria
Renovascular hypertension	Angiogram (computed tomography or magnetic resonance)

filtration rate (eGFR), and urine albumin creatinine ratio. Renovascular etiologies of RH can be worked up by either computed tomography or magnetic resonance angiogram if patients are symptomatic.

7. **What is the best pharmacologic management of RH?**

There are high-quality data from RCTs, as well as from systematic reviews that spironolactone reduces BP to a greater extent than other antihypertensive agents. However, there are no RCT data supporting a benefit of these drugs on CV outcomes or mortality. Additionally, from clinical trial data, doxazosin, bisoprolol, amiloride, and clonidine also reduce BP more than placebo in this population.

Spironolactone has been shown to be the best fourth-line agent at reducing BP in patients with RH, as shown in the Prevention And Treatment of Hypertension With Algorithm based therapY-2 (PATHWAY-2) trial. In summary, patients with RH were enrolled in a double-blind, placebo-controlled crossover study with spironolactone, bisoprolol (beta-blocker), doxazosin (alpha-1 blocker), and placebo. Patients were treated with each class of medication for 12 weeks with a forced dose up-titration at week 6 and then crossed over to another medication class. The primary outcome was a reduction in home SBP compared with placebo, which was greatest with spironolactone (-8.70 mm Hg [95% CI: -9.72 to -7.69]) as compared with doxazosin (-4.03 mm Hg [-5.04 to -3.02]) and bisoprolol (-4.48 mm Hg [-5.50 to -3.46]). BP control for spironolactone, bisoprolol, and doxazosin was 58%, 44%, and 42%, respectively. Similar serious adverse events were noted between the groups; specifically, there were no differences in gynecomastia or hyperkalemia noted. This is likely due to the short duration of exposure to spironolactone and patients with normal renal function at the time of enrollment.

Spironolactone was more effective across almost all levels of plasma renin, with the exception for those individuals with very high levels of renin. In those with very high levels of renin, bisoprolol was most effective. This suggests that the pathophysiological mechanisms of RH are driven by low renin states, suggesting excessive fluid and sodium retention. Furthermore, in patients with RH, the antihypertensive effect of spironolactone was associated with significant reduction in thoracic volume content.

In an open label extension of the PATHWAY-2 trial, patients could crossover to amiloride, a distal tubular diuretic that inhibits the aldosterone-sensitive epithelial sodium channel. Amiloride (10 mg) had similar reduction in clinic SBP (20.4 mm Hg [95% CI: 18.3 to 22.5]) compared with spironolactone (18.3 mm Hg [95% CI: 16.2 to 20.5]). Limitations of this study include the fact that it was open label, clinic BP was used instead of home BPs, and a lower number of participants were enrolled. However, amiloride seems to be as effective as spironolactone for RH.

Lastly, the Resistant Hypertension Optimal Treatment (ReHOT) trial included 187 patients with RH randomized to spironolactone compared with clonidine. At 3 months, the mean change from baseline in office BP was similar between spironolactone (-15.1 mm Hg for SBP and -7.7 mm Hg for diastolic blood pressure [DBP]) and clonidine (-13.7 mm Hg and -6.4 mm Hg), respectively. However, the decrease in 24-hour ABPM was greater with spironolactone (-11.8 mm Hg for SBP and -6.3 mm Hg for DBP) than with clonidine (-7.3 and -3.9 mm Hg, respectively).

8. **What is the role of device therapy for RH?**

As overactive SNS is a potential mechanism for RH, there is much interest in renal denervation (RDN) and baroreceptor activation therapy (BAT) as adjunctive treatment for RH; however, these interventions are still in the clinical research phase and not approved for clinical use. Ablation of sympathetic afferents in the renal artery was developed with initial pilot studies demonstrating a decrease of 20 to 30 mm Hg in office SBP in patients with RH. However, the largest sham-controlled RCT was Symplicity HTN-3, which did not report a significant difference between sham and RDN arms. Subsequent metaanalysis confirms that the pooled effect from the three sham-controlled RCTs was not different between arms. Therefore, at present, there is insufficient data to recommend the use of RDN in patients with RH.

BAT relies on the activation of the myogenic stretch reflex in the carotid body, which results in reduction in sympathetic activity and BP lowering. After the initial promising pilot RCT data, the pivotal double blind Rheos RCT did not demonstrate a significant BP lowering. Additionally, 25% of participants had procedural adverse events. Thus currently there is no evidence to support device therapy outside the setting of clinical research.

KEY POINTS

1. RH is increasing in prevalence due to higher rates of obesity, diabetes, sleep apnea, and salt intake.
2. RH represents a population at high risk of morbidity and mortality.
3. Confirmation of RH needs to be done by ensuring assessment for medication adherence, accurate BP measurement with automated office BP and out-of-office BP measurements.
4. Secondary work-up of RH should be done once the diagnosis is confirmed and if patients have symptoms.
5. The majority of RCTs, physiological data, and metaanalysis support the use of spironolactone as a fourth-line agent due to the greatest BP lowering.
6. Use of an agent from different classes (i.e., beta-blockers, alpha-1 blockers, alpha-2 agonists, amiloride) may be an alternative to spironolactone.
7. Currently, no device therapy has been shown to be useful in RH.

BIBLIOGRAPHY

Acelajado MC, Hughes ZH, Oparil S, Calhoun DA. Treatment of resistant and refractory hypertension. *Circ Res.* 2019;124:1061–1070.
Bhatt DL, Kandzari DE, O'Neill WW, et al. A controlled trial of renal denervation for resistant hypertension. *N Engl J Med.* 2014;370(15):1393–1401.
Bisognano JD, Bakris G, Nadim MK, et al. Baroreflex activation therapy lowers blood pressure in patients with resistant hypertension: results from the double-blind, randomized, placebo-controlled Rheos pivotal trial. *J Am Coll Cardiol.* 2011;58(7):765–773.
Calhoun DA, Jones D, Textor S, et al. Resistant hypertension: diagnosis, evaluation, and treatment a scientific statement from the American Heart Association Professional Education Committee of the Council for High Blood Pressure Research. *Hypertension.* 2008;51(6):1403–1419.
Krieger EM, Drager LF, Giorgi DMA, et al. Spironolactone versus clonidine as a fourth-drug therapy for resistant hypertension: the ReHOT randomized study (Resistant Hypertension Optimal Treatment). *Hypertension.* 2018;71(4):681–690.
Nerenberg KA, Zarnke KB, Leung AA, et al. Hypertension Canada's 2018 guidelines for diagnosis, risk assessment, prevention, and treatment of hypertension in adults and children. *Can J Cardiol.* 2018;34(5):506–525.
Noubiap JJ, Nansseu JR, Nyaga UF, Sime PS, Francis I, Bigna JJ. Global prevalence of resistant hypertension: a meta-analysis of data from 3.2 million patients. *Heart.* 2019;105:98–105.
Pappaccogli M, Covella M, Berra E, et al. Effective of renal denervation in resistant hypertension: A meta-analysis of 11 controlled studies. *High Blood Press Cardiovasc Prev.* 2018;25(2):167–176.
Sinnott SJ, Tomlinson LA, Root AA, et al. Comparative effectiveness of fourth-line anti-hypertensive agents in resistant hypertension: A systematic review and meta-analysis. *Eur J Prev Cardiol.* 2017;24(3):228–238.
Whelton PK, Carey RM, Aronow WS, et al. 2017 ACC/AHA/AAPA/ABC/ACPM/AGS/APhA/ASH/ASPC/NMA/PCNA guideline for the prevention, detection, evaluation, and management of high blood pressure in adults: a report of the American College of Cardiology/American Heart Association Task Force on Clinical Practice Guidelines. *Circulation.* 2018;138(17):e484–e594.
Williams B, MacDonald TM, Morant SV, et al. Endocrine and haemodynamic changes in resistant hypertension and blood pressure responses to spironolactone or amiloride: the PATHWAY-2 mechanisms substudies. *Lancet Diabetes Endocrinol.* 2018;6(6):464–475.
Williams B, MacDonald TM, Webb DJ, et al. Spironolactone versus placebo, bisoprolol, and doxazosin to determine the optimal treatment for drug-resistant hypertension (PATHWAY-2): a randomised, double-blind, crossover trial. *Lancet.* 2015;386(10008):2059–2068.
Williams B, Mancia G, Spiering W, et al. 2018 ESC/ESH guidelines for the management of arterial hypertension: the task force for the management of arterial hypertension of the European Society of Cardiology and the European Society of Hypertension: The Task Force for the management of arterial hypertension of the European Society of Cardiology and the European Society of Hypertension. *J Hypertens.* 2018;36(10):1953–2041.

CHAPTER 28

HYPERKALEMIA IN HYPERTENSION

Ryan P. Flood, DO, and John R. Montford, MD

QUESTIONS

1. Why is hyperkalemia important to understand in the management of individuals with hypertension?

   Hyperkalemia is one of the most common electrolyte disorders encountered and affects a disproportionate number of individuals with chronic hypertension. The incidence of hyperkalemia ranges from 1.9% to 38% among participants of prospectively conducted trials examining the effects of renin-angiotensin-aldosterone system (RAAS) inhibitors on blood pressure reduction.[1] In many studies, higher rates of hyperkalemia accompany patients with lower estimated glomerular filtration rate (eGFR), older age, and presence of comorbid diabetes mellitus and cardiovascular disease (CVD). Rates of hyperkalemia are particularly high among participants of trials combining angiotensin-converting enzyme inhibitors/angiotensin receptor blockers (ACEis/ARBs) with mineralocorticoid receptor antagonists (MRAs) for the treatment of heart failure.[2]

   The development of hyperkalemia is associated with higher rates of hospitalization and mortality in virtually every patient population studied. Hyperkalemia is known to confer direct cardiotoxicity (see following sections), as well as being a major cause of RAAS inhibitor de-escalation; which, in turn, is linked to increased rates of health care utilization, poor control of blood pressure, and worse survival. In general, most professional societies recommend heightened awareness when plasma potassium levels exceed 5.0 mEq/L and de-escalation or discontinuation of RAAS inhibitors with levels greater than 5.5 mEq/L. Practitioners should be aware that underlying patient characteristics such as the presence of heart failure, acute kidney injury (AKI), critical illness, and rapid hyperkalemia development appear to be at least as important as the degree of hyperkalemia at conferring poor patient outcomes.[3]

2. How does the body normally manage potassium?

   Potassium is the predominant intracellular cation with only a small percentage (1%–2%) remaining in the extracellular space. The Na^+K^+-ATPase pump, which is located in the plasma membrane of most nucleated cells in the body, is responsible for maintaining the high intracellular/low extracellular potassium concentration. The Na^+K^+-ATPase exchanges intracellular sodium for extracellular potassium and is under the influence of many physiological stimuli that serve in a coordinated fashion to buffer acute potassium loads:

   - The pancreas releases insulin in response to nutritional glucose intake, which signals for cellular glucose uptake. This upregulates the Na^+K^+-ATPase in glucose responsive tissues like skeletal muscle.
   - Catecholamine release and β_2-adrenergic receptor activation increases the activity of the Na^+K^+-ATPase.
   - Elevated plasma potassium concentrations directly stimulate aldosterone release from the zona glomerulosa of the adrenal gland, which activates mineralocorticoid receptors to upregulate Na^+K^+-ATPase activity.

   While the Na^+K^+-ATPase limits a rapid rise in extracellular potassium concentration after loading, the kidney maintains long-term balance by accomplishing net potassium excretion with only a small contribution occurring via gastrointestinal (GI) excretion (~5%–10% of daily intake). The primary site of potassium handling in the kidney occurs in the principal cells of the collecting duct of the distal nephron. Potassium excretion by this nephron segment requires adequate distal nephron sodium delivery, a high tubular flow rate, and the presence (and signaling activity) of aldosterone. A feedback loop also exists between these principal cells and the distal convoluted tubule, whereby elevated plasma potassium concentrations directly inhibit the thiazide-sensitive sodium chloride cotransporter (NCC), thus augmenting distal sodium delivery and facilitating Na^+-K^+ exchange in the more distal nephron. Consequently, any dysregulation in one or more of these processes can contribute significantly to the development of hyperkalemia.

3. Define the electrocardiographic changes associated with hyperkalemia.

   A wealth of animal studies and extreme human presentations have demonstrated a "typical" progression of myocardial toxicity with acute hyperkalemia occurring in a graded fashion past plasma potassium levels of 5.0 mEq/L. One of the earliest changes to occur is hyperexcitability, manifesting as "tented" T-waves most prominent in the precordial electrocardiogram (ECG) leads (Fig. 28.1). As hyperkalemia progresses, elongation of the PR interval and diminution of the P-wave amplitude occur. An increased QRS complex width is an ominous finding and can precede a classically described "sine-wave" pattern. Thus hyperkalemia predisposes to both cardiac hyperexcitability (ventricular tachycardia and ventricular fibrillation) and depression (bradycardia, atrioventricular block, interventricular conduction delay, and asystole), both of which can be fatal.

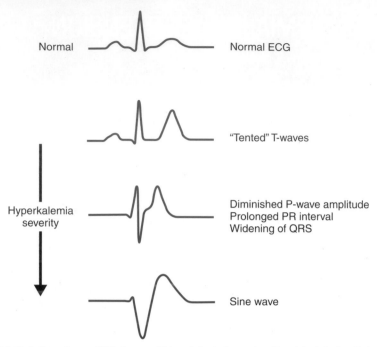

Normal	Normal ECG
	"Tented" T-waves
Hyperkalemia severity	Diminished P-wave amplitude Prolonged PR interval Widening of QRS
	Sine wave

Fig. 28.1 "Typical" electrocardiogram (ECG) changes with hyperkalemia. Progression of hyperkalemia begins with hyperpolarization of T-wave amplitude, causing a "tenting" phenomenon, followed by diminution of P-wave amplitude, prolonging of the PR interval, and widening of the QRS, ultimately progressing to a sine-wave pattern.

However, most human cases of hyperkalemia are of unknown duration and occur among individuals with different cardiometabolic risk factors, limiting the interpretability of ECG as both a diagnostic and prognostic tool. The ECG lacks sensitivity and specificity at predicting the degree of hyperkalemia, and there are a host of conditions that can mimic the ECG changes seen with hyperkalemia including sepsis, myocardial infarction, acidosis, left ventricular hypertrophy, and bundle branch blocks.[3] There are even cases of fatal or near-fatal hyperkalemia occurring in patients with normal ECGs. Ultimately, the ECG alone should not be relied upon to correctly identify which patients require immediate attention.

4. How should one approach the hypertensive patient with hyperkalemia?

The first step in approaching a hypertensive patient with hyperkalemia is to determine if the finding is artefactual. Poor phlebotomy technique and certain hematological conditions causing extreme leukocytosis and thrombocytosis should alert the clinician to the possibility of a hemolyzed specimen or pseudohyperkalemia, respectively. Although excess potassium intake is often implicated, it is usually insufficient to cause hyperkalemia unless advanced chronic kidney disease (CKD) is present (eGFR <30 mL/min) or acute loading is performed by intravenous potassium administration. Exceptions can occur in patients with distal tubular injury or dysfunction, such as occurs with urinary obstruction, connective tissue diseases, and distal (type 4) renal tubular acidosis, which can predispose to hyperkalemia despite a normal or near-normal eGFR. Disruption of the RAAS axis is the most common cause of hyperkalemia in patients with hypertension. There is often a temporal link to incipient hyperkalemia and initiation or up-titration of ACEis, ARBs, and MRAs. RAAS inhibitors cause hyperkalemia by disrupting aldosterone signaling in the distal nephron, and, in some cases, by lowering of GFR due to angiotensin-2 blockade and lower glomerular hydrostatic pressure from their antihypertensive effects. However, one must also not overlook important contributors to hyperkalemia development among hypertensive patients. For example, significant hyperkalemia resulting from a trimethoprim prescription for a soft tissue infection in a hypertensive patient with CKD on RAAS inhibition can result in dangerous synergy to engender severe hyperkalemia. Table 28.1 highlights many of the common clinical conditions and medications predisposing individuals to hyperkalemia.

5. What is the role of dietary modification in the prevention of hyperkalemia?

Despite widespread application, advising dietary potassium reduction in individuals prone to hyperkalemia, particularly those with hypertension, is not supported by evidence, and might even be harmful. Dietary sources

Table 28.1 Common Conditions Leading to Hyperkalemia

CONDITION	ETIOLOGY	MECHANISM OF ACTION
Increased intake	Intravenous K^+ Intravenous K^+-containing antimicrobials Massive blood product transfusion	Exogenous K^+ loading
Impaired redistribution	Rhabdomyolysis Hemolysis Tumor lysis syndrome Malignant hyperthermia	Endogenous K^+ turnover
	Cardiac glycoside toxicity Uremia	Impaired Na^+K^+-ATPase activity
	Metabolic acidosis Hypertonicity (hyperglycemia, mannitol)	Altered Na^+/K^+ extracellular/ intracel-lular gradient
	β^2-Adrenergic blockers	β^2-Adrenergic blockade
Reduced elimination	AKI, CKD	Low GFR
	Urinary obstruction Sickle cell crisis	Distal nephron injury
	Volume depletion Heart failure	Poor distal Na^+ delivery
	Amiloride Triamterene Trimethoprim CNIs Pentamidine	ENaC blockade
	Distal (type 4) RTA Adrenal insufficiency Diabetes mellitus Heparin RAAS inhibitors MR antagonists	Impaired aldosterone synthesis, activity, or MR blockade[a]
	Constipation, bowel obstruction	Reduced K^+ elimination from GI tract[b]

[a]Also can alter K^+ redistribution outside the kidney.
[b]Only in advanced CKD (GI elimination of K^+ upregulated with lower GFR.)
AKI, Acute kidney injury; *CKD*, chronic kidney disease; *CNIs*, calcineurin inhibitors; *ENaC*, epithelial sodium channel; *GFR*, glomerular filtration rate; *GI*, gastrointestinal; *MR*, mineralocorticoid receptor; *RAAS*, renin-angiotensin-aldosterone system; *RTA*, renal tubular acidosis.

of potassium, including meats, fruits, and legumes, are incorporated into many popular diets (such as the Dietary Approaches to Stop Hypertension [DASH] diet, Mediterranean diet, and plant-based diets) that have an evidence base supporting general health benefits. Furthermore, adequate dietary potassium intake is linked with lower blood pressure and associated with lower CVD and overall mortality in a variety of patient populations including those with hypertension heart failure, and CKD.[4] There is also a lack of published data that supports dietary potassium restriction is a particularly efficacious strategy to treat hyperkalemia. It may be reasonable to screen for, and curtail, excessive sources of dietary potassium intake in patients with hyperkalemia, but practitioners should also prioritize other aspects of cardiovascular health to tailor an individualized approach. Registered dieticians are an excellent resource; and visits are often covered by a patient's insurance. The National Kidney Foundation, Centers for Disease Control and Prevention, and American Association of Kidney Patients also have excellent online dietary resources for patients and providers relating to hyperkalemia.

6. **Define the role of proper diuretic use in mitigation of hyperkalemia.**
   Diuretics remain a front-line treatment for hypertension, yet despite the overwhelming evidence of their therapeutic efficacy, they remain under-prescribed due to concerns of electrolyte imbalances, azotemia, and other metabolic side effects. Both loop and thiazide/thiazide-like diuretics increase urinary potassium secretion largely by augmenting urinary flow and sodium delivery to the distal nephron (see Chapters 34 and 35). Often the prescription of potent K-wasting diuretic is all that is needed to counterbalance the hyperkalemic effects of RAAS inhibition. Poor compliance with a diuretic prescription, or prescription of shorter acting loop (furosemide, bumetanide) and thiazide (hydrochlorothiazide) diuretics are potential clues that inadequate distal sodium

delivery may be contributing to the perpetuation of hyperkalemia. Changing such patients to a longer acting loop (torsemide) or thiazide-like (indapamide, chlorthalidone) diuretic regimens may prove efficacious at mitigating both hyperkalemia and untreated hypertension. Often, both diuretics and RAAS inhibitors are de-prescribed due to concerns of worsening azotemia. Yet data from the Systolic Blood Pressure Intervention Trial (SPRINT) suggest that, despite an initial larger drop in eGFR with aggressive blood pressure control, participants randomized to a more aggressive antihypertensive regimen (consisting of high usage of diuretics and RAAS inhibitors) had less major cardiovascular events and all-cause mortality.[5] Furthermore, the acute reduction in GFR with aggressive blood pressure control in this trial appears to lack many features shared with other causes of AKI, such as markers of tubular damage,[6] suggesting this phenomenon results from lower intraglomerular pressure and may not be deleterious for longer term renal outcomes. The lack of hypertensive individuals with advanced CKD and diabetes might limit generalizability to this particular cohort of patients. Nevertheless, both SPRINT and other studies suggest that mild to moderate azotemia occurring after antihypertensive prescription might be tolerable in order to reduce CVD progression, which has major implications for managing hypertensive patients with higher serum potassium levels.

7. **How can newer potassium-exchange resins be used in hypertensive individuals with hyperkalemia on RAAS inhibitors?**
Patiromer is a nonabsorbable cation exchange polymer that binds free potassium in the GI tract, primarily in the distal colon, in exchange for calcium and thus enhances potassium losses in the stool. Daily use of oral Patiromer allows for successful mitigation of chronic hyperkalemia in hypertensive patients with advanced CKD and heart failure while receiving RAAS blockade.[7,8] Additionally, a recently published prospective, randomized, placebo-controlled trial of prophylactic Patiromer administration among individuals with resistant hypertension demonstrated significantly enhanced compliance with newly prescribed spironolactone versus placebo.[9] Patiromer is administered as a dry powder and may be mixed with food or liquids. Starting doses begin at 8.4 g daily up to 12.6 g twice-daily (BID), demonstrating efficacy in major clinical trials. Patiromer has a tolerable adverse effect profile consisting of nausea, diarrhea, constipation, abdominal discomfort, and rare hypomagnesemia. It is important to note that most of the studies performed using Patiromer demonstrate efficacy over a period of weeks to months, and its use as a short-term agent in the treatment of more urgent hyperkalemia has not been fully examined.

Sodium Zirconium Cyclosilicate (SZC) is a nonabsorbed silicate that captures free potassium in exchange for hydrogen and sodium along the GI tract. The molecular structure of SZC includes micropores with small diameters favorably trapping potassium, rather than larger divalent cations like magnesium and calcium and thus limiting the potential for development of hypocalcemia and hypomagnesemia. Like Patiromer, SZC has shown long-term efficacy at reducing serum potassium among individuals with hypertension and high RAAS inhibitor usage.[10,11] SZC has even shown efficacy at reducing predialysis serum potassium among patients with end-stage renal disease,[12] a population with often difficult-to-control hypertension. Furthermore, these studies have demonstrated SZC works within hours to rapidly lower serum potassium in a dose-dependent fashion. Typical doses of SZC are 5 g and 10 g BID. SZC appears to also be safe and have a tolerable safety profile similar to Patiromer. It is important to note the sodium content of one 5-g dose of SZC is 400 mg, and there have been reported instances of edema and hypertension among patients treated with higher daily doses (>15 g daily) for longer durations.

Overall, Patiromer and SZC appear to be effective therapies for the treatment of individuals with hypertension, diabetes mellitus, CKD, and CVD with hyperkalemia and those at risk of developing hyperkalemia. These newer exchange resins are rapidly replacing the role of sodium polystyrene sulfate in treating hyperkalemia due to their studied efficacy and favorable side effect profile.

KEY POINTS

1. Hyperkalemia is a common electrolyte disorder in patients with hypertension and is linked with poor outcomes including RAAS inhibitor de-escalation, hospitalization, and higher mortality.
2. Hyperkalemia results from a failure of homeostatic mechanisms that redistribute acute potassium loads in the intracellular space while simultaneously augmenting urinary excretion.
3. Acute and chronic kidney diseases, diabetes mellitus, and commonly prescribed medications can have synergistic effects to initiate and maintain hyperkalemia.
4. Knowledge of proper diuretic pharmacology serves as the cornerstone to managing and preventing hyperkalemia in hypertensive individuals.
5. Novel potassium exchange resins such as Patiromer and SZC show great promise in both the acute and chronic treatment of hyperkalemia, and might allow for better RAAS inhibitor adherence among individuals with hypertension.

REFERENCES

1. Kovesdy CP. Management of hyperkalemia in chronic kidney disease. *Nat Rev Nephrol.* 2014;10(11):653–662.
2. Tromp J, van der Meer P. Hyperkalemia: aetiology, epidemiology, and clinical significance. *Eur Heart J Supp.* 2019;21(Suppl A):A6–A11.
3. Montford JR, Linas S. How dangerous is hyperkalemia?. *J Am Soc Nephrol.* 2017;28(11):3155–3165.
4. Clase CM, Carrero JJ, Ellison DH, et al. Potassium homeostasis and management of dyskalemia in kidney diseases: conclusions from a Kidney Disease: Improving Global Outcomes (KDIGO) Controversies Conference. *Kidney Int.* 2020;97(1):42–61.
5. Wright Jr JT, Williamson JD, Whelton PK, et al. A randomized trial of intensive versus standard blood-pressure control. *N Engl J Med.* 2015;373(22): 2103–2116.
6. Malhotra R, Craven T, Ambrosius WT, et al. Effects of intensive blood pressure lowering on kidney tubule injury in CKD: a longitudinal subgroup analysis in SPRINT. *Am J Kidney Dis.* 2019;73(1):21–30.
7. Pitt B, Anker SD, Bushinsky DA, et al. Evaluation of the efficacy and safety of RLY5016, a polymeric potassium binder, in a double-blind, placebo-controlled study in patients with chronic heart failure (the PEARL-HF) trial. *Eur Heart J.* 2011;32(7):820–828.
8. Weir MR, Bakris GL, Bushinsky DA, et al. Patiromer in patients with kidney disease and hyperkalemia receiving RAAS inhibitors. *N Engl J Med.* 2015;372(3):211–221.
9. Agarwal R, Rossignol P, Romero A, et al. Patiromer versus placebo to enable spironolactone use in patients with resistant hypertension and chronic kidney disease (AMBER); a phase 2, randomized, double-blind, placebo-controlled trial. *Lancet.* 2019;394(10208):1540–1550.
10. Kosiborod M, Rasmussen HS, Lavin P, et al. Effect of sodium zirconium cyclosilicate on potassium lowering for 28 days among outpatients with hyperkalemia. *JAMA.* 2014;312(21):2223–2233.
11. Spinowitz BS, Fishbane S, Pergola PE, et al. Sodium zirconium cyclosilicate among individuals with hyperkalemia: a 12-month phase 3 study. *Clin J Am Soc Nephrol.* 2019;14(6):798–809.
12. Fishbane S, Ford M, Fukagawa M, et al. A phase 3b, randomized, double-blind, placebo-controlled study of sodium zirconium cyclosilicate for reducing the incidence of predialysis hyperkalemia. *J Am Soc Nephrol.* 2019;30(9):1723–1733.

CHAPTER 29

LIFESTYLE MODIFICATIONS FOR HYPERTENSION MANAGEMENT

Hina N. Mehta, MD, and Matthew A. Sparks, MD

QUESTIONS

1. **What is the role of lifestyle modifications in the treatment of hypertension?**

   The 2017 American College of Cardiology/American Heart Association (ACC/AHA) Guideline for the Prevention, Detection, Evaluation, and Management of High Blood Pressure in Adults recommends lifestyle changes that can reduce systolic blood pressure (SBP) by approximately 4 to 11 mm Hg in patients with hypertension. These guidelines stress the importance of maintaining a healthy diet with limited sodium intake, routine exercise, weight management, tobacco cessation, and decreased alcohol consumption (Tables 29.1 and 29.2). One of the original trials (published in 2002) that evaluated the efficacy of implementing all of these recommendations was the diet, exercise, and weight loss intervention trial (DEW-IT), which enrolled 44 adults who were overweight and had hypertension who were treated with a single blood pressure (BP) medication. DEW-IT consisted of a control group (no intervention) and a comprehensive intensive lifestyle program (Dietary Approaches to Stop Hypertension [DASH] diet and an exercise regimen that included 30 to 45 minutes of supervised moderate-intensity aerobic exercise 3 d/wk, and alcohol restriction). Five energy levels (1350, 1600, 2100, 2600, 3100 kcal/d) of the DASH

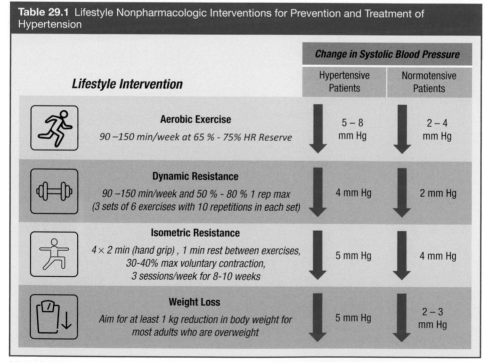

Table 29.1 Lifestyle Nonpharmacologic Interventions for Prevention and Treatment of Hypertension

Lifestyle Intervention		Change in Systolic Blood Pressure	
		Hypertensive Patients	Normotensive Patients
Aerobic Exercise *90–150 min/week at 65 % - 75% HR Reserve*		5 – 8 mm Hg	2 – 4 mm Hg
Dynamic Resistance *90–150 min/week and 50 % - 80 % 1 rep max (3 sets of 6 exercises with 10 repetitions in each set)*		4 mm Hg	2 mm Hg
Isometric Resistance *4 × 2 min (hand grip) , 1 min rest between exercises, 30-40% max voluntary contraction, 3 sessions/week for 8-10 weeks*		5 mm Hg	4 mm Hg
Weight Loss *Aim for at least 1 kg reduction in body weight for most adults who are overweight*		5 mm Hg	2 – 3 mm Hg

Adapted from Whelton PK, Carey RM, Aronow WS, et al. ACC/AHA/AAPA/ABC/ACPM/AGS/APhA/ASH/ASPC/NMA/PCNA guideline for the prevention, detection, evaluation, and management of high blood pressure in adults: a report of the American College of Cardiology/ American Heart Association task force on clinical practice guidelines. *J Am Coll Cardiol.* 2018;71:e127–248.

Table 29.2 Dietary Nonpharmacologic Interventions for Prevention and Treatment of Hypertension

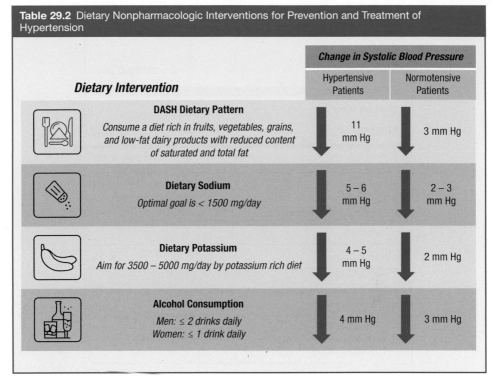

Dietary Intervention	*Change in Systolic Blood Pressure*	
	Hypertensive Patients	Normotensive Patients
DASH Dietary Pattern *Consume a diet rich in fruits, vegetables, grains, and low-fat dairy products with reduced content of saturated and total fat*	11 mm Hg	3 mm Hg
Dietary Sodium *Optimal goal is < 1500 mg/day*	5 – 6 mm Hg	2 – 3 mm Hg
Dietary Potassium *Aim for 3500 – 5000 mg/day by potassium rich diet*	4 – 5 mm Hg	2 mm Hg
Alcohol Consumption *Men: ≤ 2 drinks daily* *Women: ≤ 1 drink daily*	4 mm Hg	3 mm Hg

DASH, Dietary Approaches to Stop Hypertension.
Adapted from Whelton PK, Carey RM, Aronow WS, et al. ACC/AHA/AAPA/ABC/ACPM/AGS/APhA/ASH/ASPC/NMA/PCNA guideline for the prevention, detection, evaluation, and management of high blood pressure in adults: a report of the American College of Cardiology/American Heart Association task force on clinical practice guidelines. *J Am Coll Cardiol.* 2018;71:e127–248.

diet were used, depending on the energy requirements of each participant. The DASH diet provided 18% kcal from protein, 55% kcal from carbohydrate, and 27% kcal from fat. After 9 weeks of intervention, the lifestyle group lost an average of 5.5 kg, whereas the control group had a mean weight loss of 0.6 kg. The mean change in 24-hour SBP and diastolic blood pressure (DBP) was −10.5/−5.9 mm Hg in the lifestyle group and −1.1/−0.6 mm Hg in the control group. BP reductions of this degree are similar to those accomplished with pharmacotherapy.

2. How do you follow a low-sodium diet?
   The United States Department of Agriculture (USDA) *2015–2020 Dietary Guidelines for Americans* describe how Americans eat more sodium than recommended—an average of more than 3400 mg or 100 mEq of sodium daily! The USDA guidelines recommend limiting sodium intake to less than 2300 mg/d (roughly 1 teaspoon of salt) and patients with prehypertension or hypertension to reduce their sodium intake to 1500 mg/d. Reducing sodium intake can decrease BP by approximately 5/3 mm Hg (see Table 29.2). About 75% of dietary sodium comes from eating packaged and restaurant foods, whereas only a small portion (11%) comes from directly adding salt to food when cooking or eating. Foods such as bread, stock (broth) cubes, and breakfast cereals are often high in salt, which is often overlooked. Of note, current guidelines differ in the recommended amount of sodium intake for patients with heart failure. Observational studies uphold that sodium restriction improves heart failure outcomes, whereas other randomized controlled trials infer that dietary sodium restriction can cause hypovolemia and increased neurohormonal activation. Thus there remains controversy surrounding restricting dietary sodium content especially in regards to heart failure.

3. How do you calculate how much sodium is in foods or beverages?
   There is a misconception that "salt" and "sodium" are synonymous terms. In reality, sodium (Na) is a mineral and a chemical element with the atomic number 11. Sodium also is a chemical element (other than chloride [Cl]) found in salt (sodium chloride [NaCl]). Foods and beverages may contain no salt (NaCl), but they still may be high in sodium because of the presence of naturally occurring sodium. Salt (NaCl) contains a 1:1 ratio of Na and Cl ions. The molar mass of Na is 22.99 g/mol and of Cl is 35.45 g/mol. One mole of NaCl equals 58.44 g NaCl.

Nutrition Facts

6 Servings per container

Servings size   **1 serving (230g)**

Amount per serving

Calories   330

	% Daily Value*
Total Fat 10g	13%
Saturated Fat 1g	5%
Trans Fat 0g	
Cholesterol 20mg	7%
Sodium 700mg	**30%**
Total Carbohydrate 44g	16%
Dietary Fiber 2g	7%
Total Sugars 5g	
Includes 0g Added Sugars	0%
Protein 15g	
Vitamin D 1 mcg	6%
Calcium 267mg	20%
Iron 2mg	10%
Potassium 169mg	4%

*The % Daily Value tells you how much a nutrient in a surving of food contribute to a daily diet 2000 calories a day used for general nutrition advice.

Fig. 29.1 Typical food label.

Therefore 100 g of NaCl contains 39.34 g Na and 60.66 g Cl, thus sodium (Na) is roughly 40% of the weight of salt, and chloride is the remaining 60%. Nutritionists often suggest diminishing salt intake, but it is sodium you will see listed on food labels (Fig. 29.1). If you are cooking and want to figure out how much sodium you are adding, convert grams of salt to milligrams of sodium, then divide the amount of salt in grams by 2.5, and then finally multiply by 1000 to get milligrams. The amount of sodium in a serving of food is listed in milligrams (mg) and as a percent of the daily value on the nutrition label. The percent daily value (% daily value) for sodium gives a general idea of how much sodium a serving adds to your total daily diet. The percent daily value for sodium on the nutrition label shown here is baseline on a daily maximum value of 2300 mg.

4. How effective is the DASH diet?

The DASH diet is a widely used dietary intervention for hypertension. The DASH diet emphasizes fruits, vegetables, and low-fat dairy products with reduced intake in saturated fat and cholesterol. In terms of macronutrient

Table 29.3 Effect of DASH Diet and Sodium Reduction on Blood Pressure

DIET	SODIUM LEVELS RESTRICTION CHANGES[a]	SBP CHANGE (mm Hg)	SBP ABSOLUTE CHANGE (mm Hg)
Control diet[b]	High to intermediate	−2 mm Hg	~133–131 mm Hg
Control diet[b]	Intermediate to low	−5 mm Hg	~131–126 mm Hg
DASH diet	High to intermediate	−1 mm Hg	~126–125 mm Hg
DASH diet	Intermediate to low	−2 mm Hg	~125–123 mm Hg

[a]High sodium level = 3500 mg; intermediate sodium level = 2400 mg; low sodium level = 1500 mg.
[b]Control diet: typical of what many people in the United States eat.
DASH, Dietary Approaches to Stop Hypertension; *SBP*, systolic blood pressure.
Adapted from Sacks FM, Svetkey LP, Vollmer WM, et al. Effects on blood pressure of reduced dietary sodium and the dietary approaches to stop hypertension diet. *N Engl J Med.* 2001;344(1):3–10.

Table 29.4 Comparison of Control Diet against DASH Diet with Varying Sodium Levels

SODIUM LEVELS[a]	DIET CHANGES[b]	SBP CHANGE (mm Hg)	SBP ABSOLUTE CHANGE (mm Hg)
High	Control to DASH diet	−6 mm Hg	~133–126 mm Hg
Intermediate	Control to DASH diet	−5 mm Hg	~131–125 mm Hg
Low	Control to DASH diet	−2 mm Hg	~126–123 mm Hg

[a]High sodium level = 3500 mg; intermediate sodium level = 2400 mg; low sodium level = 1500 mg.
[b]Control diet: typical of what many people in the United States eat.
DASH, Dietary Approaches to Stop Hypertension; *SBP*, systolic blood pressure.
Adapted from Sacks FM, Svetkey LP, Vollmer WM, et al. Effects on blood pressure of reduced dietary sodium and the dietary approaches to stop hypertension diet. *N Engl J Med.* 2001;344(1):3–10.

composition, the nutrient goals of the DASH diet are as follows: total fat (27% of calories), saturated fat (6% of calories), protein (18% of calories), and carbohydrates (55% of calories). It includes a sodium goal of 2300 mg and potassium goal of 4700 mg. The original trial (Appel et al., NEJM, 1997) demonstrated the DASH diet reducing BP (reduced SBP by 11.4 mm Hg and DBP by 5.5 mm Hg) in subjects with known hypertension, but it also showed reductions in BP in subjects without hypertension (reduced SBP by 3.5 mm Hg and DBP by 2.1 mm Hg) compared to the control diet.

5. **Is the DASH diet more effective with the addition of sodium restriction?**
   Because the DASH trial was conducted independent of testing the effect of sodium restriction, a subsequent multicenter, randomized trial was conducted to examine the combined effect of the DASH diet with sodium restriction on BP. The DASH diet showed to lower BP at high (3500 mg/d; typical of current US sodium consumption), intermediate (2400 mg/d; reflecting the upper limit of current US recommendations), and lower levels (1500 mg/d; reflecting potentially optimal sodium levels) of sodium intake, but the lowest SBP and DBP were seen in patients who were on the DASH diet with the lowest amount of sodium intake (Tables 29.3 and 29.4). Thus the combined effects of low sodium intake (1500 mg/d) and DASH diet were greater than the effects of either intervention alone and they were substantial. In addition, in participants with hypertension, the effects were equal to or greater than those of single drug therapy. Although the DASH diet has been endorsed by the Joint National Committee, the American Diabetic Association, and the National Heart, Lung and Blood Institute Lifestyle Guidelines, the adherence to the DASH diet remains suboptimal across all races/ethnicities, education levels, and income levels across the United States.

6. **Can the DASH diet be used in patients with diminished kidney function to lower BP?**
   More than two thirds of US adults with chronic kidney disease (CKD) have uncontrolled hypertension. Lowering BP to recommended treatment targets slows down the progression of CKD, and the DASH diet may have an important role in BP control. In a pilot study, 11 participants with moderate CKD (epidermal growth factor receptor between 30 and 59 mL/min/1.73 m^2) were monitored after completing 1 week of reduced-sodium, run-in diet followed by a reduced-sodium DASH diet. The pilot date showed minimal acute metabolic abnormalities in adults with moderate CKD and a possible improvement in nocturnal BP. Overall, mean serum potassium was significantly higher after DASH diet week 1, but it was not significantly different from baseline after DASH diet week 2.

7. **Does the Mediterranean diet result in BP effects?**
   There have been considerable efforts to test how adoption of a Mediterranean diet impacts cardiovascular health. The Mediterranean diet consists of a diet heavy in fish, monounsaturated fats from olive oil, fruits, vegetables, whole grains, legumes, nuts, and moderate alcohol consumption. The diet can graphically be represented in

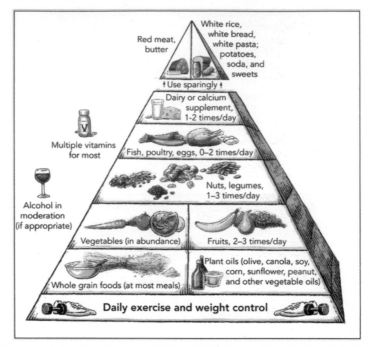

Fig. 29.2 Harvard food pyramid for the Mediterranean diet. (Copyright 2008. For more information about The Healthy Eating Pyramid, please see The Nutrition Source, Department of Nutrition, Harvard T.H. Chan School of Public Health, www.thenutritionsource.org; and Willett WC, Skerrett PJ. *Eat, Drink, and Be Healthy* New York: Free Press/Simon & Schuster; 2005.)

the Mediterranean diet pyramid, which is often considered an alternative to the USDA's original food pyramid (Fig. 29.2). It includes all food groups with adequate frequencies and quantities in the daily diet. Numerous epidemiological studies have associated the Mediterranean diet to be superior to American diets in respect to longevity and reduced risk of cardiovascular disease. A few studies have shown a positive effect of the Mediterranean diet in reducing BP in hypertensive or healthy people. However, there is not enough evidence to declare how strong this effect is.

8. **Does the Nordic diet result in BP effects?**
   The Nordic diet highlights the local and seasonal foods from Denmark, Finland, Iceland, Norway, and Sweden. It is similar to the Mediterranean diet in that it accentuates whole grains, berries, vegetables, fatty fish, and legumes, and it is low in sweets and red meat. A systematic review consisting of five randomized controlled trials with 513 participants showed the Nordic diet significantly reducing the SBP and DBP by 3.97 mm Hg and 2.08 mm Hg, respectively.

9. **Does the Ketogenic diet result in BP effects?**
   A ketogenic diet is a carbohydrate-restrictive and high-fat diet. It restricts carbohydrate intake to less than 25 to 50 g/d in an attempt to enhance tissues to use fat or ketones as fuel during caloric restriction. Ketogenic diets typically recommend that only 5% of daily calories come from carbohydrates, 75% from fat, and 20% from protein. The ketogenic diet is successful in achieving weight loss, but data on BP effects are lacking. However, it should be used in caution due to it limiting fruits and vegetables, which are emphasized in the DASH diet. Moreover, the ketogenic diet should not be used in patients with diabetes and reduced kidney function secondary to risk of developing ketoacidosis.

10. **Does intermittent fasting result in BP effects?**
    Intermittent fasting is a form of time-restricted eating (typically 16 hours fasting and 8 hours eating), which has gained popularity. Intermittent fasting shows promise as a possible new approach to weight loss and potential long-term health benefits through its antiinflammatory properties. Intermittent fasting causes an increase in brain-derived neurotrophic factor (BDNF), which results in lowering the SBP and DBP by activating the parasympathetic nervous system (PNS). PNS activation leads to decreased cardiac output via a decrease in heart rate, resulting in lower BP. Most of the data derived to determine the beneficial effects of intermittent fasting come from animal models. Only small, short-term duration studies have been performed in humans.

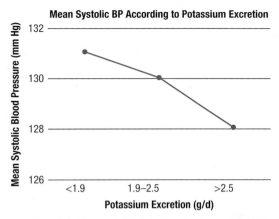

Fig. 29.3 Urinary potassium excretion and blood pressure (BP). A significant inverse association between estimated potassium excretion and systolic BP in the setting of sodium excretion 3 to 5 g/d. (Adapted from Mente A, O'Donnell MJ, Rangarajan S, et al. Association of urinary sodium and potassium excretion with blood pressure. *N Engl J Med.* 2014;371(7): 601–611.)

For example, strict alternate-day fasting (ADF) for 4 weeks in nonobese, healthy adults showed a decrease in body weight by 4.5%. In addition, cardiovascular parameters and the CVD risk are improved upon ADF.

11. **Does the high potassium diet result in BP effects?**
Population studies as well as randomized controlled trials have shown an inverse relation of potassium intake to BP (Fig. 29.3), the prevalence of hypertension, and the risk of stroke. Some have postulated that the ratio of sodium to potassium may be more important than the specific amounts of sodium or potassium that an individual consumes. The daily recommended allowance for potassium is 3500 to 4700 mg/dL per the National Academics of Sciences, Engineering, and Medicine (NASEM), preferable by consumption of a diet high in potassium-rich foods. Examples include bananas (358 potassium content/100 g), avocados (485 potassium content/100 g), prunes (732 potassium content/100 g), spinach (558 potassium content/100 g), and fat free yogurt (255 potassium content/100 g). The World Health Organization (WHO) as well suggests a potassium intake of at least 90 mmol/d (3510 mg/d) from food, with a goal to reduce BP and risk of cardiovascular disease, stroke, and coronary heart disease in adults.

12. **What are the recommendations for alcohol consumption to reduce BP?**
The 2017 ACC/AHA High Blood Pressure Guideline recommends capping daily alcohol intake to one to two drinks for men and one drink for women. One drink contains roughly 14 g of pure alcohol, which is typically found in 12 oz beer (roughly 5% alcohol), 5 oz wine (roughly 12% alcohol), and 1.5 oz of distilled spirits (usually 40% alcohol). When individuals restrict their intake per these guidelines, patients with hypertension saw a roughly −4-mm Hg drop in SBP and normotensive patients saw a roughly −3-mm Hg in SBP in randomized controls.

13. **What effect does heavy alcohol intake have on BP?**
It is well established that heavy alcohol consumption increases the risk of hypertension, especially in a binge pattern. In a systematic review and metaanalyses, which included 36 trials and 2865 participants (2464 men and 401 women), reducing alcohol intake lowered BP in a dose-dependent manner with an apparent threshold effect. A reduction in BP was seen in patients who drank more than two drinks per day, but the strongest reduction in BP was seen in patients who drank six or more drinks per day, and when they cut back roughly 50%.

14. **What role does smoking have on BP?**
Despite the known harmful effects of cigarette smoking on cardiovascular disease, epidemiological studies show that smokers have a lower BP than nonsmokers. Surprisingly, cigarette smoking does not appear to be a risk factor for hypertension alone. In contrast, cessation of smoking cigarettes increases the risk of hypertension in healthy men, and former smokers increase their risk of developing hypertension by up to 3.5-fold. The increase in BP could be a stress response involved with smoking cessation, the loss of a coping mechanism, and the associated weight gain. Nonetheless, smoking cessation is still universally recommended to prevent its other adverse effects on cardiovascular health and carcinogenesis.

15. **What is the pathophysiology of obesity-related hypertension?**

   Obesity continues to increase in prevalence with approximately 68% of adults in the United States being overweight or obese. Hypertension is associated with obesity, and weight loss is first-line therapy in the treatment of hypertension in these individuals. Adults who are obese have a 3.5-fold increased likelihood of hypertension, and the prevalence of hypertension is threefold higher in obese children than in nonobese children. Several factors have been suggested to promote obesity-associated hypertension by activating the sympathetic nervous system (SNS), including hyperinsulinemia, renin-angiotensin-aldosterone system (RAAS) activation, baroreflex dysfunction, and obstructive sleep apnea (OSA). Mechanisms involved in activation of the RAAS in obesity include SNS stimulation, synthesis of adipokines by the RAAS in visceral fat, and hemodynamic alterations. In addition, leptin, a hormone produced in fat, produces satiety and weight loss by diminishing caloric intake but can also cause hypertension by upregulating the SNS.

16. **What impact does weight loss have in reducing BP?**

   A metaanalysis of randomized controlled trials published in *Hypertension* in 2003 (Neter et al.) showed an approximately 1-mm Hg drop in SBP for each kilogram of weight lost. Net weight reductions in these studies was approximately 5 kg. Bariatric surgery, such as Roux-en-Y gastric bypass or laparoscopic sleeve gastrectomy, are the most successful approaches to sustaining weight loss in patients who failed in lifestyle and pharmacologic therapy. The data on hypertension following bariatric surgery is somewhat mixed, but the majority of evidence supports significant improvement in hypertension control with weight-reduction surgery. The majority of studies have a short follow-up period of less than 2 years.

17. **What is the role of physical exercise in hypertension?**

   Physical inactivity is believed to be solely responsible for 5% to 13% of hypertension today. Patients should be instructed to be physically active, which should include 90 to 150 minutes per week of aerobic exercise or dynamic resistance per 2017 ACC/AHA High Blood Pressure Guidelines. In a metaanalysis of 54 randomized controlled trials (2419 participants), the average reduction in SBP with aerobic exercise was approximately 2 to 4 mm Hg and 5 to 8 mm Hg in adult patients with normotension and hypertension, respectively. The 2017 ACC/AHA High Blood Pressure Guidelines recommend isometric exercise, but it should be performed with caution. Isometric exercise routines (e.g., weightlifting) may raise BP acutely and should be directed by a professional.

18. **How effective is OSA treatment in reducing BP in hypertension?**

   OSA is a common disorder that is caused by a collapse of the upper airway during sleep, which leads to metabolic and neurohormonal disturbances that have adverse cardiovascular consequences. Data shows that there is a strong association between OSA and systemic hypertension, and the use of continuous positive airway pressure (CPAP) drops SBP by roughly 2 mm Hg. However, patients with resistant hypertension show a drop of −7.21 in ambulatory BP and of −4.99 mm Hg in SBP and DBP, respectively.

19. **What alternative approaches may be beneficial in treating hypertension?**

   Extensive evidence indicates that psychosocial stress contributes to hypertension, and stress-reducing techniques have the potential to lower BP. Stress-reducing treatments like guided breathing, yoga, transcendental meditation, and biofeedback have undergone less rigorous study, but they are a potential opportunity for additional research. They currently lack strong evidence for long-term BP-lowering effect. A systematic review of published literature looking at 17 trials with 23 treatment comparisons and 960 participants demonstrated transcendental meditation and showed potential in reducing BP. Transcendental meditation allows a person to reach a peaceful level of consciousness by meditating quietly with eyes closed for 15 to 20 minutes twice a day to decrease stress and reach pure mind awareness. It resulted in the most significant weighted mean difference in BP (indicating net change relative to control groups) with SBP decreasing by 5.0 mm Hg and DBP decreasing by 2.8 mm Hg. Related data also shows improvement in other cardiovascular disease risk factors and clinical outcomes.

KEY POINTS

1. The 2017 ACC/AHA Guideline for the Prevention, Detection, Evaluation, and Management of High Blood Pressure in Adults recommends limiting dietary sodium intake (<1500 mg/d), routine exercise, weight management, tobacco cessation, and decreased alcohol consumption.
2. The DASH diet is a widely used intervention for hypertension, which emphasizes fruits, vegetables, and low-fat dairy products with reduced intake in saturated fat and cholesterol. It is most effective when combined with sodium restriction (<1500 mg/d or 65 mmol/d).
3. Population studies and trials show an inverse relationship to potassium intake to BP. The daily recommended potassium intake is 3510 mg/d or higher (90 mmol) per WHO.
4. Adults are recommended to limit daily alcohol intake to one to two drinks for men and one drink for women.
5. Obesity is associated with the development and worsening of hypertension, and the best goal is to achieve ideal body weight. Blood pressure reduction with weight loss is typically 1 mm Hg per kilogram of weight loss.
6. Adults should be instructed to include 90 to 150 minutes a week of aerobic exercise or dynamic resistance.

BIBLIOGRAPHY

Aburto NJ, Hanson S, Gutierrez H, Hooper L, Elliott P, Cappuccio FP. Effect of increased potassium intake on cardiovascular risk factors and disease: Systematic review and meta-analyses. *BMJ*. 2013;346(Apr03 3.)doi: 10.1136/bmj.f1378.

Appel LJ, Moore TJ, Obarzanek E, et al. A clinical trial of the effects of dietary patterns on blood pressure. DASH Collaborative Research Group. *N Engl J Med*. 1997 Apr 17;336(16):1117–1124. doi: 10.1056/NEJM199704173361601. PMID: 9099655.

Bonafini S, Fava C. Home blood pressure measurements: advantages and disadvantages compared to office and ambulatory monitoring. *Blood Pressure*. 2015;24(6):325–332. doi: 10.3109/08037051.2015.1070599.

Brook RD, Appel LJ, Rubenfire M, et al. American Heart Association Professional Education Committee of the Council for High Blood Pressure Research, Council on Cardiovascular and Stroke Nursing, Council on Epidemiology and Prevention, and Council on Nutrition, Physical Activity. Beyond medications and diet: alternative approaches to lowering blood pressure: a scientific statement from the American Heart Association. *Hypertension*. 2013 Jun;61(6):1360–1383. doi: 10.1161/HYP.0b013e318293645f. Epub 2013 Apr 22. PMID: 23608661.

Caligiuri SPB, Pierce GN. A review of the relative efficacy of dietary, nutritional supplements, lifestyle, and drug therapies in the management of hypertension. *Crit Rev Food Sci Nutr*. 2016;57(16):3508–3527. doi: 10.1080/10408398.2016.1142420.

Chen H, Shen FE, Tan XD, Jiang WB, Gu YH. Efficacy and safety of acupuncture for essential hypertension: a meta-analysis. *Med Sci Monit*. 2018 May 8;24:2946–2969. doi: 10.12659/MSM.909995. PMID: 29735972; PMCID: PMC5963739.

Eckel RH, Jakicic JM, Ard JD, et al. American College of Cardiology/American Heart Association Task Force on Practice Guidelines. 2013 AHA/ACC guideline on lifestyle management to reduce cardiovascular risk: a report of the American College of Cardiology/American Heart Association Task Force on Practice Guidelines. *J Am Coll Cardiol*. 2014 Jul 1;63(25 Pt B):2960–2984. doi: 10.1016/j.jacc.2013.11.003. Epub 2013 Nov 12. Erratum in: *J Am Coll Cardiol*. 2014 Jul 1;63(25 Pt B):3027-3028. PMID: 24239922.

Green MS, Jucha E, Luz Y. Blood pressure in smokers and nonsmokers: epidemiologic findings. *Am Heart J*. 1986 May;111(5):932–940. doi: 10.1016/0002-8703(86)90645-9. PMID: 3706114.

Juraschek SP, Miller 3rd ER, Weaver CM, Appel LJ. Effects of sodium reduction and the DASH diet in relation to baseline blood pressure. *J Am Coll Cardiol*. 2017 Dec 12;70(23):2841–2848. doi: 10.1016/j.jacc.2017.10.011. Epub 2017 Nov 12. PMID: 29141784; PMCID: PMC5742671.

Konerman MC, Hummel SL. Sodium restriction in heart failure: benefit or harm?. *Curr Treat Options Cardiovasc Med*. 2014;16(2)doi: 10.1007/s11936-013-0286-x.

Lee DH, Ha MH, Kim JR, Jacobs Jr DR. Effects of smoking cessation on changes in blood pressure and incidence of hypertension: a 4-year follow-up study. *Hypertension*. 2001 Feb;37(2):194–198. doi: 10.1161/01.hyp.37.2.194. PMID: 11230270.

Malinowski B, Zalewska K, Węsierska A, et al. Intermittent fasting in cardiovascular disorders—an overview. *Nutrients*. 2019 Mar 20;11(3):673. doi: 10.3390/nu11030673. PMID: 30897855; PMCID: PMC6471315.

Mente A, O'Donnell MJ, Rangarajan S, et al. PURE Investigators. Association of urinary sodium and potassium excretion with blood pressure. *N Engl J Med*. 2014 Aug 14;371(7):601–611. doi: 10.1056/NEJMoa1311989. PMID: 25119606.

Miller ER, Erlinger TP, Young D, et al. Results of the Diet, Exercise, and Weight Loss Intervention Trial (DEW-IT). *Hypertension* (Dallas, TX: 1979). 2002;40(5):612–618. https://doi.org/10.1161/01.hyp.0000037217.96002.8e.

Notor JE, Stam BE, Kok FJ, Grobbee DE, Geleijnse JM. Influence of weight reduction on blood pressure: a meta-analysis of randomized controlled trials. *Hypertension* (Dallas, TX: 1979). 2003;42(5):878–884. https://doi.org/10.1161/01.HYP.0000094221.86888.AE.

Rainforth MV, Schneider RH, Nidich SI, Gaylord-King C, Salerno JW, Anderson JW. Stress reduction programs in patients with elevated blood pressure: a systematic review and meta-analysis. *Curr Hypertens Rep*. 2007;9(6):520–528. https://doi.org/10.1007/s11906-007-0094-3.

Ramezani-Jolfaie N, Mohammadi M, Salehi-Abargouei A. The effect of healthy Nordic diet on cardio metabolic markers: a systematic review and meta-analysis of randomized controlled clinical trials. *Eur J Nutr*. 2019;58(6):2159–2174. https://doi.org/10.1007/s00394-018-1804-0.

Roerecke M, Kaczorowski J, Tobe SW, Gmel G, Hasan O, Rehm J. The effect of a reduction in alcohol consumption on blood pressure: a systematic review and meta-analysis. *Lancet Public Health*. 2017;2(2):e108–e120. https://doi.org/10.1016/S2468-2667(17)30003-8.

Sacks FM, Svetkey LP, Vollmer WM, et al. Effects on blood pressure of reduced dietary sodium and the dietary approaches to stop hypertension (Dash) diet. *New Engl J Med*. 4 Jan 2001;344(1):3–10. doi: 10.1097/00008483-200105000-00012.

Samadian F, Dalili N, Jamalian A. Lifestyle modifications to prevent and control hypertension. *Iran J Kidney Dis*. 2016;10(5):237–263.

Steinberg D, Bennett GG, Svetkey L. The DASH diet, 20 years later. *JAMA*. 2017;317(15):1529–1530. https://doi.org/10.1001/jama.2017.1628.

Svetkey LP, Sacks FM, Obarzanek E, et al. The DASH diet, Sodium Intake and Blood Pressure Trial (DASH-sodium): rationale and design. DASH-Sodium Collaborative Research Group. *J Am Diet Assoc*. 1999;99(8 Suppl):S96–S104. https://doi.org/10.1016/s0002-8223(99)00423-x.

Torres G, Sánchez-de-la-Torre M, Barbé F. Relationship between OSA and hypertension. *Chest*. 2015;148(3):824–832. https://doi.org/10.1378/chest.15-0136.

The treatment of mild hypertension study. A randomized, placebo-controlled trial of a nutritional-hygienic regimen along with various drug monotherapies. The Treatment of Mild Hypertension Research Group. *Arch Intern Med*. 1991;151(7):1413–1423. https://doi.org/10.1001/archinte.151.7.1413.

Tripolt NJ, Stekovic S, Aberer F, et al. Intermittent fasting (alternate day fasting) in healthy, non-obese adults: protocol for a cohort trial with an embedded randomized controlled pilot trial. *Adv Ther*. 2018;35(8):1265–1283. https://doi.org/10.1007/s12325-018-0746-5.

Tyson CC, Lin PH, Corsino L, et al. Short-term effects of the DASH diet in adults with moderate chronic kidney disease: a pilot feeding study. *Clin Kidney J*. 2016 Aug;9(4):592–598. doi: 10.1093/ckj/sfw046. Epub 2016 Jun 5. PMID: 27478603; PMCID: PMC4957723.

Whelton SP, Chin A, Xin X, He J. Effect of aerobic exercise on blood pressure: a meta-analysis of randomized, controlled trials. *Ann Intern Med*. 2002 Apr 2;136(7):493–503. doi: 10.7326/0003-4819-136-7-200204020-00006. PMID: 11926784.

Whelton PK, Carey RM, Aronow WS, et al. 2017 ACC/AHA/AAPA/ABC/ACPM/AGS/APhA/ASH/ASPC/NMA/PCNA guideline for the prevention, detection, evaluation, and management of high blood pressure in adults: a report of the American College of Cardiology/American Heart Association task force on clinical practice guidelines. *J Am Coll Cardiol*. 2018;71:e127–248.

WHO. *Guideline: Potassium intake for adults and children*. Geneva: World Health Organization; 2009.

Wu Y, Johnson BT, Acabchuk RL, et al. Yoga as antihypertensive lifestyle therapy: a systematic review and meta-analysis. *Mayo Clin Proc*. 2019 Mar;94(3):432–446. doi: 10.1016/j.mayocp.2018.09.023. Epub 2019 Feb 18. PMID: 30792067.

Yang J, Chen J, Yang M, et al. Acupuncture for hypertension. *Cochrane Database Syst Rev*. 2018 Nov 14;11(11):CD008821. doi: 10.1002/14651858.CD008821.pub2. PMID: 30480757; PMCID: PMC6516840.

CHAPTER 30

BLOOD PRESSURE TREATMENT GOALS

Atul Bali, MD, Uta Erdbrügger, MD, and Robert M. Carey, MD, MACP

QUESTIONS

1. **Why is a treatment goal important for hypertension?**
   Hypertension is the most important risk factor for cardiovascular disease (CVD) and stroke worldwide. Epidemiological studies demonstrate that blood pressure (BP) is continuously related to the risk of fatal stroke, ischemic heart disease (IHD), and noncardiac vascular disease well down into the normal range (beginning at 115/75 mm Hg). For example, a 20-mm Hg higher systolic blood pressure (SBP) or a 10-mm Hg higher diastolic blood pressure (DBP) associates with a doubling of the risk for a fatal cardiovascular event.

   Control of BP to an established target is critical to prevent CVD events and mortality. Specifically, suboptimal BP control (above target) is the most common attributable risk factor for death worldwide, being responsible for approximately 62% of CVD, 49% of IHD, and 7.1 million deaths annually.

   Randomized controlled trials (RCTs) have confirmed that the risk of CVD can be greatly reduced with effective antihypertensive therapy. For example, a 10-mm Hg lower SBP or a 5-mm Hg lower DBP results in approximately a 40% reduction in stroke risk and a 30% reduction in IHD risk.

   A BP treatment goal represents the average optimum BP level for CVD prevention based on current evidence and balanced against the occurrence of detrimental side effects resulting from the BP reduction itself and/or the treatment. BP treatment goals are derived from results of RCTs, which represent aggregate responses of their study populations. Therefore BP goals are intended as general guides, and, with this knowledge, individual BP goals should be set by the clinician in consultation with the patient.

2. **What was the established treatment goal up to 2017, and what was the evidence?**
   The treatment goals prior to 2017 were established in 2003 by the Joint National Committee (JNC)-7 Report. The general goal was BP less than 140/90 mm Hg and less than 130/80 mm Hg for patients with diabetes mellitus (DM) and/or chronic kidney disease (CKD). In 2003 the evidence was largely derived from the Hypertension Optimal Treatment (HOT) clinical trial (1998) and the Blood Pressure Lowering Treatment Trialists Collaboration clinical trials (2000), which recorded, for example, a 35% to 40% reduction in stroke incidence at this level of BP control. A sustained 12-mm Hg lowering of SBP resulted in 1 life saved of 11 patients treated, and this number increased to 1 in 9 if background CVD or target-organ damage was present.

3. **What new findings contributed to the establishment of new BP treatment goals in 2017?**
   In 2015 the results of the landmark Systolic Blood Pressure Intervention Trial (SPRINT) were published. SPRINT randomized over 9000 patients with hypertension of 50 years of age or older with background CVD or high CVD risk to more intensive (goal SBP <120 mm Hg) or less intensive (goal SBP <140 mm Hg) BP-lowering treatment. Patients with DM or prior stroke were excluded. The trial was halted early after the Data Safety Monitoring Board revealed a 25% lower risk of fatal and nonfatal major CVD events and a 27% lower risk of death from any cause in the intensive BP-lowering arm. The SPRINT results have been accepted worldwide as providing convincing evidence that treatment to a lower BP goal, at least in adults at high CVD risk, prevents CVD events and death.

   In addition to SPRINT, several high-quality systematic reviews and metaanalyses of RCTs bearing on BP goal were published in 2016–17 (results summarized in Table 30.1). In a metaanalysis reported by Xie et al., which did not include SPRINT, more intensive BP lowering to an average BP of 133/76 mm Hg reduced major CVD events (risk ratio [RR], 0.86; 95% confidence interval [CI], 0.78–0.96) compared to less intensive BP control (BP 140/81 mm Hg).[1] A systematic review and metaanalysis by Thomopoulos et al. stratified outcomes by BP achieved in trials that employed more versus less intense BP lowering.[2] Comparing those who achieved an SBP of less than 130 mm Hg to those achieving an SBP of 130 mm Hg or higher, the RR for stroke was 0.71 (95% CI, 0.61–0.84), for cardiovascular death was 0.80 (95% CI, 0.67–0.97), and for all-cause mortality was 0.84 (95% CI, 0.73–0.95). In a cumulative sequential metaanalysis by Verdecchia et al., more (BP 129/76 mm Hg) compared to less (BP 138/81 mm Hg) BP lowering resulted in an RR for stroke of 0.80 (95% CI, 0.67–0.95) and for myocardial infarction (MI) of 0.85 (95% CI, 0.76–0.95).[3] A network metaanalysis by Bangalore et al., restricted to 17 trials in which participants were randomly assigned to different BP targets, demonstrated progressive benefit with lower BP targets down to an SBP of less than 120 mm Hg for both CVD outcomes and mortality.[4]

   The highest quality network metaanalysis available included 42 randomized controlled two-arm trials with 144,220 adults in which the more and less intensively treated groups had an SBP that differed by 5 mm Hg or

Table 30.1 Cardiovascular Disease Risk Reduction from More vs. Less Intensive Blood Pressure Lowering in Metaanalyses of Randomized Clinical Trials (2016-2017)

FIRST AUTHOR (SEE LIST OF REFERENCES)	COMPARISONS (RANDOM)	OUTCOMES	PERCENT RISK REDUCTION
Xie	More vs. less intensive treatment	MACE	14
		Stroke	22
		MI	13
		HF	15
Thomopoulos	SBP/DBP 10/5 mm Hg lower in more intensively treated group SBP <130 mm Hg vs. SBP >130 mm Hg	MACE	25
		Stroke	29
		CHD	20
		HF	20
		Stroke	29
		CHD	14
		HF	19
Verdecchia	More vs. less intensive treatment	Stroke	20
		MI	15
		HF	25
Bangalore	SBP <120 vs. <160 mm Hg SBP <130 vs. <160 mm Hg SBP <130 vs. <140 mm Hg	Stroke	46
		MI	32
		Stroke	38
		Stroke	17
Bundy	SBP 120–124 vs. >160 mm Hg SBP 130–134 vs. >160 mm Hg SBP 130–134 vs. 140–144 mm Hg	MACE	64
		Stroke	73
		CHD	53
		CVM	66
		ACM	53
		MACE	49
		Stroke	61
		CHD	41
		CVM	49
		ACM	35
		MACE	17
		Stroke	26
		CHD	12
		CVM	19
		ACM	18

ACM, All-cause mortality; *CHD,* chronic heart disease; *CVM,* cardiovascular mortality; *DBP,* diastolic blood pressure; *HF,* heart failure; *MACE,* major adverse cardiovascular event; *MI,* myocardial infarction; *SBP,* systolic blood pressure.

more in randomized comparisons.[5] A progressive reduction in CVD risk was observed at lower levels of achieved SBP, including major CVD events, stroke, IHD, and all-cause mortality. Similar findings were observed when direct metaanalysis was employed and in sensitivity analyses with the SPRINT results excluded.

Finally, the independent Evidence Review Committee (ERC) for the 2017 American College of Cardiology/American Heart Association (ACC/AHA) BP guideline conducted a thorough systematic review and metaanalysis of more versus less intensive BP lowering in RCTs. The metaanalysis demonstrated a consistent pattern of benefit of intensive BP lowering for all CVD outcomes and all-cause mortality. Intensive BP lowering significantly reduced the risk of major adverse cardiovascular events (MACE) (RR, 0.81; 95% CI, 0.70–0.94) as well as MI, stroke, and heart failure. To identify the optimal target for BP reduction, the ERC examined the risk reduction of these outcomes for RCTs with an SBP target of less than 130 mm Hg in the lower BP target group and again found a significantly reduced risk of stroke (RR, 0.82; 95% CI, 0.70–0.96) and MACE (RR, 0.84; 95% CI, 0.73–0.99) with marginally significant reductions in risk of MI (RR, 0.85; 95% CI, 0.73–1.00) and all-cause mortality.

4. What is the new general BP treatment goal for hypertension?
The new general BP treatment goal is less than 130/80 mm Hg, as recommended by the 2017 ACC/AHA guideline. These BP goals are intended as general guides, and, with this knowledge, individual BP goals should be set by the clinician in consultation with the patient.

5. **Is there additional evidence for a goal of less than 130/80 mm Hg since publication of the 2017 ACC/AHA BP guideline?**

   Yes, a systematic review and metaanalysis by Sakima et al., restricted to 19 trials in which adults with hypertension were randomly assigned to a different BP target, reported a significant reduction in major CVD events, MI, and stroke in those assigned to more versus less intensive treatment and, in subgroup analysis, identified a BP target of less than 130/80 mm Hg as optimal for CVD protection.[6]

6. **What is the current BP treatment goal for adults of 65 years of age or older and why?**

   The current BP treatment goal for adults of 65 years or older is SBP less than 130 mm Hg, as recommended by the 2017 ACC/AHA guideline. DBP is not included in the recommendation because many older adults have lower DBP values due to vascular stiffness with aging.

   SPRINT included 2636 community-dwelling adults age 75 years or older (28% of the total study population). This subgroup experienced a 34% lower risk of developing the primary composite CVD outcome and a 33% lower risk of all-cause mortality with intensive versus standard treatment. The results did not differ for those who were frail or had impaired gait speed. Most importantly, there was no difference in serious adverse events including falls or in self-assessed quality of life, irrespective of frailty status.

   During trial follow-up, the incidence of mild cognitive impairment (MCI) was significantly reduced in the SPRINT intensive compared to standard treatment group (hazard ratio [HR], 0.83; 95% CI, 0.70–0.99). During extended trial and posttrial follow-up (median of 5.1 years), the composite of MCI and dementia was significantly less common in those randomized to the intensive compared to standard treatment (0.85 [95% CI, 0.74–0.97]).

   During a median follow-up of 4 years, a magnetic resonance imaging (MRI) substudy conducted in 670 SPRINT participants reported significantly less progression of cerebral small vessel ischemic disease as indicated by white matter lesions, characteristically associated with Alzheimer disease, in the intensive compared to standard treatment group. A similar benefit was noted during intensive BP treatment in the ACCORD-BP trial and more recently in the INFINITY trial. Taken together, these findings provide confidence that intensive BP-lowering therapy is at least safe with respect to brain function in ambulatory noninstitutionalized older adults.

   Recently, the beneficial effect on major CVD events, MCI, and death was reaffirmed in SPRINT participants age 80 years or older. Although the risk of changes in kidney function was increased in the intensive treatment group, the clinical and biological importance of these findings is unknown. There was no difference in the incidence of injurious falls, a major source of morbidity in this advanced age group. As recognized by the SPRINT and SPRINT MIND investigators, the results of SPRINT are not generalizable to institutionalized older adults or those with clinical dementia, limited life expectancy, or a high burden of comorbidities.

7. **What is the current BP treatment goal for patients with CKD/end-stage kidney disease and why?**

   The 2017 ACC/AHA guideline identified special populations with comorbid conditions associated with an increased risk of adverse outcomes. In these populations, the goal of antihypertensive therapy is primary or secondary prevention of CVD and other targets of hypertension-mediated end-organ damage. A summary of recent guideline BP goal recommendations according to comorbidities for the US and international sources is presented in Table 30.2.

   In patients with CKD, the recommended BP goal is less than 130/80 mm Hg.

   The ACC/AHA writing committee noted that, although CKD is not considered in atherosclerotic CVD (ASCVD) risk assessment, most patients with CKD should be categorized as high risk for ASCVD. Based on recent systematic reviews and metaanalyses that include patients with CKD in SPRINT, although no significant benefit in the primary renal outcomes is noted, the reduction in CVD events is sufficient to support the above recommendation.

   Due to the paucity of studies evaluating hypertension and CVD events in patients with end-stage kidney disease, the 2017 ACC/AHA guidelines have not defined a BP target in this population.

   The KDIGO, kidney disease improving global outcomes (KDIGO) provided commentary on the 2017 ACC/AHA hypertension guidelines in April 2019. All patients with CKD stage 3 with or without albuminuria greater than 300 mg/d (albumin-to-creatinine ratio) and all patients with CKD stages 1 and 2 with albuminuria should be treated to maintain a BP goal of less than 130/80 mm Hg. Additionally, the 2021 updated KDIGO guidelines recommend a BP goal of less than 120/80 in patients with CKD.

8. **What is the current BP treatment goal for patients with diabetes and why?**

   In diabetic patients, the recommended BP goal is less than 130/80 mm Hg.

   The ACCORD trial, a 2:2 factorial study that was underpowered, demonstrated no significant difference in CVD composite between standard therapy (<140 mm Hg) and intensive therapy (<120 mm Hg), even though there was a small risk reduction in stroke and greater reduction in left ventricular hypertrophy with intensive therapy. A subsequent metaanalysis suggested a significant reduction in stroke risk with SBP of less than 130 mm Hg, although not for MI risk. A target BP of 133/76 mm Hg, when compared to 140/81mm Hg, resulted in significant reductions in MACE, MI, stroke, albuminuria, and progression of retinopathy. Additionally, a subset of patients in SPRINT with prediabetes appeared to have a similar benefit to nonprediabetic enrollees with intensive BP control.

Table 30.2 BP Goals According to Comorbidities by ACC/AHA and Subsequent International Blood Pressure Guidelines

		ACC/AHA	ESC/ESH	ISH
	YEAR OF PUBLICATION	**2017**	**2018**	**2020**
Blood pressure target based on comorbidity	CKD[a]	<130/80	<65 years: 130–139/70–79 ≥65 years: 130–139/70–79	Essential <140/90 Optimal <130/80 Elderly <140/80
	DM	<130/80	<65 years: 120–130/70–79 ≥65 years: 130–139/70–79	Essential <140/90 Optimal <130/80 Elderly <140/80
	Stroke	<130/80[b]	<65 years: 120–130/70–79 ≥65 years: 130–139/70–79	Essential <140/90 Optimal <130/80 Elderly <140/80
	CAD	<130/80	<65 years: 120–130/70–79 ≥65 years: 130–139/70–79	Essential <140/90 Optimal <130/80 Elderly <140/80
	CHF	<130/80	<65 years: 120–130/70–79 ≥65 years: 130–139/70–79	Essential <140/90 Optimal <130/80 (but >120/70)

[a]The 2021 KDIGO guidelines recommend a BP target of <120/80 in CKD as well.
[b]Target not recommended for those with no established diagnosis of hypertension who have had a stroke.
ACC/AHA, American College of Cardiology/American Heart Association; *BP*, blood pressure; *CHF*, chronic heart failure; *CKD*, chronic kidney disease; *DM*, diabetes mellitus; *ESC/ESH*, European Society of Cardiology/European Society of Hypertension; *ISH*, International Society of Hypertension.

9. **What is the current BP treatment goal for patients who have had a stroke?**
   In patients with known hypertension who have suffered a stroke, resumption of antihypertensive therapy with a target BP of less than 130/80 mm Hg is recommended.
   In patients without an established diagnosis of hypertension who have suffered a stroke who meet the criteria for stage 2 hypertension (SRP ≥140 or DBP ≥90 mm Hg), initiation of antihypertensive therapy with a target BP less than 130/80 mm Hg is recommended.
   The SPS3 study, a multicentric, randomized, open-label trial, demonstrated that patients randomized to the lower BP target arm (SBP <130 mm Hg) showed a lower risk of intracerebral bleeding and nonstatistically significant reductions in all strokes, disabling or fatal strokes, and composite CVD outcome (MI, vascular death).
   In patients without an established diagnosis of hypertension who have suffered a stroke, the benefit of initiating antihypertensive therapy is unclear. Post-hoc analysis of an RCT suggested that the benefit of antihypertensive therapy for secondary stroke prevention decreases as initial baseline BP declines, leading to this recommendation.

10. **What is the current BP treatment goal for patients with coronary artery disease and heart failure?**
    In hypertensive patients with stable coronary artery disease (CAD), the recommended BP goal is less than 130/80 mm Hg.
    In the INVEST study, which was a post-hoc analysis of the PROBE trial, the intervention group (SBP <140 mm Hg) was noted to have lower risk of cardiovascular mortality, total MI, nonfatal MI, total stroke, and nonfatal stroke.
    In hypertensive patients with chronic heart failure (both with preserved and reduced ejection fraction), the recommended BP goal is less than 130/80 mm Hg.
    Whereas the guideline writing committee acknowledged that there was a significant reduction in CVD composite outcome (including heart failure) with an SBP goal less than 120 mm Hg noted in SPRINT due to the limited body of evidence and less compelling results noted in other RCTs, the less stringent target of less than 130/80 mm Hg was recommended.

11. **Is there a risk of reducing BP to or below goal in some patients?**
    Despite the significant deleterious impact of hypertension, emerging evidence suggests "too tight" BP control may also be harmful. The so-called "J-curve" (or U-curve) has been documented in several observational studies showing an inverse relationship between DBP and coronary heart disease. The J-curve seems to occur at levels of DBP considered as physiological (e.g., 70–80 mm Hg). In contrast to observational studies, in SPRINT, the benefit of DBP was seen in all quintiles of baseline DBP, even the lowest one with a mean DBP of 61 ± 5 mm Hg.

In patients with CKD, most studies have shown a J-curve for cardiovascular morbidity and mortality. However, there is no evidence that a stricter BP target (<130/70 mm Hg) can improve renal outcomes, although it improves cardiovascular outcomes. The intensive control of BP may even lead to an unintended reduction of renal function (as documented in SPRINT); this is likely due to a renal hemodynamic effect and is usually reversible. However, the significance of lowering glomerular filtration rate on long-term clinical outcomes is unknown. Additionally, the J-curve pattern does not hold for stroke, and more evidence is needed for patients with a high pulse pressure.

12. **Is there benefit of lowering BP even though the goal may not be met?**
The relationship between BP and the increased risk of CVD is continuous and starts as low as 115/75 mm Hg. Several trials show that antihypertensive therapy reduces relative risk of cardiovascular events by approximately 25% to 30%, irrespective of pretreatment BP. Even BP lowering of as little as 5 mm Hg can lead to a 14% mortality risk reduction for stroke and 9% for MI. Nevertheless, about 50% of patients continue to be inadequately treated currently.

13. **How can I overcome therapeutic inertia?**
Failure of the health care provider to initiate or intensify antihypertensive therapy despite elevated BP levels is termed *therapeutic or clinical inertia*, which is due to factors (Table 30.3) such as reduced access to health care, complex comorbidities, polypharmacy, and intolerance to medications. Often, only one BP measurement is available. Thus uncertainty of the presence of hypertension often prevents intervention. Strategies to overcome inertia include team-based care employing nonphysician personnel, effective BP screening, and self-management for available and affordable therapy. Availability of single-pill formulations of drug combinations most commonly recommended currently allows simplification of treatment regimens and increases medication adherence.

14. **What is the best way to monitor the BP goal?**
Hypertension is usually asymptomatic. Therefore BP needs to be monitored both in a clinical office and in out-of-office settings (Table 30.4). However, it is still not known if hypertension management improves by basing treatment strategies on serial unattended automated office BP measurements, out-of-office (home or ambulatory) BP

Table 30.3 Causes of Therapeutic Inertia in Lowering Blood Pressure to Goal

PATIENT CHARACTERISTICS	PROVIDER CHARACTERISTICS
Older age; lower life expectancy	Lack of knowledge of appropriate goals
Multiple comorbidities, especially psychiatric conditions	High patient volume
Patient "near target"	Time constraints
Patient at acceptable physician-defined target	Another physician taking care of cardiovascular disease risk factors
Inadequate access to follow-up visits	Attitude that blood pressure is not an important risk factor
History of intolerance to medications for other conditions	Suspicion of poor medication adherence

Table 30.4 Optimal Methods for Monitoring Progress toward Blood Pressure Goal Achievement

BP MONITORING METHOD TO ADJUST THERAPY	ADVANTAGES/DISADVANTAGES
Standard office blood pressure measurement	Requires regular office follow up visits; used by most randomized clinical trials; does not reflect out-of-office BP readings; cannot detect the white coat effect or masked uncontrolled hypertension.
Unattended automated office blood pressure (AOBP)	Eliminates the white coat effect; does not detect masked uncontrolled hypertension; more accurate reflection of central BP than standard office BP measurement.
Home blood pressure monitoring (HBPM)	Reflects BP in usual home environment; more accurate reflection of average daily BP; identifies the white coat effect; identifies masked uncontrolled hypertension
Ambulatory blood pressure monitoring (ABPM)	Requires computer download; reflects nighttime BP, including nocturnal dipping; can cause insomnia; identifies the white coat effect; documents masked uncontrolled hypertension

BP, Blood pressure.

monitoring, or traditional office BP measurements. Out-of-office measurements have been increasingly employed including home BP monitoring (HBPM) and ambulatory BP monitoring (ABPM). HBPM refers to BP measurement by an individual outside the clinic setting (commonly at home) on a regular basis. ABPM refers to BP measurement at regular intervals (every 20–30 minutes), often for 24-hours including activities and sleep. Thus HBPM and ABPM can identify distinct BP types including white coat (isolated clinic) and masked (isolated ambulatory) hypertension. HBPM with titration of treatment improves BP in the short term, but evidence for a long-term effect is lacking. It is also not known if HBPM improves medication adherence. Nevertheless, largely because of its convenience and low cost, HBPM is recommended as the best currently available monitoring method for adjustment of antihypertensive drugs and dosages.

Patients require education to properly measure their BP at home. The patient should sit quietly for 5 minutes before a BP reading is obtained and the BP cuff should be at heart level and of correct size. An average of two to three BP measurements obtained on at least two to three separate occasions per week provides an accurate basis for estimation of BP for medication titration. Patients using HBPM should use a device that is validated, is fully automated, and has an upper arm cuff (not a wrist monitor).

KEY POINTS

1. Substantial evidence from RCTs supports a general BP goal of less than 130/80 mm Hg for most adults and a systolic BP goal of less than 130 mm Hg in adults aged 65 years or older.
2. The BP goal for patients with comorbidities (DM, CDK, stroke, IHD, and/or heart failure) is also less than 130/80 mm Hg.
3. Progress to achieve BP goal in hypertensive patients should be monitored with a combination of regular office and out-of-office BP measurements that are used to make periodic adjustments that will optimize antihypertensive therapy over time.
4. Overcoming therapeutic inertia is important because every millimeter of mercury reduced in BP toward BP goal can prevent CVD events and death.

REFERENCES

1. Xie X, Atkins E, Lv J. Effects of intensive blood pressure lowering on cardiovascular and renal outcomes: updated systematic review and meta-analysis. *Lancet.* 2016;387:435–443.
2. Thomopoulos C, Parati G, Zanchetti A. Effects of blood pressure lowering on outcome incidence in hypertension. 7. Effects of more or less intense blood pressure lowering and different achieved blood pressure levels – updated overview and meta-analysis of randomized trials. *J Hypertens.* 2016;34:613–622.
3. Verdecchia P, Angelli F, Gentile G, Reboldi G. More versus less intensive blood pressure lowering strategy: cumulative evidence and trial sequential analysis. *Hypertension.* 2016;68:642–653.
4. Bangalore S, Toklu B, Gianos E, et al. Optimal systolic blood pressure target after SPRINT: insights from a network meta-analysis of randomized trials. *Am J Med.* 2017;130:707–719.
5. Bundy JD, Li C, Stuchlik P, et al. Systolic blood pressure reduction and risk of cardiovascular disease and mortality: a systematic review and network meta-analysis. *JAMA Cardiol.* 2017;2:775–781.
6. Sakima A, Satonaka H, Nishida N, Yatsu K, Arima H. Optimal blood pressure target for patients with hypertension: a systematic review and meta-analysis. *Hypertens Res.* 2019;42:483–495.

BIBLIOGRAPHY

Beddhu S, Chertow GM, Cheung AK, et al. Influence of baseline diastolic blood pressure on effects of intensive compared with standard blood pressure control. *Circulation.* 2018;137(2):134–143.

Carey RM, Muntner P, Bosworth HB, Whelton PK. Prevention and control of hypertension. JACC Health Promotion Series. *J Am Coll Cardiol.* 2018;72:1278–1293.

Cheung AK, Chang TI, Cushman WC, et al. KDIGO 2021 clinical practice guideline for the management of blood pressure in chronic kidney disease. *Kidney Int.* 2021;99(3):S1–87.

Chobanian AV, Bakris GL, Black HR, et al. Seventh report of the Joint National Committee on prevention, detection, evaluation, and treatment of high blood pressure. *Hypertension.* 2003;42:1206–1252.

Muntner P, Shimbo D, Carey RM, et al. Measurement of blood pressure in humans: a scientific statement of the American Heart Association. *Hypertension.* 2019;73:e35–e66.

Pajewski NM, Berlowitz DR, Bress AP, et al. Intensive vs standard blood pressure control in adults 80 years or older: a secondary analysis of the Systolic Blood Pressure Intervention Trial. *J Am Geriatr Soc.* 2020;68:496–504.

Reboussin DM, Allen NB, Griswold ME, et al. Systematic review for the 2017 ACC/AHA/AAPA/ABC/ACPM/AGS/APhA/ASH/ASPC/NMA/PCNA guideline for the prevention, detection, evaluation and management of high blood pressure in adults: a report of the American College of Cardiology/American Heart Association Task Force on Clinical Practice Guidelines. *Hypertension.* 2018;71:e116–e135.

Research Group SPRINT., Wright Jr JT, Williamson JD, et al. A randomized trial of intensive versus standard blood-pressure control. *N Engl J Med.* 2015;373:2003–2016.

SPRINT MIND Investigators for the SPRINT Research Group, Williamson JD, Pajewski NM, et al. Effect of intensive versus standard blood pressure control on possible dementia: a randomized clinical trial. *JAMA.* 2019;321:553–561.

SPRINT MIND Investigators, Williamson JD, Supiano MA, et al. Association of intensive versus standard blood pressure control with cerebral white matter lesions. *JAMA.* 2019;322:524–534.

Unger T, Borghi C, Charchar F, et al. 2020 International Society of Hypertension global hypertension practice guidelines. *Hypertension.* 2020;75(6):1334–1357.

Whelton PK, Carey RM, Aronow WS, et al. A guideline for the prevention, detection, evaluation and management of high blood pressure. A report of the American College of Cardiology/American Heart Association Task Force on Clinical Practice Guidelines. *Hypertension.* 2018;71:e13–e115.

Williams B, Mancia G, Spiering W, et al. 2018 ESC/ESH Guidelines for the management of arterial hypertension. *Eur Heart J.* 2018;39(33):3021–3104.

Williamson J, Williamson JD, Supiano MA, et al. Intensive versus standard blood pressure control and cardiovascular disease outcomes in adults ≥ years: a randomized clinical trial. *JAMA.* 2016;86:1206–1216.

ANGIOTENSIN-CONVERTING ENZYME INHIBITORS AND ANGIOTENSIN RECEPTOR BLOCKER

Sarah Gilligan, MD, and Nirupama Ramkumar, MD, MPH

QUESTIONS

1. Describe the mechanism of action of antiogensin-converting enzyme inhibitors and angiotensin receptor blockers?

   The renin-angiotensin-aldosterone system plays an essential role in the maintenance of blood pressure, and hence drugs that target this system are effective antihypertensive agents. In this system, the substrate, angiotensinogen, is cleaved by renin to generate angiotensin-I. Angiotensin-converting enzyme (ACE) converts angiotensin-I to angiotensin-II which then increases blood pressure through effects on angiotensin type 1 receptor by mediating vasoconstriction, sodium reabsorption in the renal tubule, stimulating aldosterone synthesis, and activating the sympathetic nervous system. ACE inhibitors competitively inhibit the conversion of angiotensin-I to angiotensin-II, whereas angiotensin receptor blockers (ARBs) prevent binding of angiotensin-II to angiotensin type 1 receptor (Fig. 31.1). In contrast to the effect on angiotensin type 1 receptor, binding of angiotensin-II to angiotensin type 2 receptor causes vasodilation and sodium excretion.

2. What differences are seen with regard to the renin-angiotensin-aldosterone system with ACE inhibitors and ARBs? How is it clinically important?

   Both ACE inhibitors and ARBs increase plasma levels of renin and angiotensin-I. ARBs increase plasma angiotensin-II levels, whereas ACE inhibitors decrease plasma angiotensin-II levels. Hence, ACE inhibitors reduce the effect on angiotensin type 1 and 2 receptors. ACE inhibitors also prevent degradation of bradykinin, leading to increased kinin levels, which may be responsible for the cough commonly seen in patients taking ACE inhibitors but not ARBs.

3. What is the effect of an ACE inhibitor or ARB on glomerular filtration rate?

   The effects of ACE inhibitors on glomerular filtration rate (GFR) depend on two factors—angiotensin-II levels and autoregulation of GFR. In patients with primary hypertension with normal renal function, there is elevated renal perfusion pressure as a result of autoregulation. In that case, angiotensin-II levels are not altered, and treatment with ACE inhibitor does not cause any changes to GFR. On the other hand, in patients with kidney disease or renal artery stenosis, there is compensatory increase in angiotensin-II levels to maintain renal perfusion pressure and GFR. Thus treatment with an ACE inhibitor will blunt the effects of angiotensin-II and reduce both glomerular pressure and GFR. It is also important to note that angiotensin-II causes vasoconstriction of both afferent and efferent arterioles but preferentially increases efferent vascular resistance. In patients with established glomerular disease whose afferent arterioles are already dilated to maintain GFR, ACE inhibitor treatment will reduce efferent vascular resistance and decrease glomerular pressure and GFR. These effects are generally seen within the first few days of starting therapy and should be monitored by measuring serum creatinine levels. Although the effect of ARBs on GFR has not been studied as extensively as ACE inhibitors, it is widely believed that ARBs exert similar effects on GFR.

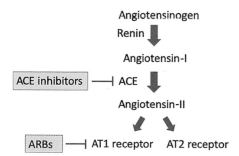

Fig. 31.1 Overview of the renin angiotensin system and mechanism of action for angiotensin-converting enzyme *(ACE)* inhibitors and angiotensin receptor blockers *(ARBs)*. *AT1*, Angiotensin type 1 receptor; *AT2*, angiotensin type 2 receptor.

Table 31.1 Commonly Used ACE Inhibitors and ARBs

MEDICATION NAME	DOSE RANGE (DAILY TOTAL)
ACE Inhibitors	
Benazepril	5–40 mg
Captopril	12.5–150 mg
Enalapril	2.5–40 mg
Fosinopril	10–40 mg
Lisinopril	2.5–40 mg
Moexipril	3.75–30 mg
Perindopril	2–16 mg
Quinapril	5–80 mg
Ramipril	2.5–20 mg
Trandolapril	1–4 mg
ARBs	
Candesartan	8–32 mg
Eprosartan	600–800 mg
Irbesartan	150–300 mg
Losartan	25–100 mg
Olmesartan	20–40mg
Telmisartan	20–80 mg
Valsartan	40–320 mg

ACE, Angiotensin-converting enzyme; *ARBs,* angiotensin receptor blockers.

4. **In which patient populations is there a proven benefit of using ACE inhibitors or ARBs?**
   ACE inhibitors and ARBs are highly effective in lowering blood pressure and should be considered as first- or second-line therapy in hypertension along with thiazide diuretics and calcium channel blockers. Commonly used ACE inhibitors and ARBs and their doses are listed in Table 31.1. There are several populations in which there is particular benefit; in these groups they should typically be initiated in the absence of contraindications. Benefits include reduction in albuminuria, progression to end-stage kidney disease (ESKD), and death, and these effects occur independent of the effect on blood pressure.
   - Patients with chronic kidney disease and hypertension: Several trials have demonstrated that ACE inhibitors and ARBs are beneficial in slowing down the progression of kidney disease.
   - Patients with type I or type II diabetes mellitus: Multiple studies demonstrate a reduction in albuminuria in patients with diabetes and moderately increased albuminuria. The Reduction of Endpoints in NIDDM with the Angiotensin II Antagonist Losartan (RENAAL) study patients with type 2 diabetes and nephropathy had a 28% reduction in progression to ESKD when taking losartan versus placebo in addition to their other antihypertensive therapy. Similarly, in patients with type 1 diabetes with moderate albuminuria, treatment with captopril lowered progression of albuminuria and ESKD.
   - Patients with moderate to severe albuminuria: Patients with nondiabetic proteinuric kidney disease have also been shown to derive benefit from ACE inhibitors and ARBs. The African American Study of Kidney Disease and Hypertension (AASK) study showed a benefit in patients with nonproteinuric kidney disease in terms of significant decrease in GFR and ESKD or death. There is also data to suggest that ACE inhibitors and ARBs may be associated with slower increase in creatinine and albuminuria in normotensive patients with moderately increased albuminuria.
   - Patients with systolic heart failure: The Cooperative North Scandinavian Enalapril Survival Study (CONSENSUS) and Studies of Left Ventricular Dysfunction (SOLVD) trials compared patients with systolic heart failure taking enalapril versus placebo and showed benefit in mortality and hospitalizations, particularly those related to heart failure. Subsequent trials have replicated these results using both other ACE inhibitors and ARBs.
   - Patients with acute myocardial infarction: Current recommendations are to start ACE inhibitors/ARBs in all patients with an acute myocardial infarction.
   - Finally, although the condition is rare, ACE inhibitors are the treatment of choice in patients with scleroderma renal crisis.

5. **What is the effect of an ACE inhibitor or ARB on proteinuria?**
ACE inhibitors and ARBs reduce proteinuria by approximately 30% to 35% primarily via reduction in glomerular pressure. The candesartan and lisinopril microalbuminuria (CALM) study demonstrated that candesartan and lisinopril were associated with 30% and 46% reduction in albuminuria in patients with type 2 diabetes, moderately increased albuminuria, and hypertension. Similarly, the RENAAL study demonstrated a 35% decline in proteinuria in patients with type 2 diabetes and diabetic nephropathy. In a trial of patients with type 2 diabetes, hypertension, and moderately increased albuminuria, patients taking an ARB had lower risk of progression of microalbuminuria. This occurred independently of blood pressure effects.

6. **What are the potential adverse effects of ACE inhibitors or ARBs?**
For both medications, the most common adverse reactions are hypotension, dizziness, acute kidney injury, and hyperkalemia. Acute kidney injury must be distinguished from the expected rise in creatinine that occurs as a result of decreased efferent arteriolar pressure leading to decreased GFR. A rise in serum creatinine of up to 30% is tolerated; a rise of more than 30% should typically prompt a change in treatment.
   The possibility of developing hyperkalemia requires close monitoring of laboratory values at the initiation of therapy with ACE inhibitors and ARBs. Risk factors for the development of hyperkalemia include chronic kidney disease, diabetes, and concomitant use of mineralocorticoid receptor antagonists or epithelial sodium channel (ENaC) inhibitors, such as triamterene or amiloride. ACE inhibitors and ARBs should not be used in combination as this can lead to life-threatening hyperkalemia as shown in the Ongoing Telmisartan Alone and in Combination with Ramipril Global Endpoint Trial (ONTARGET). Less common adverse reactions shared by both medication classes include syncope and gastrointestinal side effects.
   In addition, ACE inhibitors but not ARBs are associated with cough (incidence of 3%–4%). This tends to occur within the first few weeks of starting therapy and resolves in 1 to 4 weeks after stopping therapy likely due to increased kinin levels that cause bronchial irritation. Angioedema is also a rare side effect that occurs most commonly with the first dose but can occur at any time during treatment.
   Despite early reports suggesting an association between ACEi or ARB use and cancer, there is no increased risk of cancer with use of ARBs.

7. **In which patient populations should these medications be used with caution?**
In patients with acute kidney injury, ACE inhibitors and ARBs are not used to avoid further rise in serum creatinine and are withheld if a patient was taking them previously. Additionally, in patients with advanced renal failure who are close to needing dialysis, these medications are typically not initiated (though may be continued) in patients with progressive kidney failure.
   Both classes of medications should be avoided in pregnancy due to teratogenic effects, especially in the second trimester. Other conditions in which use of these medications can be problematic are aortic stenosis, ascites, and bilateral renal artery stenosis.

8. **Is there any benefit to combined ACE inhibitor and ARB therapy?**
The ONTARGET trial examined effects of ramipril, telmisartan, and combined therapy in over 25,000 patients and found increased risk of adverse effects in the combined therapy group with regards to hypotension, syncope, renal dysfunction, and hyperkalemia. In addition, there was also a trend toward increased risk of death and cancer in the combined therapy group. Similar results were reported in the Veterans Affairs Nephropathy in Diabetes (VA NEPHRON-D) trial, which included about 1500 patients with diabetic kidney disease. The trial did not show any benefit and indeed had to be stopped early because of increased rates of serious adverse events, hyperkalemia, and acute kidney injury in the combination arm. Hence, combined ACE inhibitor/ARB therapy is not recommended for hypertension or any other indications.

KEY POINTS

1. ACE inhibitors and ARBs are highly effective antihypertensive drugs that also have proven benefit in reducing albuminuria, progression to kidney disease, and death.
2. Both ACE inhibitors and ARBs reduce GFR. A rise in serum creatinine of up to 30% is tolerated; a rise of more than 30% should typically prompt a change in treatment.
3. Common side effects of ACE inhibitors and ARBs are hypotension, dizziness, acute kidney injury, and hyperkalemia. ACE inhibitors can also cause cough, which does not occur with ARBs.
4. Avoid using ACE inhibitors and ARBs in pregnancy, volume depletion, aortic stenosis, ascites, and bilateral renal artery stenosis.
5. Avoid using combined therapy with ACE inhibitors and ARBs due to increased adverse events.

BIBLIOGRAPHY

Brenner BM, Cooper ME, de Zeeuw D, et al. (RENAAL) Effects of losartan on renal and cardiovascular outcomes in patients with type 2 diabetes and nephropathy. *N Engl J Med*. 2001;345:861–869.

Consensus Trial Study GroupEffects of enalapril on mortality in severe congestive heart failure. Results of the Cooperative North Scandinavian Enalapril Survival Study (CONSENSUS). *N Engl J Med*. 1987;316(23):1429–1435.

Mann JF, Schemieder RE, McQueen M, et al. Renal outcomes with telmisartan, ramipril or both, in people at high vascular risk (the ONTARGET study): a multicenter, randomized, double-blind, controlled trial. *Lancet*. 2008;372(9638). 547-543.

Messerli FH, Bangalore S, Bavishi C, Rimoldi SF. Angiotensin converting enzyme inhibitors in hypertension – to use or not to use?. *J Am Coll Cardiol*. 2018;71(13):1474–1482.

Mogensen CE, Neldam S, Tikkanen I, et al. Randomized controlled trial of dual blockade of renin-angiotensin system in patients with hypertension, microalbuminuria, and non-insulin dependent diabetes: the candesartan and lisinopril microalbuminuria (CALM) study. *Br Med J*. 2000;321(7274):1440–1444.

Parving HH, Lehnert H, Brochner-Mortensen J, Gomis R, Andersen S, Arner P. Irbesartan in patient with type 2 diabetes and microalbuminuria study group. The effect of irbesartan on the development of diabetic nephropathy in patients with type 2 diabetes. *N Engl J Med*. 2001;345(12):870.

Sano T, Hotta N, Kawamura T, et al. Effects of long-term enalapril treatment on persistent microalbuminuria in normotensive type 2 diabetic patients: results of a 4-year, prospective, randomized study. *Diabet Med*. 1996;13(2):120–124.

Slomowitz LA, Bergamo R, Grosvenor M, Kopple JD. Enalapril reduces albumin excretion in diabetic patients with low levels of microalbuminuria. *Am J Neph*. 1990;10(6):457–462.

The SOLVD Investigators. Effect of enalapril on survival in patients with reduced left ventricular ejection fractions and congestive heart failure. *N Engl J Med*. 1991;325:293–302.

Taylor AA, Siragy HM, Nesbitt S. Angiotensin receptor blockers: pharmacology, efficacy and safety. *J Clin Hypertens*. 2011;13(9): 677–686.

Wright Jr JT, Bakris G, Greene T, et al. Effect of blood pressure lowering and antihypertensive drug class on progression of hypertensive kidney disease: results from the AASK trial. *JAMA*. 2002;288(19):2421–2431.

CHAPTER 32

CALCIUM CHANNEL BLOCKERS

Nashat Imran, MD, FASN, FACP, Ali Ayesh, MD, and Hillel Sternlicht, MD

QUESTIONS

1. **How do calcium channel blockers exert their antihypertensive effect?**
   Among the many calcium channels found throughout the body, the "L-type" remains the most clinically relevant. All calcium channel blockers (CCBs), whether classified as a dihydro pyridine (e.g., nifedipine, felodipine, amlodipine) or a nondihydropyridine (e.g., diltiazem, verapamil), bind this channel at various sites, thereby preventing cellular calcium entry.

   Calcium channel inhibitors lower blood pressure (BP) by preventing calcium influx into cells. This impairs myocyte contraction, particularly in the vascular smooth muscle of the peripheral and coronary beds and thus leads to decreases in vascular resistance and BP. These agents also induce a modest diuresis and interfere with the renin-angiotensin-aldosterone system (RAAS).

   Dihydropyridines are more effective antihypertensives than the nondihydropyridines as they preferentially disrupt the calcium influx into peripheral smooth muscle tissue. Nondihydropyridines exert lesser effects on arterial vascular beds. Rather, they are selective for cardiac myocytes and slow sinoatrial (SA) and atrioventricular (AV) nodal conduction. This lowers the heart rate and prevents the propagation of supraventricular arrhythmias.

2. **Explain the classification system for dihydropyridine-CCBs.**
   Calcium antagonists are best understood according to their "generation" (see Table 32.1). This system groups agents according to their pharmacologic properties rather than an agent's date of approval. First-generation agents such as nifedipine immediate-release (IR) are characterized by their rapid onset and short duration of action (6–8 hours). Most second-generation agents are molecularly identical to their predecessors (e.g., nifedipine extended-release [ER] and IR, respectively) but reformulated to extend their duration of action (12–24 hours), principally by slowing their absorption from the gastrointestinal tract. Isradipine and nimodipine, however, are novel molecules but, because their duration of action is comparable to the previously mentioned agents, they are also considered second-generation CCBs. Third generation agents (e.g., amlodipine) are unique molecules that are inherently longer acting (24–36 hours) and bind to cellular calcium channels at a different location than earlier generation dihydropyridines.

3. **Nifedipine and amlodipine are often used interchangeably. What are the clinically relevant differences between them?**
   Both sustained release (SR) nifedipine (referred to as "nifedipine" herein) and amlodipine are long-acting dihydropyridines. The half-life of ER nifedipine is 6 hours with a duration of action of approximately 22 hours. Amlodipine's half-life and duration of action are 30 to 50 hours and less than 30 hours, respectively. Thus amlodipine is an ideal outpatient medication because of its extended antihypertensive effect. However, it is a poor choice for inpatient BP control because the onset of action is 1 to 2 days. Conversely, because nifedipine's duration of action is less than 24 hours, it provides inadequate BP control in the ambulatory setting. By contrast, it lowers BP within 6 to 8 hours, thus lending itself to use in the hospital setting where a prompt antihypertensive effect is sought.

Table 32.1 Dihydropyridine Calcium Channel Blockers by Generation

GENERATION	COMMONLY ENCOUNTERED AGENTS
First	Nifedipine Immediate-Release (IR) Nicardipine IR
Second	Nifedipine Extended-Release (ER) Nifedipine Gastro-Intestinal Therapeutic System (GITS) Felodipine ER Isradipine Nimodipine
Third	Amlodipine Lacidipine (unavailable in the US) Cilnidipine (unavailable in the US)

The gradual nature of amlodipine's effect (i.e., arterial vasodilation) minimizes reflex sympathetic activity and tachycardia. Whereas short-term nifedipine use among those with heart failure and reduced ejection fraction (HFrEF) is associated with worse long-term outcomes, amlodipine is safe in this population. Studies that involve nifedipine ER in patients with HFrEF have not been conducted.

Amlodipine is available in multiple combination tablets, decreasing patient pill burden. These include amlodipine-atorvastatin, amlodipine-olmesartan, amlodipine-benazepril, and amlodipine-olmesartan-hydrochloro-thiazide, to name but a few. Combination tablets with ER nifedipine do not exist.

One caveat is that when administering dihydropyridine CCBs via enteral tube route, amlodipine may be the right option as it can be crushed (as opposed to nifedipine).

4. **Name key trials that support the efficacy and safety of CCBs.**
Both randomized controlled trials (Table 32.2) and metaanalyses support the safety and efficacy of *long-acting* CCBs. A Cochrane metaanalysis demonstrated calcium channel inhibitors to be comparable to diuretics, angioten-sin-converting enzyme inhibitors (ACEis), angiotensin receptor blockers (ARBs), and beta-blockers with respect to decreasing rates of all-cause mortality, myocardial infarction, and stroke. CCBs offer comparable levels of BP reductions to diuretics and modestly greater antihypertensive effect than ACEi, ARBs, and beta-antagonists. Based on this evidence, the 2017 American College of Cardiology/American Heart Association (ACC/AHA) Guidelines recommended dihydropyridines as first line therapy for hypertension.

It should be emphasized that the aforementioned data are drawn from trials of calcium blockers with extended durations of action such as amlodipine, cilnidipine, and nifedipine ER or gastrointestinal therapeutic system (GITS) formulations. IR nifedipine, particularly sublingual, is associated with an elevated risk of myocardial infarction. Therefore it is contraindicated in hypertensive crises. More broadly, no short-acting CCBs should be prescribed for the management of hypertension.

5. **Can dihydropyridine (e.g., amlodipine) and nondihydropyridine (e.g., diltiazem) be prescribed in combination?**
Traditionally the use of two drugs from the same class is inadvisable and can be harmful (e.g., concomitant ACEi and ARB administration). However, because dihydro- and nondihydro agents bind the calcium channel at different sites, an additive effect is plausible. Trial data confirms this enhanced antihypertensive effect with dual CCB ther-apy, achieving a further reduction in systolic BP of 5 to 10 mm Hg. However, the studies cited are of low-quality, lacking placebo arms, randomization, or a large subject number (average n of 25). Furthermore, bradycardia with concomitant beta-blocker use and alterations in CYP450 by nondihydropyridines (detailed later) limit this practice.

6. **Are there indications for CCBs apart from hypertension?**
Angina Pectoris: Both dihydro pyridines and nondihydropyridines can alleviate cardiac angina. They promote coronary artery vasodilation, thereby improving myocardial perfusion. However, only verapamil and diltiazem exert negative inotropic and chronotropic effects, which further decreases myocardial oxygen demand.

Table 32.2 Calcium Channel Blockers: Trials of Importance

TRIAL	STUDY DESIGN	ENDPOINT	INTERVENTION	OUTCOME
ALLHAT n ≈ 33,000	Randomized, double-blind	Adverse cardiovascular events	Treatment with chlorthalidone, amlodipine, or lisinopril	No difference in endpoint between agents
ASCOT-BPLA n ≈ 19,000	Randomized, open label	Adverse cardiovascular events	Treatment with amlo- dipine-benazepril or atenolol-thiazide	Amlodipine- benazepril superior
ACCOMPLISH n ≈ 11,500	Randomized, double-blind	Adverse cardiovascular events	Treatment with amlodipine combined with either benazepril or hydrochlorothiazide	Amlodipine- benazepril superior
Grimaldi-Bensouda et al. n ≈ 865,000	Cohort, retrospective	Association between CCB use and cancer	Assessed cancer risk among those receiv- ing CCBs, alternative antihypertensives, or no therapy	CCB exposure not associated with excess risk of malignancy

CCB, Calcium channel blocker.
From Grimaldi-Bensouda L, Klungel O, Kurz X, de Groot MC, Maciel Afonso AS, de Bruin ML, Reynolds R, Rossignol M. Calcium channel blockers and cancer: a risk analysis using the UK Clinical Practice Research Datalink (CPRD). BMJ Open. 2016 Jan 8;6(1):e009147.

Arrhythmia: Verapamil and diltiazem are class IV antiarrhythmics prescribed for supraventricular tachycardias. Each inhibits calcium influx into the SA and AV nodal tissue.

Cerebral Vasospasm: Nimodipine preferentially distributes within the cerebral vasculature and improves neurological outcomes in patients with subarachnoid hemorrhage. Its mechanism of effect is unclear.

Migraine Headache: Although calcium channel therapy can provoke headache, verapamil has been found to reduce migraine and cluster headache frequency. The mechanism of effect is not understood, but it may be the result of antagonism of P/Q type (rather than L-type) calcium channels.

Proteinuria Reduction: Trials consistently show that nondihydropyridines reduce proteinuria by 25% to 50%, perhaps by decreasing glomerular permeability to filtered serum proteins. Even so, the literature demonstrating that suppression of proteinuria slows the progression of kidney disease (as occurs with ACEIs/ARBs) is lacking. Dihydropyridines modestly (<10%) increase urinary protein excretion. However, the ACCOMPLISH trial found that those randomized to amlodipine-benazepril experienced *lesser* declines in renal function compared to those receiving hydrochlorothiazide, even though the latter combination produced *greater* reductions in proteinuria.

Raynaud Phenomenon: Calcium antagonists suppress digital vasospasm and decrease attacks by 50%. Nifedipine has classically been the agent of choice, but amlodipine appears effective. Verapamil and diltiazem are effective.

7. Discuss the potential advantages of CCBs compared to other classes of antihypertensives.
   Whereas RAAS blockers, diuretics, and beta-blockers lower BP to variable degrees as a function of the patient's comorbidities, calcium channel inhibitors provide a uniform hypotensive effect across all populations.

   CCBs vs Diuretics: In contrast to diuretics, CCBs are "metabolically neutral" and therefore do not produce glucose intolerance or predispose to diabetes mellitus. Electrolyte abnormalities are absent as are the risks of hyperuricemia and gout flair precipitation. Acute kidney injury (as a result of diuretic-induced volume depletion) does not occur.

   CCBs vs RAAS Blockers: ACEIs, ARBs, and spironolactone promote hyperkalemia in those with advanced chronic kidney disease or receiving nonsteroidals or trimethoprim ("Bactrim"); CCBs do not. Cough and angioedema are not reported with calcium antagonists. Gynecomastia is noted with higher doses of spironolactone.

   CCBs vs Beta-Blockers: Dihydropyridines do not cause hypoglycemic unawareness among diabetics and are not associated with the (modestly) heightened risk of depression and sexual dysfunction accompanying beta-blocker use. Decompensation of asthma or obstructive lung disease is associated with nonselective beta-blocker therapy but not CCBs. Apart from carvedilol and nebivolol, weight gains of 1 to 3 kg and worsening glycemic control are well-established adverse effects of beta-antagonists. CCBs are metabolically neutral.

8. In which populations should CCBs be prescribed with caution?
   Heart Failure: Given their negative inotropic effects, nondihydropyridines, particularly verapamil, should be avoided in those with HFrEF. Early generation dihydropyridines (nifedipine IR, nifedipine SR) heighten sympathetic tone and thus precipitate reflex tachycardia. Because of its gradual onset of action, amlodipine is well-tolerated in those with HFrEF.

   Symptomatic Aortic Stenosis: Because the hallmark of aortic stenosis is inability of the left ventricle to increase cardiac output in response to falls in systemic vascular resistance (afterload reduction), CCB-induced vasodilation can limit coronary perfusion.

   AV Block: High-grade AV block or sick sinus syndrome are contraindications to nondihydropyridines. Their negative dromotropic effects are further magnified in the presence of beta-blockers.

9. Describe the common adverse effects of CCBs.
   In research trials, calcium channel antagonists tend to be among the best-tolerated classes of agents. Symptomatic side effects (detailed later), if present, are often dose-dependent and relieved with either dosage de-escalation or, if necessary, agent discontinuation. Attendant laboratory abnormalities are nearly nonexistent.

   Peripheral Edema: The hallmark side effect of dihydropyridines is a dose-dependent edema of the ankle and shins. CCBs preferentially dilate the precapillary vessels such that a greater transcapillary pressure gradient is generated. This promotes the extravasation of fluid into the interstitium. It appears within months of therapy initiation with an incidence of 10% at low doses and perhaps 40% at full doses. It is significantly less common with verapamil and diltiazem. As it is not the result of fluid retention, diuretics are ineffective. Because it is dose-dependent, down-titration ameliorates or resolves its appearance. Therapy withdrawal results in edema resolution. Concurrent ACEi or ARB therapy decreases the incidence by one-third to one-half by dilating postcapillary beds, thereby minimizing the transcapillary gradient.

   Gingival Hyperplasia: Often overlooked, gingival overgrowth begins within several months of therapy initiation and is not dose-dependent. Its strongest association is with nifedipine but other agents have been implicated. Although poorly understood, it is thought to be the result of excess connective tissue deposition. Resolution occurs with CCB cessation, but dramatic hyperplasia requires surgical removal of the superfluous tissue.

Constipation and Nausea: Largely encountered with nondihydropyridines, it is the result of reduced peristalsis throughout the gastrointestinal tract, a consequence of the inhibition of calcium-dependent smooth muscle contraction.

Headache and Flushing: Both are reported with all agents. Although attributed to the vasodilatory properties of these agents, the lack of publications limits our understanding of these complications. They may be less common with longer acting preparations.

SA and AV Node Block: Both verapamil and diltiazem can precipitate or exacerbate bradycardia via SA node depression. AV blocks are regularly reported among those on the previously mentioned agents.

10. **With which commonly prescribed medications do CCBs interact?**
Nondihydropyridines are more likely to interfere with the metabolism of other drugs than dihydropyridines. They are moderate inhibitors of the CYP3A4 hepatic enzyme. Consequently, medications metabolized through this pathway are subject to alterations (generally elevations) in serum concentration when administered with nondihydropyridines. The CYP3A4 protein is also responsible for CCB metabolism. Thus medications that interact with CYP3A4 enhance the potency of calcium antagonists.

Statins: The incidence of statin myopathy is higher among those taking simvastatin with diltiazem or verapamil as simvastatin is metabolized by CYP3A4. Myopathy has been reported with atorvastatin but is less common. Rosuvastatin is well tolerated.

Methylprednisolone: The coadministration of diltiazem and methylprednisolone can result in greater than a twofold increase in serum methylprednisolone levels because this steroid is metabolized by CYP3A4.

Digitalis: Diltiazem, verapamil, and, to a lesser extent, nifedipine can potentiate the potency of digitalis by up to 50%. It appears these nondihydropyridines reduce its renal clearance.

Grapefruit Juice: Grapefruit juice depresses CYP3A4 function, thereby increasing CCB serum concentrations. Consumption of large amounts—6 glasses—of grapefruit juice can lead to hypotension.

Protease Inhibitors: Robust CYP3A4 inhibition is a class effect and, in routine practice, is seen with darunavir and atazanavir. Clinically, this amplifies the potency of calcium antagonists such that a lower dose is sufficient to achieve a given response in BP.

Azoles: Apart from fluconazole, these antifungals are potent inhibitors of CYP3A4 and accordingly augment the antihypertensive effect of all CCBs. Although the converse is true—that CCBs lessen hepatic clearance of azoles—untoward effects are less common.

Calcineurin Inhibitors: Diltiazem, verapamil, and nicardipine increase cyclosporine and tacrolimus concentrations (levels) by 25% to 100% (both are substrates of CYP3A4). By contrast, nifedipine and isradipine do not interact with calcineurin inhibitors.

Amiodarone: Because amiodarone, diltiazem, and verapamil possess AV nodal properties, the additive effects can exacerbate sick sinus syndrome and AV block. Amiodarone's inhibition of CYP3A4 further heightens nondihydropyridine levels and the potential for bradycardia.

Erythromycin and Clarithromycin: Both serve as the substrate of CYP3A4 such that diltiazem and verapamil raise the risk of macrolide-induced QTc prolongation. The liver metabolizes azithromycin but not via the P450 enzyme family. It is therefore well tolerated.

KEY POINTS

1. CCBs primarily lower BP by inhibition of the L-type calcium channel found in vascular smooth muscle.
2. Calcium channel antagonists lack the adverse metabolic effects of beta-blockers and diuretics and are not associated with the kidney injury or hyperkalemia seen with renin-angiotensin-aldosterone inhibitors.
3. Advanced heart block is a contraindication to nondihydropyridine use. IR and ER CCB use should be minimized in those with HFrEF.
4. Diltiazem and verapamil are CYP3A4 inhibitors. Concomitant medications that are metabolized through this pathway should be used judiciously because of the risk of toxicity.
5. CCB edema is dose-dependent and can be further reduced with ACEis.

BIBLIOGRAPHY

Bakris GL, Fonseca V, Katholi RE, et al. Metabolic effects of carvedilol vs metoprolol in patients with type 2 diabetes mellitus and hypertension: a randomized controlled trial. *JAMA.* 2004;292(18):2227–2236.

Chen N, Zhou M, Yang M, et al. Calcium channel blockers versus other classes of drugs for hypertension. *Cochrane Database Syst Rev.* 2010;(8):CD003654.

de Vries RJ, van Veldhuisen DJ, Dunselman PH. Efficacy and safety of calcium channel blockers in heart failure: focus on recent trials with second-generation dihydropyridines. *Am Heart J.* 2000;139(2 Pt 1):185–194.

Jamerson K, Weber MA, Bakris GL, et al. Benazepril plus amlodipine or hydrochlorothiazide for hypertension in high-risk patients. *N Engl J Med.* 2008;359(23):2417–2428.

Livada R, Shiloah J. Calcium channel blocker-induced gingival enlargement. *J Hum Hypertens.* 2014;28(1):10–14.

Lüscher TF, Cosentino F. The classification of calcium antagonists and their selection in the treatment of hypertension. A reappraisal. *Drugs*. 1998;55(4):509–517.

Makani H, Bangalore S, Romero J, Wever-Pinzon O, Messerli FH. Effect of renin-angiotensin system blockade on calcium channel blocker-associated peripheral edema. *Am J Med*. 2011;124(2):128–135.

Neuvonen PJ, Niemi M, Backman JT. Drug interactions with lipid-lowering drugs: mechanisms and clinical relevance. *Clin Pharmacol Ther*. 2006;80(6):565–581.

Rirash F, Tingey PC, Harding SE, et al. Calcium channel blockers for primary and secondary Raynaud's phenomenon. *Cochrane Database Syst Rev*. 2017;12:CD000467.

CHAPTER 33

DIRECT VASODILATORS

Ibrahim A. AlQassas, MD, and George K. Dresser, MD, PhD, FRCPC

QUESTIONS

DIRECT SMOOTH MUSCLE ARTERIAL VASODILATORS

1. What is a direct smooth muscle arterial vasodilator?
   Direct arterial vasodilators are blood pressure–lowering medications characterized by a decrease in peripheral resistance mediated by relaxation of smooth muscle in arterioles. Two medications commonly recognized in this class include hydralazine and minoxidil.

2. What is the mechanism of action of direct arterial vasodilators?
   Hydralazine acts on the arterial vessels, causing vasodilation and reduction of vascular resistance and blood pressure. The intracellular mechanisms mediating smooth muscle relaxation are not completely understood, but recent ex vivo studies suggest that the primary action is inhibition of inositol triphosphate (IP3) induced release of calcium from the sarcoplasmic reticulum.

   Minoxidil produces smooth muscle relaxation by opening energy-dependent adenosine triphosphate (ATP) potassium channels, allowing potassium efflux to cause smooth muscle relaxation.

   Direct vasodilators have minimal effect on nonvascular smooth muscle and the venous circulation or any direct effect on cardiomyocyte function.

3. What are the hemodynamic changes associated with direct vasodilators?
   The reduction in afterload associated with direct vasodilators results in activation of the sympathetic nervous system with an increase in heart rate, cardiac contractility, stroke volume, and cardiac output (Fig. 33.1). Hydralazine

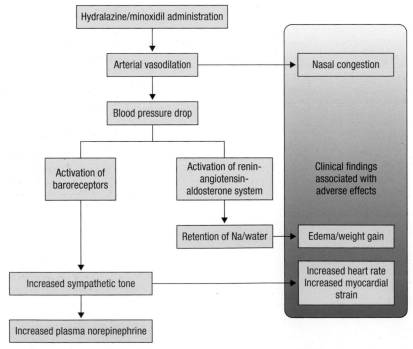

Fig. 33.1 Compensatory hemodynamic response to direct vasodilators.

can decrease peripheral resistance by up to 75%, but the resultant hypotensive effect is offset by an increase in cardiac output of 50% to 75%. This counterproductive compensatory effect can be mitigated by coadministration of beta-blockers and diuretics.

4. **What are the important pharmacokinetic parameters of direct vasodilators?**

Hydralazine is metabolized in the intestine and liver via N-acetyltransferase-2 (NAT2)–mediated acetylation. The metabolized form and unchanged drug are excreted in urine and feces. Renal insufficiency has been associated with higher plasma concentrations of hydralazine.

Oral hydralazine is initially administered three to four times daily at a dose of 12.5 to 25 mg. The dose can be increased to achieve target blood pressure but preferably not more than 200 mg to avoid side effects. The peak concentration of the oral dose occurs at 20 to 40 minutes, and the duration of effect is 2 to 6 hours. Oral availability of hydralazine ranges from 10% to 50%, dependent on the dose of oral drug and intrinsic NAT2 acetylator status. Approximately one-third of individuals are rapid acetylators and will achieve lower plasma concentrations and correspondingly less blood pressure lowering.

With the intravenous form, the peak concentration and hypotensive effect occur within 5 to 30 minutes and lasts 2 to 6 hours. It is recommended that an initial test bolus of 5 mg IV be given. Depending on response, subsequent boluses of 5 to 10 mg can be repeated at 30-minute intervals to a maximum of 40 mg within any 6-hour interval. It is recommended to switch to the oral dose as soon as possible.

Minoxidil has oral absorption of approximately 90% with peak concentrations and effect occurring at 1 hour. It is metabolized in the liver and excreted by the kidney with a half-life of approximately 4 hours.

5. **What are the side effects of direct vasodilators?**

Side effects can be categorized as those associated with the primary mechanism of action (vasodilation and afterload reduction) or unique to the chemical entity. Common side effects of hydralazine and minoxidil associated with the primary mechanism of action include headache, nausea, flushing, edema, palpitations, reflex tachycardia, dizziness, and angina (Table 33.1). With minoxidil, volume expansion and edema can be clinically dramatic.

Whereas reductions in renal resistance vessels have been associated with an increase in total renal blood flow, glomerular filtration rate (GFR) is reported to be unchanged in patients taking hydralazine. Despite the maintenance of GFR, activation of the renin-angiotensin-aldosterone system (RAAS) is observed with resultant exacerbation of peripheral edema. Side effects secondary to sympathetic activation can be minimized by coadministering beta-blockers, whereas side effects related to activation of the RAAS can be minimized by coadministration of loop diuretics.

Hydralazine is associated with toxicities mediated by an antipyridoxine effect (peripheral neuropathy) and by immune system activation (Fig. 33.2). The peripheral neuropathy may be mitigated by pyridoxine supplementation and tends to occur in those with higher overall exposure. It is estimated that 30% to 60% of patients with higher exposure may develop antinuclear antibodies (ANAs). Patients who become ANA-positive while taking hydralazine do not necessarily develop immune-related disease. One survey reported that 7% to 13% of patients with higher

Table 33.1 Adverse Reactions Associated with Direct-Acting Arterial Vasodilators

DRUG	DIRECTLY RELATED TO MECHANISM OF ACTION	OTHERS
Hydralazine	Headache, nasal congestion, tachycardia, palpitations, flushing, fluid retention, and edema	Sweating, drug-induced lupus, fever, anemia, purpura, peripheral neuropathy
Minoxidil	Headache, nasal congestion, tachycardia, palpitations, flushing, fluid retention, and edema	Hirsutism, nausea, breast pain, echocardiogram T-wave depression or inversion

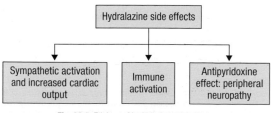

Fig. 33.2 Etiology of hydralazine side effects.

overall exposure developed lupus-like clinical findings. These clinical findings include arthralgia, myalgia, fever, arthritis, pleuritis, blood dyscrasias, and hepatitis.

All of these side effects appear to be exposure-dependent. Total exposure is determined by dose, duration, and NAT2 acetylator status. Chronic hydralazine doses of greater than 200 mg/day are more commonly associated with side effects, although in slow acetylators, they can be seen at lower doses. Discontinuation of hydralazine has been reported to improve both immune and nonimmune side effects.

The primary drug-specific side effect of minoxidil is abnormal hair growth. All patients using this agent should be educated about this effect. The only treatment for hypertrichosis is removal of the hair or discontinuation of the drug. Excess hair growth reverses several months after discontinuation of the offending agent.

6. What monitoring is required for patients taking vasodilators?
Patients should be examined for the presence of edema. It is recommended that patients receiving hydralazine have their complete blood count (CBC) and ANA titer monitored. In the absence of high-quality data supporting any specific recommendation, it is suggested that the CBC be checked when initiating dosing with a follow-up measurement within a month and periodically thereafter. In patients considered for longer term dosing with hydralazine, the ANA should be checked prior to initiation and at yearly intervals. More frequent monitoring of ANA might be indicated if the patient exhibits features of lupus.

7. When are direct vasodilators contraindicated?
Patients who may not tolerate the significant drop in afterload or the attendant increase in sympathetic activity and cardiac output should not be treated with these agents. Examples include myocardial ischemia, aortic or mitral stenosis, and high output heart failure. These agents increase shear stress in the aorta and should not be used in patients with acute aortic dissection. They are relatively contraindicated in patients with aortic aneurysm or healed aortic dissection. Patients with immune-mediated, lupus-like illness should not receive hydralazine.

8. What is the level of evidence for using direct smooth muscle arterial vasodilators?
The evidence supporting the use of the direct vasodilators is limited. Phase 2 studies have examined the blood pressure lowering and safety of these agents. Contemporary use of these agents is limited because of the inconvenient dosing and frequent side effects, and the availability of better options for the majority of patients (Table 33.2).

Hydralazine has some evidence from phase 3 and 4 studies in specific populations. The Veterans Administration Cooperative Study Group Trials showed that hydralazine in combination with hydrochlorothiazide and reserpine decreased morbidity and mortality in patients with moderate to severe hypertension.

A multicenter trial showed that in patients already started on a beta-blocker and diuretic, hydralazine was the most suitable third add-on agent in patients with severe hypertension. The other agents included in the study were labetalol, prazosin, methyldopa, and placebo.

Table 33.2 Hydralazine Clinical Scenarios					
	ACUTE SYMPTOMATIC HYPERTENSION WITH PARENTERAL ACCESS AND INTENSIVE BP MONITORING	**RESISTANT HYPERTENSION DESPITE ACEI, CCB, AND DIURETIC**	**HFREF ON MAXIMAL GDMT WITH NYHA CLASS III-IV SYMPTOMS OR INTOLERANT TO ACEI/ARB (IN COMBINATION WITH NITRATES)**	**HYPERTENSION IN PREGNANCY**	**ADVANCED CKD OR ESRD**
Good option	10–20 mg IV q30 min	25–50 mg PO q6 h	25–50 mg PO q6 h	25–50 mg PO q6 h	25–50 mg PO q6 h
Consider	25–50 mg PO q6 h	NA	NA	5–10 mg IV q6 h as needed	NA
Contraindications	Aortic dissection	NA	Myocardial ischemia Aortic stenosis Mitral stenosis	NA	NA

ACEi, Angiotensin-converting enzyme inhibitor; *ARB*, angiotensin receptor blocker; *BP*, blood pressure; *CCB*, calcium channel blocker; *CKD*, chronic kidney disease; *ESRD*, end-stage renal disease; *GDMT*, goal-directed medical therapy; *HFrEF*, heart failure with reduced ejection fraction; *NA*, not applicable; *NYHA*, New York Heart Association, *PO*, by mouth (per os); *q*, every.

The Vasodilator Heart Failure Trial (V-HEFT) trial showed a clear benefit for decreasing morbidity and mortality when hydralazine was combined with isosorbide dinitrate in patients with congestive heart failure (New York Heart Association [NYHA]) class III-IV on appropriate standard heart failure therapy or who were intolerant to it.

9. **What is the role of hydralazine in the critical care setting?**
Adequate evidence supporting the use of any parenteral antihypertensive drug in preference to any other are lacking. Given the range of 5 to 30 minutes for onset of action, hydralazine is often used when rapid reduction of blood pressure is indicated. Patients dependent on parenteral hydralazine should be monitored using continuous intraarterial BP measurement if this is available. Given the variable duration of action from 2 to 6 hours, these patients require constant bedside nursing support.

Hydralazine is one of the most widely used medications in treating hypertensive urgencies and emergencies. Although it can be administered orally or intravenously as a bolus or continuous infusion, no studies have provided guidance on which administration method may be preferred. Clinical data indicates that one-third of patients admitted to the emergency room receive IV hydralazine without appropriate justification. There is also data indicating potentially inappropriate use for controlling hypertension among inpatients.

10. **How is hydralazine used in managing hypertension in pregnancy and during lactation?**
Hydralazine is pregnancy risk class C. In rats it was found to cause malformations of cranial and facial bones as well as cleft palate. Despite this, it has a long history of safe use during pregnancy and breast-feeding. To date there have been no teratogenic or toxic effects caused by hydralazine in this setting. Hydralazine bolus (5–10 mg, repeated every 30 minutes as needed) has been reported to be more effective and safer than continuous hydralazine infusion (0.5–10 mg/h) in managing hypertension emergencies in pregnancy. It is comparable to intravenous labetalol in this regard.

Hydralazine concentrations in breast milk are approximately 50% of that in maternal plasma. It has been estimated that breast-feeding children would be exposed to less than 25 μg as an oral dose. Hydralazine is not detectable in the plasma of breast-feeding children of mothers taking hydralazine doses up to 200 mg/day due to levels below the limit of quantification for the assay.

11. **What is the benefit of hydralazine in combination with nitrates in the treatment of patients with congestive heart failure?**
The V-HEFT trial showed a mortality benefit when hydralazine was combined with isosorbide dinitrate in patients with congestive heart failure with reduced left ventricular ejection fraction (HFrEF) NYHA class III-IV. Adding the combination to standard heart failure treatment, which included ACEis, beta-blockers, and mineralocorticoid receptor antagonists but not sacubitril-valsartan has been shown to improve survival and decrease hospitalization in Black patients. Morcover, the combination is useful in symptomatic patients with HFrEF who cannot tolerate ACEis or ARBs. The combination remains underused in Black patients.

12. **What is the role of hydralazine in patients with renal dysfunction?**
Hydralazine is used to control blood pressure in patients with advanced chronic kidney disease or in patients on dialysis in which ACEis and ARBs are ineffective or contraindicated. As hydralazine is metabolized by the liver, dose adjustment is not needed in renal impairment.

KEY POINTS

1. Direct arterial vasodilators lower blood pressure by relaxation of smooth muscles in arterioles.
2. The reduction in afterload associated with direct vasodilators results in activation of the sympathetic nervous system with an increase in heart rate, cardiac contractility, stroke volume, and cardiac output. These effects can be mitigated by the concomitant administration of beta-blockers and diuretics.
3. Hydralazine combined with nitrates conferred a mortality benefit in a selected group of patients with heart failure in the V-HEFT trial.
4. Hydralazine is pregnancy risk class C. It is not detectable by conventional assays in the serum of breastfed babies of mothers receiving less than 200 mg of hydralazine per day.
5. Hydralazine can be safely used in patients with chronic kidney disease.
6. Parenterally administered hydralazine has a rapid onset of action (5–10 minutes) accounting for its utilization in situations in which acute blood pressure control is desired.
7. Administration of hydralazine is contraindicated in patients with conditions sensitive to the significant drop in afterload or the attendant increase in sympathetic activity and cardiac output. Examples include myocardial ischemia, aortic or mitral stenosis, and high output heart failure.

BIBLIOGRAPHY

ACOG Committee Opinion No. 767 Summary: Emergent therapy for acute-onset, severe hypertension during pregnancy and the postpartum period. Obstet Gynecol. 2019;133(2):409-412.

ACOG Practice Bulletin No. 202: Gestational hypertension and preeclampsia. Obstet Gynecol. 2019;133(1):e1-e25.

ACOG Practice Bulletin No. 203: Chronic hypertension in pregnancy. Obstet Gynecol. 2019; 133(1):e26-e50.

Ahuja K, Charap MH. Management of perioperative hypertensive urgencies with parenteral medications. *J Hosp Med.* 2010;5(2):E11–16.

Al-Mohammad A. Hydralazine and nitrates in the treatment of heart failure with reduced ejection fraction. *ESC Heart Fail.* 2019;6(4):878–883.

Amjad W, John G, Gulru S. Hydralazine-induced autoimmune hepatitis precipitated by the blood transfusion. *Am J Ther.* 2018;25(4):e514–e516.

Aronow WS. Current treatment of heart failure with reduction of left ventricular ejection fraction. *Expert Rev Clin Pharmacol.* 2016;9(12):1619–1631.

Begum MR1, Quadir E, Begum A, et al. Management of hypertensive emergencies of pregnancy by hydralazine bolus injection vs continuous drip--a comparative study. *Medscape Womens Health.* 2002;7(5):1.

Borchers AT, Keen CL, Gershwin ME. Drug-induced lupus. Ann NY Acad Sci. 2007;1108:166–182.

Campbell P, Baker WL, Bendel SD, et al. Intravenous hydralazine for blood pressure management in the hospitalized patient: its use is often unjustified. *J Am Soc Hypertens.* 2011;5(6):473–477.

Chen TK, Knicely DH, Grams ME. Chronic kidney disease diagnosis and management: a review. *JAMA.* 2019;322(13):1294–1304.

Cheung AK, Chang TI, Cushman WC, et al. Blood pressure in chronic kidney disease: conclusions from a Kidney Disease: Improving Global Outcomes (KDIGO) Controversies Conference. *Kidney Int.* 2019;95(5):1027–1036.

Delgado De Pasquale S, Velarde R, Reyes O, et al. Hydralazine vs labetalol for the treatment of severe hypertensive disorders of pregnancy. *A randomized, controlled trial. Pregnancy Hypertens.* 2014;4(1):19–22.

Ellershaw DC1, Gurney AM. Mechanisms of hydralazine induced vasodilation in rabbit aorta and pulmonary artery. *Br J Pharmacol.* 2001;134(3):621–631.

He Y, Sawalha AH. Drug-induced lupus erythematosus: an update on drugs and mechanisms. *Curr Opin Rheumatol.* 2018;30(5):490–497.

Herman LL, Tivakaran VS. Hydralazine. In: StatPearls [Internet]. Treasure Island (FL). *StatPearls Publishing.* 2019;. Available at: https://www.ncbi.nlm.nih.gov/books/NBK470296/. Updated October 7.

Kirsten R, Nelson K, Kirsten D, et al. Clinical pharmacokinetics of vasodilators. *Part I. Clin Pharmacokinet.* 1998;34(6):457–482.

Kirsten R, Nelson K, Kirsten D, et al. Clinical pharmacokinetics of vasodilators. *Part II. Clin Pharmacokinet.* 1998;35(1):9–36.

Kumar B, Stroude J, Swee M, et al. Hydralazine-associated vasculitis: overlapping features of drug-induced lupus and vasculitis. *Semin Arthritis Rheum.* 2018;48(2):283–287.

Lamont RF, Elder MG. Transfer of hydralazine across the placenta and into breast milk. *J Obstet Gynaecol.* 1986;7:47–48.

McAreavey D, Ramsey LE, Latham L, et al. Third drug" trial: comparative study of antihypertensive agents added to treatment when blood pressure remains uncontrolled by a beta blocker plus thiazide diuretic. *Br Med J (Clin Res Ed).* 1984;288(6411):106–111.

McComb MN, Chao JY, Ng TM. Direct vasodilators and sympatholytic agents. *J Cardiovasc Pharmacol Ther.* 2016;21(1):3–19.

Miller JB, Arter A, Wilson SS, et al. Appropriateness of bolus antihypertensive therapy for elevated blood pressure in the emergency department. *West J Emerg Med.* 2017;18(5):957–962.

Olson-Chen C1, Seligman NS. Hypertensive emergencies in pregnancy. *Crit Care Clin.* 2016;32(1):29–41.

Pettinger WA. Minoxidil and the treatment of severe hypertension. N Engl J Med. 1980;303(16):922–926.

Rhoney D, Peacock WF. Intravenous therapy for hypertensive emergencies, part 2. Am J Health Syst Pharm. 2009;66(16):1448–1457.

Salgado DR, Silva E, Vincent JL. Control of hypertension in the critically ill: a pathophysiological approach. *Ann Intensive Care.* 2013;3:17.

Santhi R, Worthley LI. Hypertension in the critically ill patient. *Crit Care Resusc.* 2003;5(1):24–42.

Sarafidis PA, Georgianos PI, Malindretos P, et al. Pharmacological management of hypertensive emergencies and urgencies: focus on newer agents. *Expert Opin Investig Drugs.* 2012;21(8):1089–1106.

Sica DA, Gehr TWB. Direct vasodilators and their role in hypertension management: minoxidil. *J Clin Hypertension.* 2001;3(2):110–114.

Thomas G. Hypertension management in chronic kidney disease and diabetes: lessons from the systolic blood pressure intervention trial. *Cardiol Clin.* 2019;37(3):307–317.

Tran TP, Khoynezhad A. Current management of type B aortic dissection. *Vasc Health Risk Manag.* 2009;5:53–63.

Whelton PK, Carey RM, Aronow WS, et al. 2017 ACC/AHA/AAPA/ABC/ACPM/AGS/APhA/ASH/ASPC/NMA/PCNA Guideline for the prevention, detection, evaluation, and management of high blood pressure in adults: a report of the American College of Cardiology/American Heart Association task force on clinical practice guidelines. *Hypertension.* 2018;71(6):e13–e115.

Zeisberg EM, Zeisberg M. A rationale for epigenetic repurposing of hydralazine in chronic heart and kidney failure. *J Clin Epigenet.* 2016;2:1.

Ziaeian B, Fonarow GC, Heidenreich PA. Clinical effectiveness of hydralazine-isosorbide dinitrate in African-American patients with heart failure. *JACC Heart Fail.* 2017;5(9):632–639.

CHAPTER 34

LOOP AND THIAZIDE DIURETICS

Andrew Terker, MD PhD, and David Ellison, MD

QUESTIONS

1. **What is the mechanism of action of thiazide diuretics?**

   Thiazide diuretics act primarily by inhibiting the sodium chloride cotransporter (NCC) along the distal convoluted tubule, which is responsible for reabsorbing 5% to 10% of the filtered sodium load (Fig. 34.1). They initially require secretion into the nephron lumen via organic anion transporters (OATs) along the proximal convoluted tubule (PCT). NCC inhibition occurs via competition for the chloride binding site and results in decreased sodium and chloride reabsorption and therefore increases urinary sodium and water losses. Thiazides may also have smaller, yet significant, natriuretic effects along the cortical collecting duct via inhibition of the sodium dependent chloride bicarbonate exchanger. Initially, this natriuresis and diuresis cause modest reductions in plasma volume and cardiac output, leading to decreased blood pressure.[1] Longer term observations with thiazides demonstrate return of plasma volume and cardiac output toward baseline accompanied by a reduction in vascular resistance; the latter has been attributed to whole body autoregulation, although the underlying mechanisms remain unclear.

2. **What is the mechanism of action of loop diuretics?**

   Loop diuretics act by inhibiting the sodium potassium 2 chloride cotransporter (NKCC2), isoform 2, along the thick ascending limb (TAL) of Henle's loop (see Fig. 34.1). Similar to thiazides, also require secretion along the PCT via OATs. As the TAL is responsible for reabsorbing approximately 25% of the filtered sodium load, they have a much greater natriuretic and diuretic effect than thiazides. Similar to thiazides, the increased sodium and water losses result in reduced plasma volume and cardiac output and therefore decreased blood pressure. In general, loop diuretics are used primarily to treat edematous states, as is seen in patients with heart failure, liver disease, and nephrotic syndrome, to reduce excess total body fluid. In the treatment of hypertension, they are not a first-line agent and are most commonly used in patients with chronic kidney disease and glomerular filtration rates less than 30 mL/min. Loop diuretics may also be required to control fluid retention induced by potent vasodilators, such as minoxidil.

   Loop diuretics also inhibit the NKCC2 isoform 1, which is thought to mediate the ototoxicity and acute effects on reducing pulmonary edema.

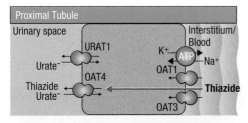

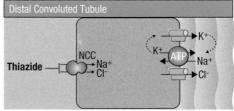

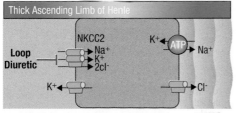

Fig. 34.1 Mechanism of action of thiazide and loop diuretics. Along the proximal tubule, thiazide and loop diuretics are secreted from the interstitial space into the urinary space by organic anion transporters *(OATs)*. Once in the tubular lumen, they are delivered to sites of action. Loops inhibit the Na⁺-K⁺-2Cl⁻ cotransporter *(NKCC2)* along the thick ascending limb. Thiazides inhibit the Na⁺-Cl⁻ cotransporter *(NCC)* along the distal convoluted tubule. URAT1, urate transporter 1.

3. Why are thiazides more effective at reducing blood pressure than loop diuretics?
Thiazides, being better antihypertensive agents than loop diuretics, may seem counterintuitive as these are both natriuretic diuretics, and loop diuretics have a higher natriuretic ceiling than thiazides do. Studies have not been performed to compare all of the commonly used loop and thiazide diuretics; however, in general, thiazides have been found to be more effective at reducing blood pressure in essential hypertension when compared with loop diuretics.[2-4] In particular, studies have shown hydrochlorothiazide to be more effective than furosemide. Although the exact reason for this is not entirely clear, it is thought the longer duration of action of thiazides contributes to their greater efficacy. It should be noted that studies comparing thiazides and torsemide, a long-acting loop diuretic, have not been performed. Additionally, chronic loop diuretic use results in hypertrophy of more distal nephron segments and increased downstream sodium reabsorption, which blunts their diuretic effect.

4. What are the most commonly used loop diuretics and how are they dosed?
See Table 34.1. Another notable difference includes widely variable oral absorption for furosemide (40%–90%), whereas bumetanide and torsemide are more consistently highly bioavailable.

5. What are the most commonly used thiazide diuretics and how are they dosed?
See Table 34.2.

Table 34.1 Loop Diuretics

MEDICATION	INDICATION	DOSE	HALF-LIFE (HOURS)
Furosemide	Edema, ascites, alternative agent in hypertension usually in volume-dependent hypertension in setting of CKD	10 mg once daily up to a maximum total daily dose of 600 mg divided into 3–4 doses. For ascites, dosed in a 40-mg furosemide to 100-mg spironolactone ratio	6–8
Bumetanide	Edema, alternative agent in hypertension usually in volume-dependent hypertension in setting of CKD	0.5 mg daily up to a maximum total daily dose of 10 mg divided in 1–2 doses	4–6
Torsemide	Edema, alternative agent in hypertension usually in volume-dependent hypertension in setting of CKD	5 mg daily up to a maximum of 200 mg once daily	6–8
Ethacrynic acid	Edema, alternative agent in hypertension in patients with contraindication to sulfonamides (e.g., allergy)	50 mg daily up to a maximum total daily dose of 400 mg divided in 1–2 doses	12

CKD, Chronic kidney disease.

Table 34.2 Thiazide Diuretics

MEDICATION	INDICATION	DOSE	HALF-LIFE (HOURS)
Chlorthalidone	Essential hypertension, refractory edema, calcium nephrolithiasis	Usually 12.5–25 mg once daily but can be used up to 100 mg once daily	45–60
Hydrochlorothiazide	Essential hypertension, refractory edema, calcium nephrolithiasis	12.5–25 mg once daily. Previously used at higher doses (50–100 mg daily), but side effects were greater	8–15
Metolazone	Edema	2.5–20 mg once daily	8–14
Indapamide	Essential hypertension, edema, calcium nephrolithiasis	1.25–5 mg once daily	14–25

6. **Do outcomes differ between different thiazide diuretics?**

   Chlorthalidone has been shown to have superior antihypertensive effects and decrease cardiovascular events and mortality when compared with hydrochlorothiazide.[5–7] Despite this, hydrochlorothiazide has traditionally been much more widely prescribed than chlorthalidone. The 2017 American College of Cardiology/American Heart Association hypertension guidelines recommend chlorthalidone as the preferred initial choice for a thiazide due to its longer half-life and demonstrated reduction of cardiovascular disease in clinical trials.

7. **What are common side effects of loop diuretics?**

   The most common side effects of loop diuretics are electrolyte imbalance, volume depletion, hypotension, ototoxicity, muscle cramping, gout, and kidney stones. Electrolyte imbalance including hypokalemia, hypocalcemia, hypomagnesemia, and hypochloremic metabolic alkalosis occurs because inhibition of NKCC2 not only increases sodium excretion, but also increases excretion of potassium, calcium, magnesium, and chloride. Notably, loop diuretics do not typically cause hyponatremia like thiazides do. The more common sodium abnormality with loop diuretics is hypernatremia. Hyperuricemia and gout are caused by direct effects on the proximal tubule via increasing OAT reabsorption of urate and by indirectly stimulating proximal tubule urate reabsorption secondary to volume depletion. Ototoxicity occurs from inhibition of NKCC1 in the inner ear. Kidney stones are caused by increased calcium excretion.

8. **What are common side effects of thiazide diuretics?**

   The most common side effects of thiazide diuretics are electrolyte imbalance, hyperglycemia, hyperlipidemia, volume depletion, hypotension, muscle cramping, gout, sexual dysfunction, and sleep disturbances. Electrolyte imbalance is similar to the loop diuretic side effect profile with some notable differences. Like loop diuretics, thiazidediuretics also cause hypokalemia, hypomagnesemia, hyperuricemia, and hypochloremic metabolic alkalosis. Additionally, they also commonly cause hyponatremia and can cause hypercalcemia due to their hypocalciuric effect. Compared with loop diuretics and other antihypertensive agents, thiazides are associated with increased glucose, cholesterol, and triglycerides. Despite some of these adverse metabolic complications, thiazides have proven to reduce cardiovascular mortality in high-risk patients with hypertension. Thiazides were previously used in much higher doses that they are today, but studies have found lower doses to be as effective at reducing blood pressure and have fewer side effects. Higher doses are associated with greater side effects and increased incidence of sudden cardiac death.[8] Additionally, side effects are greater with chlorthalidone than with hydrochlorothiazide or indapamide.

9. **Why do thiazide diuretics cause hypercalcemia?**

   The mechanism by which thiazide diuretics increase urinary calcium reabsorption is complex and remains an active area of investigation but likely involves indirect and direct actions of thiazide diuretics. Diuretic-induced volume depletion increases proximal calcium reabsorption by increasing proximal tubule sodium reabsorption accompanied by increased calcium reabsorption. Thiazidediuretics also increase calcium reabsorption in the distal nephron, which is not dependent on volume status. Although these effects are not dependent on parathyroid hormone, thiazides may provoke hypercalcemia due to previously unrecognized primary hyperparathyroidism. Approximately 24% of patients with thiazide-associated hypercalcemia are found to have underlying primary hyperparathyroidism.[9] In the remaining patients, hypercalcemia may not normalize regardless of thiazide discontinuation, suggesting another underlying calcium disorder. In the absence of overt hypercalcemia, the effects of thiazide diuretics on calcium handling may have beneficial effects, such as reduction in nephrolithiasis and increased bone mineral density.

10. **Why do thiazide diuretics cause hyponatremia more often than loop diuretics?**

    Hyponatremia is a potentially life-threatening complication of thiazide diuretics and requires frequent monitoring of electrolytes. The incidence of thiazide-associated hyponatremia may be as high as 9%, although severe hyponatremia is less common. Cross-sectional studies suggest that thiazide-induced hyponatremia is independent of antidiuretic hormone but have identified genetic defects in prostaglandin E_2 reuptake that predispose individuals to this complication.[10] Diuretic-induced volume depletion also stimulates thirst and water drinking. Whereas loop diuretics reduce the maximal medullary interstitial accumulation of sodium chloride and other solutes, thiazide diuretics do not impair this concentrating ability. Therefore water can be reabsorbed in the distal nephron to a greater extent with thiazide use, likely contributing to the incidence of hyponatremia during treatment.

11. **Why do diuretics increase the risk of gout?**

    Uric acid is reabsorbed primarily via urate-anion exchange in the proximal tubule Fig. 34.1, which is frequently targeted by the uricosuric drug probenecid. Thiazide diuretics are also secreted into the urinary lumen via OAT4, which can reabsorb urate in exchange during thiazide secretion.[11] Therefore secretion of thiazides is accompanied by urate reabsorption, which can worsen hyperuricemia and gout. Diuretics also activate the renin-angiotensin-aldosterone system, which, in turn, increases the reabsorption of urate.

KEY POINTS

1. Thiazide diuretics, such as chlorthalidone, are among the most effect antihypertensive agents and have proven to reduce cardiovascular events and death in hypertension trials despite some adverse metabolic effects.
2. Loop diuretics may be required for control of edematous states but are generally less effective antihypertensive agents than thiazide diuretics in patients with normal kidney function.
3. Loop and thiazide diuretics cause volume depletion, hypokalemia, and hyperuricemia, whereas thiazides cause hyponatremia, hypercalcemia, hyperglycemia, and dyslipidemia.
4. Thiazide treatment my provoke hypercalcemia, which indicates primary hyperparathyroidism in a significant proportion of cases.

REFERENCES

1. Shah S, Khatri I, Freis ED. Mechanism of antihypertensive effect of thiazide diuretics. *Am Heart J.* 1978;95:611–618.
2. Araoye MA, Chang MY, Khatri IM, Freis ED. Furosemide compared with hydrochlorothiazide. Long-term treatment of hypertension. *JAMA.* 1978;240:1863–1866.
3. Holland OB, Gomez-Sanchez CE, Kuhnert LV, Poindexter C, Pak CY. Antihypertensive comparison of furosemide with hydrochlorothiazide for black patients. *Arch Intern Med.* 1979;139:1015–1021.
4. Finnerty Jr FA, Maxwell MH, Lunn J, Moser M. Long-term effects of furosemide and hydrochlorothiazide in patients with essential hypertension a two-year comparison of efficacy and safety. *Angiology.* 1977;28:125–133.
5. Mortality after 10 1/2 years for hypertensive participants in the Multiple Risk Factor Intervention Trial. *Circulation.* 1990;82:1616-1628.
6. SHEP cooperative research group. Prevention of stroke by antihypertensive drug treatment in older persons with isolated systolic hypertension. Final results of the systolic hypertension in the elderly program (SHEP). *JAMA.* 1991;265:3255-3264.
7. ALLHAT Officers and Coordinators for the ACRGTA, Lipid-Lowering Treatment to Prevent Heart Attack Trial. Major outcomes in high-risk hypertensive patients randomized to angiotensin-converting enzyme inhibitor or calcium channel blocker vs diuretic: the Antihypertensive and Lipid-Lowering Treatment to Prevent Heart Attack Trial (ALLHAT). *JAMA.* 2002;288:2981-2997.
8. Siscovick DS, Raghunathan TE, Psaty BM, et al. Diuretic therapy for hypertension and the risk of primary cardiac arrest. *N Engl J Med.* 1994;330:1852–1857.
9. Griebeler ML, Kearns AE, Ryu E, et al. Thiazide-associated hypercalcemia: Incidence and association with primary hyperparathyroidism over two decades. *J Clin Endocrinol Metab.* 2016;101:1166–1173.
10. Ware JS, Wain LV, Channavajjhala SK, et al. Phenotypic and pharmacogenetic evaluation of patients with thiazide-induced hyponatremia. *J Clin Invest.* 2017;127:3367–3374.
11. Palmer BF. Metabolic complications associated with use of diuretics. *Semin Nephrol.* 2011;31:542–552.

CHAPTER 35

POTASSIUM-SPARING DIURETICS

Juan P. Arroyo, MD, PhD, and James M. Luther, MD, MSCI

QUESTIONS

1. **How do potassium-sparing diuretics work?**
   Potassium-sparing diuretics block the reabsorption of sodium through the epithelial sodium channel (ENaC) in exchange for potassium in the connecting tubule (CNT) and collecting duct (CD). Traditional potassium-sparing diuretics (amiloride, triamterene) directly block ENaC, and others block the mineralocorticoid receptor (MR [e.g., spironolactone, eplerenone]). Because a major action of the MR is to increase ENaC activity, MR antagonism acts indirectly by decreasing ENaC activity.

   These diuretics may also have kidney-independent effects. ENaC is present in extra renal tissues such as the vascular endothelium, although the clinical effects of vascular ENaC are unclear. The MR is distributed throughout the body, and MR antagonists may contribute to cardiovascular protection via actions in the heart and vasculature.

2. **Why is this class of diuretics called potassium-sparing diuretics?**
   Unlike diuretics that inhibit sodium transport in the proximal convoluted tubule, loop of Henle, or the distal convoluted tubule, potassium-sparing diuretics inhibit sodium reabsorption in the CNT and the CD. In the CNT and CD, sodium reabsorption occurs mainly via ENaC. As sodium is reabsorbed, the lumen becomes negative. The negative

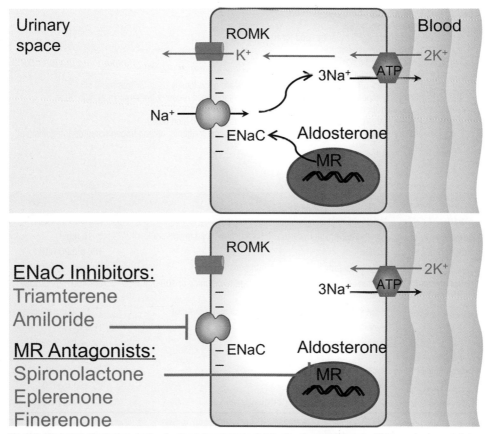

Fig. 35.1 Mechanism of potassium-sparing diuretics in the principal cell. MR, mineralocorticoid receptor. ROMK, renal outer medullary potassium channel. ATP, adenosin triphosphate. ENaC, epithelial sodium channel..

intraluminal voltage then favors potassium secretion from the cells of the CNT and CD to maintain electroneutrality (Fig. 35.1). If sodium reabsorption in the CNT and CD is impaired, then potassium secretion is also impaired. Therefore diuretics that block the movement of sodium in the CNT and CD and decrease potassium secretion are called *potassium-sparing diuretics*.

3. What are the generic names for potassium-sparing diuretics?
   Amiloride and triamterene directly block ENaC and are therefore the classic "potassium-sparing" diuretics. Spironolactone is a steroidal MR antagonist, which is considered a potassium-sparing diuretic. Spironolactone does not directly inhibit ENaC but blocks the effect of aldosterone at the MR and decreases the synthesis of new ENaC channels. Eplerenone is also a steroidal MR antagonist, and finerenone is a nonsteroidal MR antagonist that has been shown to reduce the risk of chronic kidney disease (CKD) progression and cardiovascular risk in CKD associated with type 2 diabetes.

4. What are common indications for potassium-sparing diuretics?
   Triamterene, used in combination with a thiazide to prevent hypokalemia, is the most commonly used potassium-sparing diuretic. Resistant hypertension is the most common indication for spironolactone. Spironolactone is the most effective additive treatment in patients with resistant hypertension.[1] Spironolactone is commonly used to treat fluid overload due to a variety of conditions, including heart failure or liver failure. Spironolactone has been shown to reduce cardiovascular mortality in patients with systolic heart failure, and eplerenone reduces mortality in patients after acute myocardial infarction.[2–4] Spironolactone also has off-target effects including progesterone receptor activation and androgen receptor inhibition, which are sometimes utilized to treat other conditions that are listed later. Eplerenone and the developing nonsteroidal MR antagonists (e.g., finerenone) are more specific for the MR and are therefore not useful for these other conditions.
   Triamterene and amiloride also are used occasionally for treatment of:
   - Liddle syndrome
   - Meniere disease
   - Lithium-induced polyuria
   - Cystic fibrosis
   MR antagonists are frequently used for treatment of:
   - Cirrhosis with ascites
   - Systolic heart failure
   - Proteinuric renal disease
   Spironolactone's off-target steroid receptor effects are occasionally used for treatment of:
   - Hirsutism, especially polycystic ovary syndrome (androgen receptor antagonism at high dose)
   - Acne (androgen receptor antagonism at high dose)
   - Female pattern hair loss (androgen receptor antagonism at high dose)
   - Male-to-female gender transition (progesterone receptor agonist and androgen receptor antagonism at high dose)

Table 35.1 Potassium-Sparing Diuretics

MEDICATION	INDICATION	DOSE PER DAY
Amiloride	Adjunct therapy in hypertension or fluid overload to prevent low K+	5–10 mg
Triamterene	Edema	100 mg PO BID
	Adjunct therapy in hypertension to prevent low K+	50–100 mg PO qDay
Spironolactone	Ascites—usual ratio of spironolactone/furosemide of 100 mg: 40 mg	50–400 mg PO qDay
	Heart failure with reduced ejection fraction (EF <45%)	12.5–50 mg PO qDay
	Hypertension—adjunct therapy	12.5–50 mg PO qDay
	Primary aldosteronism	12.5–200 mg PO qDay
Eplerenone	Hypertension, Heart Failure	25–50 mg BID
	Primary aldosteronism	25-150 mg BID
Finerenone	CKD associated with type 2 diabetes	10-20 mg PO qDay

BID, Twice daily; *CKD*, chronic kidney disease; *K+*, potassium; *PO*, by mouth (per os); *q*, every.

Table 35.2 Side Effect Profile Comparison for Antihypertensive Diuretics

	LOOP	THIAZIDE	Potassium-Sparing Diuretics		
			AMILORIDE	SPIRONOLACTONE	EPLERENONE
Sodium	↔	↓↓	↓	↓	↓
Potassium	↓	↓↓	↑	↑	↑
Bicarbonate	↑	↑	↓	↓	↓
Calcium	↔/↓	↑	↔	↔	↔
Magnesium	↓	↓↓	↔	↔	↔
Uric acid	↑↑	↑↑	↑	↑	↑
Glucose	↔/↑	↑	↔	↔/↑	↔/↑
Cholesterol	↑	↑			
Triglycerides	↑	↑			
Kidney stones	↑	↓	↔	↔	↔
Ototoxicity	Yes	No	No	No	No
Cramping	Yes	Yes	Yes	Yes	Yes
Gynecomastia	No	No	No	Yes	No
Erectile dysfunction	No	No	No	Yes	No

arrows indicate increased (↑), decreased (↓), or neutral (↔) effect of the drug on relevant concentration.

5. How are potassium-sparing diuretics dosed?
   See Table 35.1 for typical doses of commonly used potassium-sparing diuretics.

6. What are the most common side effects and contraindications to the use of potassium-sparing diuretics?
   Hyperkalemia (K^+ >5.0 mEqL) is the single most common contraindication for potassium-sparing diuretics, and most recommend not starting therapy if serum potassium is greater than 4.7 mEq/L. Severe kidney disease (estimated glomerular filtration rate <30 mL/min) is a relative contraindication given the increased risk of hyperkalemia in patients with renal disease. Diuretics may also have reduced efficacy in advanced kidney disease.
   Spironolactone is structurally similar to progesterone and may produce off-target effects through other steroid receptors, such as gynecomastia or breast tenderness, amenorrhea (progesterone receptor activation), and reduced libido or impotence (androgen receptor antagonism). The risk of gynecomastia in men is dose- and duration-dependent with an occurrence of 5% to 10% after 1 year of taking spironolactone 25 mg daily. Eplerenone is MR-selective and does not produce these side effects more often than placebo. Chronic triamterene use is associated with a high incidence of eosinophiluria, the significance of which is unclear. Common side effects and contraindications are shown in Table 35.2.

7. What drug interactions should be considered before using potassium-sparing diuretics?
   Hyperkalemia is the most dangerous complication of potassium-sparing diuretics. Therefore potassium-sparing diuretics in combination with medications that can increase potassium should be taken with caution or avoided altogether. Several medications, such as trimethoprim and pentamidine, block ENaC as an off-target effect (see Fig. 35.1) and markedly increase the risk of hyperkalemia when used with other drugs that block the renin-angiotensin-aldosterone system.[5]
   Drug concentrations of eplerenone and finerenone may be increased if used with drugs that inhibit CYP3A4. Use of finerenone with strong CYP3A4 inhibitors is contraindicated.

KEY POINTS

1. Potassium-sparing diuretics act by blocking ENaC or by blocking activation of the mineralocorticoid receptor.
2. The potassium-sparing diuretics spironolactone and amiloride are effective agents for treating resistant hypertension.
3. All potassium-sparing diuretics carry a risk of hyperkalemia, and special attention should be given to drug interactions, diet, and electrolyte monitoring when prescribing these medications.
4. Spironolactone is associated with off target hormonal effects such as gynecomastia and erectile dysfunction in men and dysmenorrhea in women.

REFERENCES

1. Williams B, MacDonald TM, Morant S, et al. Spironolactone versus placebo, bisoprolol, and doxazosin to determine the optimal treatment for drug-resistant hypertension (PATHWAY-2): a randomised, double-blind, crossover trial. *Lancet.* 2015;. doi: 10.1016/S0140-6736(15)00257-3.
2. Zannad F, McMurray JJ, Krum H, et al. Eplerenone in patients with systolic heart failure and mild symptoms. *N Engl J Med.* 2011;364(1):11–21.
3. Pitt B, White H, Nicolau J, et al. Eplerenone reduces mortality 30 days after randomization following acute myocardial infarction in patients with left ventricular systolic dysfunction and heart failure. *J Am Coll Cardiol.* 2005;46(3):425–431.
4. Pitt B, Zannad F, Remme WJ, et al. The effect of spironolactone on morbidity and mortality in patients with severe heart failure. Randomized Aldactone Evaluation Study Investigators. *N Engl J Med.* 1999;341(10):709–717.
5. Antoniou T, Gomes T, Juurlink DN, Loutfy MR, Glazier RH, Mamdani MM. Trimethoprim-sulfamethoxazole-induced hyperkalemia in patients receiving inhibitors of the renin-angiotensin system: a population-based study. *Arch Intern Med.* 2010;170(12):1045–1049.

CHAPTER 36

ALPHA ANTAGONISTS

Bilal Munir MD, FRCPC, and George K. Dresser MD, PhD, FRCPC

QUESTIONS

1. **How do alpha adrenergic receptors contribute to blood pressure regulation?**

   Alpha adrenergic receptors are G protein coupled receptors (GPCR) that are found in various locations in the human body. In the context of hypertension their most important peripheral locations are on smooth muscle cells (Table 36.1 and Fig. 36.1). There are two main types, alpha-1 and alpha-2, both of which have multiple subtypes. The alpha-1 receptors are Gq type receptors, which activate phospholipase C, in turn, increasing inositol triphosphate and diacylglycerol, which leads to increased intracellular calcium concentrations. This serves two main purposes: smooth muscle contraction and glyconeogenesis. Alpha-1 receptors can be activated by catecholamines (norepinephrine and epinephrine). As a consequence, these receptors are activated by hypoperfusion (i.e., in settings of low cardiac output or decreased systemic vascular resistance as would occur in shock). Common alpha-1 agonists include doxazosin, terazosin, and prazosin.

   Alpha-2 receptors are allosteric inhibitors through Gi function, leading to the inhibition of adenylyl cyclase which lowers the availability of cyclic adenosine monophosphate (cAMP), cytoplasmic calcium, and neurotransmitter release culminating in a central vasodilatory effect. This reduces sympathetic outflow centrally and leads to an increased vagal (parasympathetic) tone. Common alpha-2 agonists include clonidine, guanfacine, and methyldopa.

   Whereas alpha agonists activate central alpha-2 receptors in either a selective or nonselective fashion, alpha-1 antagonists bind receptors in the peripheral vasculature to prevent catecholamine binding in smooth muscle cells with a resultant vasodilatory effect that results in lower blood pressure.[1]

2. **Why are quinazoline-derived selective alpha-1 receptor antagonists preferred in modern hypertension management over nonselective alpha antagonists?**

   Quinazoline-derived alpha antagonists include doxazosin, terazosin, and prazosin. They belong to the N-containing heterocyclic compounds which have diuretic, antihistamine, analgesic, lipid lowering, and antiinflammatory properties in addition to their antihypertensive actions.[2] These alpha antagonists decrease vascular resistance without changing cardiac output and have minimal effect on renin release, as well as a long duration of action. They reduce both pre-load and after-load while causing minimal alterations to renal blood flow and glomerular filtration rate (GFR).[3] Unlike nonselective alpha antagonists, selective alpha antagonists generate less reflex tachycardia due to their inhibition of norepinephrine release. As with other antihypertensive agents, quinazoline alpha antagonists have been associated with left ventricular hypertrophy (LVH) regression, although this effect is less pronounced compared to other classes of antihypertensive agents. One advantage of nonselective alpha

Table 36.1 Alpha Adrenergic Receptor Types, Tissue Distribution, Physiological Effects, and Endogenous and Xenobiotic Agonists and Antagonists

RECEPTOR	TISSUE DISTRIBUTION	PHYSIOLOGICAL EFFECTS	AGONIST	ANTAGONIST
α1	Smooth muscle	Gluconeogenesis Smooth muscle contraction Vasoconstriction Mydriasis Urinary and gastro-intestinal sphincter contraction	Epinephrine Midodrine Norepinephrine Phenylephrine	Alfuzosin Antipsychotics Doxazosin Hydroxyzine phentolamine Phenoxybenzamine Trazodone Tricyclic antidepressants
α2	Ciliary epithelium Nerve endings Pancreas Platelets Salivary glands	Inhibition of neurotransmitter release Platelet activation	Clonidine Dexmedetomidine	Antipsychotics Phentolamine Trazodone Yohimbine

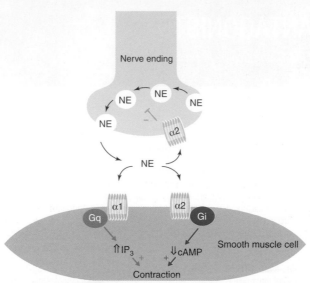

Fig. 36.1 Alpha adrenergic receptors and the action of neurotransmitter norepinephrine *(NE)* at the neuromuscular junction. Norepinephrine is released from storage granules at the presynaptic sympathetic nerve endings and can bind to either alpha-1 adrenergic receptor ($\alpha1$) or alpha-2 adrenergic receptor ($\alpha2$) on the cell membrane of smooth muscle cells. $\alpha1$ Receptors mediate calcium release and cellular contraction via the inositol triphosphate (*IP³*) intracellular signaling pathway, whereas $\alpha2$ receptors do the same via the cyclic adenosine monophosphate (*cAMP*) intracellular signaling pathway. The $\alpha2$ receptor on the presynaptic nerve ending functions in a negative feedback loop to inhibit further release of norepinephrine. *Gq* and *Gi*, G-Protein coupled receptor subtype.

antagonists is targeting of smooth muscle in the bladder and prostate which allows for use as treatment in patients with benign prostatic hyperplasia (BPH).

Selective quinazoline alpha antagonists have the additional advantage of not interrupting the local regulatory mechanisms of the prejunctional alpha receptors in the neurovascular junction, leading to a decrease in the accumulation and leakage of catecholamines into the circulation as seen with alpha-2 antagonists.[4]

In some health jurisdictions a gastrointestinal therapeutic system (GITS) formulation of doxazosin and prazosin are available to provide a more refined pharmacokinetic profile.[4]

3. **Why is doxazosin preferred over other quinazoline-derived alpha antagonists? What are the important pharmacokinetic parameters for this drug?**
Alpha antagonists are generally well absorbed and have excellent oral bioavailability. After oral consumption, alpha antagonists are absorbed into the blood stream and undergo extensive hepatic metabolism via CYP3A4 and CYP2D6 (CYP2C9 to a lesser extent).[4] Elimination is biphasic and occurs by O-demethylation of the quinazoline nucleus or hydroxylation of the benzodioxan moiety with subsequent excretion in the feces (63% of a radiolabeled dose) and urine (9%).[5] Only 4.8% of the parent drug is eliminated unchanged in urine and feces.[5] The main difference between quinazoline alpha antagonists is the half-life of elimination. Doxazosin is a competitive inhibitor of postsynaptic alpha-1 adrenergic receptors and has a longer half-life than prazosin with an oral bioavailability of 62% to 69%.[6] Doxazosin has linear (first order) pharmacokinetics within an oral dose range of 2 mg to 8 mg per day. Peak plasma concentrations occurred 1.7 to 3.6 hours after oral consumption and maximum reduction in blood pressure occurred 2 to 6 hours after ingestion.[5] Administration with food reduced the rate but not the extent of absorption.[7] Within the dose range of 2 to 8 mg per day, the half-life, volume of distribution, clearance and degree of protein binding (98% bound) was stable.[5,7] The terminal half-life of doxazosin is 16 to 22 hours and is not dependent on renal function,[6] in comparison with prazosin which has a half-life 4 to 7 times shorter. Doxazosin has an affinity for alpha-1 receptors that is 400 times greater than its affinity for alpha-2 receptors.[8] This longer duration of action allows for once daily dosing with doxazosin, whereas the other selective alpha antagonists require more frequent dosing. Doxazosin and terazosin are less lipid soluble with lower affinity for alpha-1 receptors compared with other options, which results in a more gradual onset of action which mitigates the first-dose hypotension seen with other agents.[9]

When compared with other alpha antagonists and classes of antihypertensives, doxazosin has a favorable effect on lipid profile, insulin resistance, and glucose metabolism.[3] The mechanism by which this occurs is unknown but one proposed mechanism is thought to be due to the blocking of Monocyte chemoattractant protein-1 (MCP-1 directed monocyte migration by inhibition of Matrix metallopeptidase 9 (MMP-9) and upregulation of Tissue Inhibitor of MetalloProteinase-1 (TIMP-1) production.[2] Doxazosin is the only antihypertensive to demonstrate a lowering of total cholesterol and low-density lipoproteins by 5% and triglycerides by 10%. There have also been some studies that demonstrate an increase in high-density lipoproteins.[3] Conversely, prazosin has not shown any significant lipid lowering effect.

4. How should doxazosin be dosed in typical antihypertensive patients?

The most widely used formulation for hypertension is the immediate release. Some degree of tachyphylaxis occurs. Initial dosing should start at 1 mg once daily and be titrated to response up to a maximum of 16 mg/day. If therapy is interrupted, doxazosin should be restarted at the introductory dose, to account for loss of tolerance.

There are no dose adjustments recommended in the labelling for doxazosin when this drug is used in patients with renal or hepatic impairment. Nevertheless, caution is appropriate in patients with Child-Pugh class A and B and use should be avoided in Child-Pugh class C hepatic failure. Although the C_{max} increased by 27% and the area under the curve (AUC) by 34% in the geriatric population, the standard dosing regimen should be used in this age group.

5. What clinical outcomes can be expected in patients using doxazosin for hypertension control?

A pooled analysis of hypertension studies (placebo-controlled) showed that doxazosin in doses of 1 to 16 mg/day lowered blood pressure on average by 10/8 mm Hg in the standing position and 9/5 mm Hg when supine.[5] Given that the Blood Pressure Lowering Treatment Trialists' Collaboration (BPLTTC) data suggests that for each 6 mm Hg reduction in systolic blood pressure (SBP), coronary heart disease (CHD) is reduced by 14% and stroke by 18%,[10] it is reasonable to expect that successful treatment with doxazosin would be associated with a 23% reduction in CHD events and a 30% reduction in stroke.

6. What clinical trial data support the use of alpha antagonists?

The Major Outcomes in High-Risk Hypertensive Patients Randomized to Angiotensin-Converting Enzyme Inhibitor or Calcium Channel Blocker versus Diuretic The Antihypertensive and Lipid-Lowering Treatment to Prevent Heart Attack Trial (ALLHAT) trial by Wright, et al. was a multicenter, multinational double blind, parallel group randomized control trial published in 2002 with a total of 42,418 participants. This trial looked at the efficacy of varying classes of antihypertensives in lowering the incidence of cardiovascular events. The doxazosin arm ($n = 9061$) was not included in the final analysis as it was prematurely terminated due to a significantly increased risk of heart failure compared to chlorthalidone in the interim analysis. Blood pressure was lower throughout the follow-up period in the chlorthalidone-treated patients. After a median of 3.3 years, 4% of patients in both groups had an outcome event. Heart failure occurred in 8.1% versus 4.5% of patients assigned to doxazosin versus chlorthalidone. Had the blood pressures been better matched during follow-up, or the doxazosin patients received diuretics where appropriate, it is possible that the outcomes in the doxazosin arm of the trial might have allowed for completion of this arm of the trial. However, most hypertension guidelines now recommend against doxazosin as initial therapy based on this trial.

In the Anglo-Scandinavian Cardiac Outcomes Trial-Blood Pressure Lowering Arm (ASCOT-BPLA) doxazosin GITS had benefit as an add-on to either amlodipine/perindopril or atenolol/bendroflumethiazide based strategies as the third drug in the up-titration algorithm.[4] Because it was used as add-on therapy in both arms of the trial, a randomized comparison with placebo is not possible. However, of 19,257 participants in the ASCOT- BPLA study, 10,069 patients were prescribed doxazosin and had valid BP data before and after receiving the drug. Within these patients, mean BP fell from 159/89 to 147/82 over a 9-month treatment period. Only 7.5% of patients experienced an adverse event that resulted in discontinuation of the alpha antagonist. Of these, the most common adverse events were dizziness (29%), vertigo (9%), fatigue (13%), headache (9%), or edema (8%). Within the entire ASCOT follow-up period, heart failure only occurred in 1.5% of patients, a rate that did not differ between those who received doxazosin and those who did not.[10]

A Cochrane review published in 2012 aiming to determine the effects of alpha antagonists on blood pressure found a total of 10 trials which looked at dose-associated lowering of blood pressure with alpha antagonists with a total of 1175 participants. They found no difference among the four alpha antagonists studied in efficacy of lowering blood pressure.[11]

The Spironolactone versus Placebo, Bisoprolol, and Doxazosin to determine the optimal treatment for drug-resistant hypertension Prevention And Treatment of Hypertension With Algorithm based therapY-2 (PATHWAY-2) trial was a randomized, double blind crossover trial that examined the impact of adding a fourth drug to patients with resistant hypertension who were already receiving a thiazide diuretic, a calcium channel blocker, and an inhibitor of the renin-angiotensin system. The primary result was that spironolactone was the most effective add-on therapy in the patients studied. Spironolactone was associated with an average reduction in home SBP of 12.8 mm Hg, whereas doxazosin had an average reduction of 8.7 mm Hg when used in this context. Doxazosin was used at 4 or 8 mg/day. Increasing the dose of doxazosin from 4 mg to 8 mg only resulted in a 0.55 mm Hg drop in SBP, suggesting that for most patients, the dose of 4 mg should be adequate. It was well tolerated without any significant side-effects, although postural dizziness and muscle spasms were reported by some patients. In contrast to some older trials, the rate of fatigue was similar to placebo. In contrast to the other agents in this trial, sodium, potassium, and creatinine were not impacted by doxazosin therapy.[12]

7. **When would alpha antagonists be a preferred treatment option?**

   At present, alpha antagonists in the treatment of hypertension are recommended as add-on or alternative therapy after inadequate blood pressure lowering or intolerance to a first line agent. Consideration can be given to those with concurrent BPH on a case-by-case basis. Given the lack of effect on electrolytes, renal function, or heart rate, patients who are most likely to benefit from alpha antagonist treatment are those with tenuous renal function, previous problems with potassium homeostasis, acute kidney injury, or bradycardia in association with treatment using alternative first line agents.

   Given the difficulty in acquiring noncompetitive alpha antagonists such as phenoxybenzamine, doxazosin is often used in the preoperative management of patients with pheochromocytoma. However, other options, such as calcium channel blockade, have also been used successfully.

8. **When should alpha antagonists not be used? And what are the side-effects or adverse events to anticipate in patients using alpha antagonists?**

   Alpha antagonists should not be used as initial or monotherapy for hypertension control. They should also be avoided in patients with known sensitivity to quinazolines. Alpha antagonists should be avoided in patients with significant orthostatic hypotension and standing BP should be assessed in patients using alpha antagonists for hypertension. There is a "first dose" effect that can occur at the start of therapy and when dosage is increased, or when re-initiation of therapy occurs after interruption. Patients naive to alpha antagonists should be counselled to avoid a situation in which syncope could lead to danger or injury. In the ALLHAT study, pedal edema and congestive heart failure were limiting adverse events occurring in patients randomized to doxazosin. Priapism is a rare complication occurring in less than one in several thousand patients treated with alpha antagonists, but it can lead to permanent impotence if not treated in a timely fashion.

   In another study cited by the Food and Drug Administration, doxazosin was administered to 4000 patients for the indication of hypertension and, though minor adverse events occurred frequently, only 7% lead to the discontinuation of the drug. Most patients discontinued alpha antagonist therapy for postural symptoms, fatigue, edema and heart rate disturbances.[5]

   Post marketing adverse reactions of gynecomastia, hypoesthesia, priapism, vomiting, allergy, bradycardia, leukopenia, thrombocytopenia, hepatitis, aggravation of bronchospasm, urticaria, intraoperative floppy iris syndrome, cataracts, hematuria, and nocturia have been reported.[5] Caution should be advised in the concurrent use of other venodilators or arteriodilators, for example phosphodiesterase inhibitors, or in those with autonomic instability.[1,10]

9. **Where do alpha antagonists fit in the contemporary management of hypertension?**

   Doxazosin is generally considered as add-on therapy for management of difficult to control hypertension after inadequate response or intolerance to first line agents (Fig. 36.2). Doxazosin is not recommended as first line therapy in the treatment of primary hypertension after the early termination of the doxazosin arm in the ALLHAT trial because of significantly higher rates of heart failure and cardiac events compared to chlorthalidone, amlodipine, and lisinopril. Doxazosin should be considered in patients receiving maximally tolerated doses of angiotensin-converting enzyme (ACE) inhibitors or angiotensin blockers, calcium channel blockers, thiazide-like diuretics, and spironolactone, who continue to have uncontrolled BP. If spironolactone is not tolerated due to hyperkalemia or renal impairment, doxazosin may become the preferred fourth line agent for resistant hypertension. Likewise, if bradycardia is a clinical concern, doxazosin may be preferred over beta-blocker therapy.

10. **Are there any drug interactions with doxazosin?**

    Given metabolism by CYP3A4 and CYP2D6, it would be anticipated that interactions would occur with inhibitors of these metabolic pathways. Altough doxazosin is highly protein bound, there is no in vitro data to demonstrate that it influences the protein binding of warfarin, digoxin, indomethacin, and phenytoin.[5] Interestingly, there are no significant cytochrome P450 mediated interactions reported in the literature. It is speculated that even at low oral doses of doxazosin, there is near maximal saturation of peripheral alpha receptors such that the increased plasma concentrations achieved with concurrent use of inhibitors of metabolism do not result in any additional pharmacodynamic effects.

KEY POINTS

1. Alpha antagonists lower blood pressure by reducing adrenergically mediated smooth muscle contraction in arterioles.
2. Doxazosin is the preferred alpha antagonist for use in patients with hypertension.
3. Due to lack of clinical outcome data supporting the use of alpha-blockers, they should be considered only as additional therapy in patients with resistant hypertension receiving maximally tolerated doses of diuretics, inhibitors of the renin-angiotensin system, and calcium channel blockers.

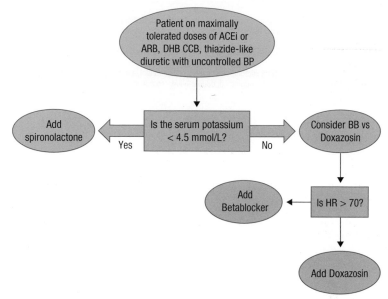

Fig. 36.2 Place of doxazosin in management of resistant hypertension. Most guidelines suggest that alpha antagonists be used only if blood pressure *(BP)* is uncontrolled after initial treatment with diuretics, inhibitors of the renin-angiotensin system, and calcium channel blockers *(CCBs)*. If hyperkalemia limits the use of spironolactone, and bradycardia limits the use of beta-blockers *(BBs)*, doxazosin becomes a preferred add-on therapy. *ACEi,* Angiotensin-converting enzyme inhibitor; *ARB,* angiotensin receptor blocker; *DHP,* dihydro-pyridine; *HR,* heart rate.

REFERENCES

1. Taylor BN, Cassagnol M. Alpha Adrenergic Receptors. [Updated 2019 Dec 20]. In: StatPearls [Internet]. Treasure Island (FL). *StatPearls Publishing.* 2020 Jan;. https://www.ncbi.nlm.nih.gov/books/NBK539830/?report=classic.
2. Heran BS, Galm BP, Wright JM. Blood pressure lowering efficacy of alpha blockers for primary hypertension. *Cochrane Database of Systematic Reviews.* 2012;(8):CD004643. doi: 10.1002/14651858.CD004643.pub3.
3. Reid JL, Vincent J. Clinical pharmacology and therapeutic role of prazosin and related alpha-adrenoceptor antagonists. *Cardiology.* 1986;73:164–174. doi: 10.1159/000174002.
4. Cardura. US Food & Drug Administration. https://www.accessdata.fda.gov/drugsatfda_docs/label/2009/019668s021lbl.pdf. Published January 12, 2016.
5. Rahman MU, Rathore A, Siddiqui AA, Parveen G, Shahar Yar M. Synthesis and antihypertensive screening of new derivatives of quinazolines linked with isoxazole. *Biomed Res Int.* 2014;2014:739056. doi:10.1155/2014/739056.
6. Fulton B, Wagstaff AJ, Sorkin EM. Doxazosin. *Drugs.* 1995;49:295–320. https://doi-org.proxy1.lib.uwo.ca/10.2165/00003495-199549020-00011.
7. Cubeddu LX, Fuenmayor N, Caplan N, Ferry D. Clinical pharmacology of doxazosin in patients with essential hypertension. *Clinical Pharmacology & Therapeutics.* 1987;41:439–449. doi: 10.1038/clpt.1987.54.
8. Cubeddu L, Pool J, Bloomfield R, et al. Effect of doxazosin monotherapy on blood pressure and plasma lipids in patients with essential hypertension. *American Journal of Hypertension.* 1988;1(2):158–167. https://doi-org.proxy1.lib.uwo.ca/10.1093/ajh/1.2.158.
9. Kaplan M. Alpha-blockers in the treatment of hypertension. *Nefrología (English Edition).* 2000;20:35.
10. Chapman N, Chang CL, Dahlöf B, et al. Effect of doxazosin gastrointestinal therapeutic system as third-line antihypertensive therapy on blood pressure and lipids in the Anglo-Scandinavian Cardiac Outcomes Trial. *Circulation.* 2008;118(1):42–48.
11. Bryson CL, Psaty BM. A review of the adverse effects of peripheral alpha-1 antagonists in hypertension therapy. *Curr Control Trials Cardiovasc Med.* 2002;3(1):7. doi:10.1186/1468-6708-3-7.
12. Salam A, Atkins E, Sundstrom J. Effects of blood pressure lowering on cardiovascular events, in the context of regression to the mean: a systematic review of randomized trials. *J Hypertension.* 2019;37(1):16–23.

BIBLIOGRAPHY

Carlson RV, Bailey RR, Begg EJ, Cowlishaw MG, Sharman JR. Pharmacokinetics and effect on blood pressure of doxazosin in normal subjects and patients with renal failure. *Clin Pharmacol Ther.* 1986;40:561–566. doi: 10.1038/clpt.1986.224.
Elliot H, Alpha adrenoreceptor antagonists. Lip G, et al. ed. *Comprehensive Hypertension.* Philadelphia, PA: Mosby Elsevier; 2007:1019–1027.
Elliott H, Meredith P, Reid J. Pharmacokinetic overview of doxazosin. *Am J Cardiol.* 1987;59(14):G78–G81.
Kintscher U, Wakino S, Kim S, Kon D, Hsueh WA, Law RE. Doxazosin inhibits MCP-1 directed migration of human monocytes. *Hypertension.* 2000;36:704–705.

LiverTox: Clinical and Research Information on Drug-Induced Liver Injury [Internet]. Bethesda (MD): National Institute of Diabetes and Digestive and Kidney Diseases; 2012-. Alpha 1 Adrenergic Receptor Antagonists. [Updated 2018 Jan 8]. https://www.ncbi.nlm.nih.gov/books/NBK548719/.

Sica DA. Alpha1 adrenergic blockers: current usage considerations. *J Clin Hyperten.* 2005;7:757–762. doi: 10.1111/j.1524-6175.2005.05300.x.

Williams B, MacDonald TM, Morant S, et al. Spironolactone versus placebo, bisoprolol, and doxazosin to determine the optimal treatment for drug-resistant hypertension (PATHWAY-2): a randomised, double-blind, crossover trial. *Lancet.* 2015;386(10008):2059–2068. doi:10.1016/S0140-6736(15)00257-3.

CHAPTER 37

BETA-BLOCKERS

Panagiotis I. Georgianos, MD, PhD, and Rajiv Agarwal, MD, MS

QUESTIONS

1. **What is the clinical pharmacology of β-adrenergic receptor blockers?**
   β-Adrenergic receptor blockers (beta-blockers) competitively inhibit the β-adrenergic receptors and by doing so act as antihypertensive drugs.[1] Although the exact mechanisms through which these agents lower systemic blood pressure (BP) remain unclear, it is the blockade of the $β_1$-adrenergic receptor that appears to be the predominant mechanism by which these drugs reduce heart rate, cardiac output, and peripheral vascular resistance and thereby lower BP.[1]

2. **How are individual β-adrenergic receptor blockers different from each other?**
   Beta-blockers represent a heterogeneous class of antihypertensive compounds. As shown in Fig. 37.1, these agents differ substantially in their $β_1$/ $β_2$-adrenergic receptor selectivity, intrinsic sympathomimetic activity, and vasodilatory properties.[2] Based on this diversity, beta-blockers have been classified into first-, second- and third-generation. First-generation includes non-cardioselective beta-blockers with equal affinity for $β_1$ and $β_2$ adrenergic receptors. Second-generation beta-blockers, also referred to as cardioselective beta-blockers, are characterized by greater affinity for $β_1$ than for $β_2$ adrenergic receptors.[2] Neither of these two traditional categories exerts vasodilatory actions, which is an intrinsic property of third-generation beta-blockers.[2]

3. **What are common adverse effects seen with use of β-blockers?**
   The use of beta-blockers has been associated with a variety of side effects. Commonly reported side effects of these agents include the following: fatigue, diminished exercise ability, aggravation of symptoms of peripheral occlusive vascular disease, erectile dysfunction, slight elevation in serum potassium levels, impaired concentration and memory, worsening of depression, and psoriasis.[2] The use of non-cardioselective beta-blockers is contraindicated in patients with asthma, where these agents exert adverse metabolic effects, such as worsening of insulin sensitivity and impairment of serum lipid profile, notably elevation in serum triglycerides and reduction in high-density-lipoprotein (HDL)-cholesterol levels.[3] In addition, beta-blockers have been associated with higher incidence of new-onset diabetes, particularly when they are administered in combination with thiazide-type diuretics.[4] It has to be noted, however, that clinical studies on third-generation beta-blockers, such as nebivolol and carvedilol, have shown that these agents do not impair glucose tolerance or glycemic control and have a more favorable side effect profile as compared with traditional beta-blockers.[5–7]

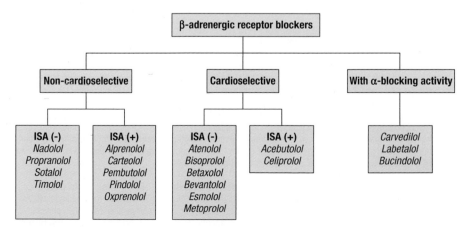

Fig. 37.1 Classification of beta-blockers according to their cardioselectivity and intrinsic sympathomimetic activity *(ISA)*.

4. **How has the recommendation for beta-blockers changed with time for hypertension?**
Beta-blockers together with diuretics were the cornerstone of the pharmacological management of hypertension, but this treatment strategy has been reappraised. Based both on US (the 2017 American Heart Association/American College of Cardiology [AHA/ACG]) and the European (2018 European Society of Hypertension/European Society of Cardiology [ESH/ESC]) guidelines, beta-blockers are no longer recommended as first-line agents in pharmacotherapy of uncomplicated hypertension.[8,9] Both guidelines recommend that beta-blockers should be considered for the management of hypertension in patients with specific indications for their use, such as among patients with concomitant heart failure (HF), angina, and atrial fibrillation or after an acute myocardial infarction.[8,9]
In the following sections of this chapter, we provide a critical evaluation of the available randomized trials that investigated the efficacy and safety of beta-blockers and reported outcomes in hypertensive patients with or without chronic kidney disease (CKD). We discuss gaps in the existing evidence and conclude with clinical practice recommendations and directions for future research in this important area.

5. **What is the clinical trial evidence for beta-blockers use in hypertension?**
The efficacy and safety of beta-blockers as first-line agents in pharmacotherapy of uncomplicated hypertension was explored in an updated 2017 Cochrane metaanalysis of 13 randomized trials comparing beta-blockers either with placebo or with active-treatment.[10] Beta-blockers were not superior to placebo (relative risk [RR]: 0.99; 95% confidence interval [CI]: 0.88–1.11) or active-treatment with diuretics (RR:1.04; 95% CI: 0.91–1.19) and renin-angiotensin-system (RAS)-blockers (RR: 1.10; 95% CI: 0.98–1.24) in reducing all-cause mortality; in contrast, all-cause mortality risk was higher when beta-blockers were compared with calcium-channel-blockers (CCBs) (RR: 1.07; 95% CI: 1.0–1.14).[10] Compared with placebo, beta-blockers provoked a 12% reduction in the risk of cardiovascular events (RR: 0.88; 95% CI: 0.79–-0.97), a benefit that was driven mainly by a favorable effect of beta-blockers on the incidence of stroke (RR: 0.80; 95% CI: 0.66–0.96). There was no difference between beta-blockers and diuretics (RR: 1.13; 95% CI: 0.99–1.28) or between beta-blockers and RAS-blockers (RR: 1.0; 95% CI: 0.72–1.38) in the risk of cardiovascular events. However, the risk of cardiovascular events was higher when beta-blockers were compared with CCBs (RR: 1.18; 95% CI: 1.08–1.29). Once again, this difference was driven by the inferiority of beta-blockers to improve the incidence of stroke (RR: 1.24; 95% CI: 1.11–1.4).[10] With respect to safety outcomes, the likelihood of drug discontinuation due to adverse events was higher when beta-blockers were compared with RAS-blockers (RR: 1.41; 95% CI: 1.29–1.54), but discontinuation rates did not differ when beta-blockers were compared with placebo, diuretics, or CCBs.[10]
This metaanalytic evidence suggests that initial treatment with beta-blockers confers modest improvement in the risk of cardiovascular morbidity and little to no benefit on all-cause mortality, providing support to current international guidelines that do not recommend beta-blockade as first-line drug therapy of uncomplicated hypertension.[8,9] It has to be noted, however, that these findings should be interpreted within the context of some methodological limitations.[11] First, all trials included in this metaanalysis provided add-on medications to the initial antihypertensive regimen, implying that the reported outcomes might have been affected by between-arm differences in add-on treatment. Second, atenolol was the agent that was used as a comparator in the majority of the trials included in this metaanalysis, limiting the generalizability of the results to the overall class of beta-blockers. Third, there were no trials to evaluate the efficacy of third-generation vasodilating beta-blockers on "hard" cardiovascular outcomes. Therefore, the certainty of evidence for most of the outcomes tested in this metaanalysis was qualified as low-to-moderate.[11] Future trials are clearly warranted to elucidate the comparative effectiveness of newer versus traditional beta-blockers in pharmacotherapy of uncomplicated hypertension.

6. **What is the evidence for beta-blockers use for preventing progression of kidney failure?**
In the AASK (African-American Study of Kidney Disease and Hypertension) trial,[12] 1094 African-Americans with hypertensive nephrosclerosis were randomized to a lower versus a standard mean BP target (<92 mm Hg versus 102–107 mm Hg) and to initiate antihypertensive therapy with metoprolol (50–200 mg/day), ramipril (2.5–10 mg/day), or amlodipine (5–10 mg/day) in a 2 × 3 factorial design. Open-label, add-on therapy was administered to achieve the assigned BP targets. The average on-treatment systolic BP was 135 ± 13 mm Hg in the metoprolol group, 135 ± 14 mm Hg in the ramipril group and 133 ± 12 mm Hg in the amlodipine group.[12] Thus, a beta-blocker-based regimen was equally effective with other antihypertensive regimens in controlling BP among African-Americans with hypertensive kidney disease. It has to be noted, however, that compared with metoprolol, therapy with ramipril lowered by 22% (*P* = .04) the composite kidney outcome of greater than 50% decline in glomerular filtration rate (GFR), end stage kidney disease, or death.[12] Compared with amlodipine, therapy with ramipril was even more clinically efficacious as it lowered these end-points by 38% (*P* = .004).

7. **What is the evidence for beta-blockers use for management of heart failure in CKD?**
The cardioprotective action of beta-blockers among patients with CKD was investigated in a metaanalysis by Badve et al.[13] Despite the absence of stringent selection criteria, this metaanalysis included only 6 placebo-controlled trials (incorporating data from 5972 CKD participants). All these trials enrolled patients with HF and reduced left ventricular (LV) ejection fraction. This systematic review identified two additional trials that were

conducted in non-HF patients, but these studies were not eligible in quantitative data synthesis due to incomplete outcome reporting. Among CKD patients with systolic HF, treatment with beta-blockers was superior to placebo in lowering the risk of all-cause death RR 0.72; 95% CI: 0.64–0.80) and in reducing the risk of cardiovascular death (RR: 0.66; 95% CI: 0.49–0.89).[13] However, this benefit on survival was paralleled with a 4.92-fold elevation in the incidence of bradycardia (RR: 4.92; 95% CI: 3.20–7.55) and a 5.08-fold higher risk of hypotension (RR: 5.08; 95% CI: 3.48–7.41).[13] These adverse events associated with beta-blockade use occur more commonly in HF patients with than without CKD. An earlier metaanalysis exploring the safety and tolerability of these agents in the general HF population showed that compared with placebo, beta-blockers were associated with a 3.62-fold relative increase in the incidence of bradycardia (RR: 3.62; 95% CI: 2.48–5.28) and with only 41% higher risk of hypotension (RR: 1.42; 95% CI: 0.96–2.06).[14] The metaanalysis of Badve et al.[13] highlights the lack of direct evidence on the efficacy of beta-blockers in the CKD population, as five out of six eligible studies were post-hoc analyses of trials reporting mortality outcome data in subgroups of participants with CKD at baseline.

8. What is the evidence for beta-blockers use in management of hypertension in dialysis?

Evidence on the comparative effectiveness of different antihypertensive drug classes among patients on dialysis was provided by the HDPAL (Hypertension in Hemodialysis treated with Atenolol or Lisinopril) trial.[15] In this trial, 200 hypertensive dialysis patients with LV hypertrophy were randomized to open-label lisinopril or atenolol, each administered on a thrice-weekly regimen immediately postdialysis. All participants were treated to the same monthly monitored home BP target of less than 140/90 mm Hg following a prespecified algorithm that included firstly, the dose titration of the study drugs and then, intensification of background antihypertensive therapy, sodium restriction, and dry-weight reduction.[15] Contrary to the original hypothesis that a lisinopril-based regimen would be superior to atenolol in causing regression of LV hypertrophy, both drugs were equally effective in reducing LV mass index during the 12-month-long follow-up of the trial. In addition, atenolol appeared to be more effective in improving BP control, as monthly monitored home BP was consistently lower in the atenolol group, despite a greater need for intervention in the lisinopril group; in lisinopril-treated participants, antihypertensive therapy and more aggressive dry-weight adjustment was required.[15] Due to cardiovascular safety reasons, the trial was terminated early. Serious adverse cardiovascular events occurred more commonly in the lisinopril than in the atenolol group (incidence rate ratio [IRR]: 2.36; 95% CI: 1.36–4.23). The risk of hospitalization for HF was also higher in lisinopril-treated than in atenolol-treated participants (IRR: 3.13; 95% CI: 1.08–10.99).[15] A secondary analysis of the HDPAL trial showed that compared with lisinopril, atenolol provoked a greater proportional reduction in aortic pulse wave velocity over the first 6 months of follow-up (between-drug difference: 14.8%; 95% CI: 1.5% to 28.5%).[16]

Therefore, atenolol appears to be more effective than lisinopril in improving BP control, in causing regression of aortic stiffness and possibly, in reducing the occurrence of serious adverse cardiovascular events among hypertensive dialysis patients.[15] In contrast to the previously mentioned guidelines that do not recommend the use of beta-blockers as first-line antihypertensive therapy,[8,9] the surprising results of the HDPAL trial support the notion that beta-blockers, and particularly atenolol administered 3 times per week postdialysis, may be the preferred choice in pharmacotherapy of hypertension in dialysis patients. Undoubtedly, the potential superiority of beta-blockers over other antihypertensive drug classes in this particular population warrants confirmation in future clinical trials.

9. What are the practical aspects in the use of beta-blockers for management of hypertension in CKD?

Taken together, although beta-blockers are no longer recommended as first-line therapy of uncomplicated hypertension,[8,9] these agents continue to be commonly prescribed in daily clinical practice, particularly in patients with advanced CKD.[17,18] In the absence of solid and robust clinical-trial evidence to guide the use of beta-blockers in this setting, we do not prescribe beta-blockers as first-line antihypertensive therapy to our patients with CKD who are not on dialysis.[1] However, based on the results of the HDPAL trial and in the absence of other trials to provide head-to-head comparisons between agents from different antihypertensive classes, the beta-blocker atenolol is our first-line choice in pharmacotherapy of hypertension for our dialysis patients without specific indication for other treatment. Because atenolol is a hydrophilic beta-blocker with high dialyzability, we prescribe this agent on a thrice-weekly regimen immediately postdialysis. This dosing regimen of atenolol is effective in controlling 44-hour interdialytic ambulatory BP.[19] The use of beta-blockers as second-line agents for those with other specific cardiovascular indications (i.e., HF) appears reasonable and is often necessary due to the need for multiple antihypertensive drugs to control hypertension in these patients. The signal of cardioprotection with beta-blockade from randomized trials among patients with eGFR less than 30 mL/min/1.73m^2 or those on dialysis is weak.[20] However, pharmacoepidemiologic studies from Canada suggest that a mortality benefit of beta-blocker use exists, even among patients with stage 4 CKD.[20,21] Although scientific gap necessitates the design of randomized trials to specifically investigate the efficacy and safety of beta-blockers in this high-risk patient population, we continue to prescribe and use these drugs liberally among patients with CKD, including those on dialysis.

KEY POINTS

1. Although the exact mechanisms through which beta-blockers lower systemic blood pressure remain unclear, it is the blockade of the β_1-adrenergic receptor that appears to be the predominant mechanism by which these drugs reduce heart rate, cardiac output, and peripheral vascular resistance and thereby lower BP.
2. Beta-blockers differ substantially in their β_1/β_2-adrenergic receptor selectivity, intrinsic sympathomimetic activity, and vasodilatory properties.
3. Beta-blockers are no longer recommended as first-line agents in pharmacotherapy of uncomplicated hypertension but should be considered for the management of hypertension in patients with specific indications for their use, such as among patients with concomitant heart failure, angina, and atrial fibrillation, or after an acute myocardial infarction.
4. Beta-blockers do appear to be more effective in improving BP control, and possibly in reducing the occurrence of serious adverse cardiovascular events, among hypertensive dialysis patients.

Disclosures: R.A. has the following disclosures:

Member data safety monitoring committees: Astra Zeneca, Ironwood Pharmaceuticals;

Member steering committees of randomized trials: Akebia, Bayer, Janssen, Glaxo Smith Cline, Relypsa, Sanofi and Genzyme US Companies;

Member adjudication committees: Bayer, Boehringer Ingelheim, Janssen;

Member scientific advisory board or consultant: Celgene, Daiichi Sankyo, Inc, Eli Lilly, Relypsa, Reata, Takeda Pharmaceuticals, USA, ZS Pharma.

Financial support: R.A. is supported by NIH 5 R01 HL126903-04 and a grant from VA Merit Review I01CX001753.

REFERENCES

1. Sinha AD, Agarwal R. Clinical pharmacology of antihypertensive therapy for the treatment of hypertension in CKD. *Clin J Am Soc Nephrol.* 2019;14(5):757–764.
2. Ripley TL, Saseen JJ. Beta-blockers: a review of their pharmacological and physiological diversity in hypertension. *Ann Pharmacother.* 2014;48(6):723–733.
3. Sarafidis PA, Bakris GL. Metabolic effects of beta-blockers: importance of dissociating newer from conventional agents. *J Hypertens.* 2007;25(1):249–252.
4. Elliott WJ, Meyer PM. Incident diabetes in clinical trials of antihypertensive drugs: a network meta-analysis. *Lancet.* 2007;369(9557):201–207.
5. Ayers K, Byrne LM, DeMatteo A, Brown NJ. Differential effects of nebivolol and metoprolol on insulin sensitivity and plasminogen activator inhibitor in the metabolic syndrome. *Hypertension.* 2012;59(4):893–898.
6. Bakris GL, Fonseca V, Katholi RE, et al. Metabolic effects of carvedilol vs metoprolol in patients with type 2 diabetes mellitus and hypertension: a randomized controlled trial. *JAMA.* 2004;292(18):2227–2236.
7. Kampus P, Serg M, Kals J, et al. Differential effects of nebivolol and metoprolol on central aortic pressure and left ventricular wall thickness. *Hypertension.* 2011;57(6):1122–1128.
8. Whelton PK, Carey RM, Aronow WS, et al. 2017 ACC/AHA/AAPA/ABC/ACPM/AGS/APhA/ASH/ASPC/NMA/PCNA Guideline for the prevention, detection, evaluation, and management of high blood pressure in adults: a report of the American College of Cardiology/American Heart Association task force on clinical practice guidelines. *J Am Coll Cardiol.* 2018;71(19):e127–e248.
9. Williams B, Mancia G, Spiering W, et al. 2018 ESC/ESH Guidelines for the management of arterial hypertension: the task force for the management of arterial hypertension of the European Society of Cardiology and the European Society of Hypertension: the task force for the management of arterial hypertension of the European Society of Cardiology and the European Society of Hypertension. *J Hypertens.* 2018;36(10):1953–2041.
10. Wiysonge CS, Bradley HA, Volmink J, Mayosi BM, Opie LH. Beta-blockers for hypertension. *Cochrane Database Syst Rev.* 2017;1:CD002003.
11. Wiysonge CS, Bradley HA, Volmink J, Mayosi BM. *Heart.* 2018;104(4):282–283.
12. Wright JT, Bakris G, Greene T, et al. Effect of blood pressure lowering and antihypertensive drug class on progression of hypertensive kidney disease: results from the AASK trial. *JAMA.* 2002;288(19):2421–2431.
13. Badve SV, Roberts MA, Hawley CM, et al. Effects of beta-adrenergic antagonists in patients with chronic kidney disease: a systematic review and meta-analysis. *J Am Coll Cardiol.* 2011;58(11):1152–1161.
14. Ko DT, Hebert PR, Coffey CS, et al. Adverse effects of beta-blocker therapy for patients with heart failure: a quantitative overview of randomized trials. *Arch Intern Med.* 2004;164(13):1389–1394.
15. Agarwal R, Sinha AD, Pappas MK, Abraham TN, Tegegne GG. Hypertension in hemodialysis patients treated with atenolol or lisinopril: a randomized controlled trial. *Nephrol Dial Transplant.* 2014;29(3):672–681.
16. Georgianos PI, Agarwal R. Effect of lisinopril and atenolol on aortic stiffness in patients on hemodialysis. *Clin J Am Soc Nephrol.* 2015;10(4):639–645.
17. Frankenfield DL, Weinhandl ED, Powers CA, Howell BL, Herzog CA, St Peter WL. Utilization and costs of cardiovascular disease medications in dialysis patients in Medicare Part D. *Am J Kidney Dis.* 2012;59(5):670–681.
18. Ku E, McCulloch CE, Vittinghoff E, Lin F, Johansen KL. Use of antihypertensive agents and association with risk of adverse outcomes in chronic kidney disease: focus on angiotensin-converting enzyme inhibitors and angiotensin receptor blockers. *J Am Heart Assoc.* 2018;7(19):e009992.

19. Agarwal R. Supervised atenolol therapy in the management of hemodialysis hypertension. *Kidney Int.* 1999;55(4):1528–1535.
20. Agarwal R, Rossignol P. Beta-blockers in heart failure patients with severe chronic kidney disease-time for a randomized controlled trial?. *Nephrol Dial Transplant.* 2020;35(5):728–731.
21. Molnar AO, Petrcich W, Weir MA, Garg AX, Walsh M, Sood MM. The association of beta-blocker use with mortality in elderly patients with congestive heart failure and advanced chronic kidney disease. *Nephrol Dial Transplant.* 2020;35(5):782–789.

CHAPTER 38

ALPHA-2 AGONISTS

Christin Giordano McAuliffe, MD, and J. Matt Luther, MD MSCI

QUESTIONS

1. **How do alpha-2 agonists reduce blood pressure?**
   Norepinephrine activates the alpha-2 adrenergic receptor in the brain, which serves as a negative feedback mechanism to suppress the sympathetic nervous system. Drugs with alpha-2 agonist activity mimic this effect centrally, resulting in suppression of peripheral norepinephrine release and subsequently lowering blood pressure.
      As a result, efficacy of these drugs is reflected by the suppression of circulating norepinephrine. This effect is also used in the clonidine-suppression test to establish autonomous catecholamine secretion by pheochromocytomas, which do not suppress catecholamine secretion in response to clonidine.

2. **Which medications act primarily as alpha-2 agonists?**
   Clonidine, guanfacine, and methyldopa are the most commonly used alpha-2 agonists for the management of hypertension (Table 38.1). Guanfacine is also used in the treatment of attention deficit/hyperactivity disorder. In addition, several medications used for other indications act primarily at the alpha-2 receptor including dexmedetomidine, which is commonly used for sedation in intensive care units (Table 38.2). Lofexidine is approved for treatment of opioid withdrawal.[1]

3. **When prescribing an alpha-2 agonist, what are the usual doses?**
   - See Table 38.2 for usual doses of the most commonly used alpha-2 agonists.
   - Note that, in most cases, the minimal dosing period is 12 hours.

Table 38.1 Dosing of Commonly Used Alpha-2 Agonists

| MEDICATION | TYPICAL DOSE RANGE | Dosage Adjustment for Impaired: | | CONSIDERATIONS |
		KIDNEY FUNCTION	LIVER FUNCTION	
Clonidine	0.1–0.3 mg three times daily	Reduce dose and/or frequency	None	Half-life ~12 hours Prolonged half-life in renal failure
Guanfacine	1–4 mg once daily	None	Use with caution CYP3A4 substrate	Half-life ~17 hours
Methyldopa	250–1000 mg two to three times daily	Reduce dose and/or frequency	None	Rare autoimmune reactions (+ANA, hemolytic anemia) and abnormal liver tests Active metabolites are renally cleared
Moxonidine	0.2–0.6 mg once daily	Reduce dose and/or frequency	None	Available outside the United States Contraindicated in heart failure Prolonged half-life in renal failure
Tizanidine	4–32 mg every 4–6 hours	Reduce dose and/or frequency	Contraindicated	Markedly increased during CYP1A2 inhibitors

ANA, Antinuclear antibody.

Table 38.2 Medications with Alpha-2 Agonist Effects	
MEDICATION	**NOTES**
Apraclonidine eye drops	For glaucoma
Brimonidine eye drops	For glaucoma
Clonidine	Most commonly used for hypertension
Dexmedetomidine	Used primarily for sedation
Guanfacine	Approved for attention deficit/hyperactivity disorder; long half-life
Guanabenz	
Lofexidine	Approved for opioid withdrawal
Methyldopa	Historically used in pregnancy
Moxonidine	Available outside of the United States An imidazoline receptor antagonist
Tizanidine	Used as nonopioid pain relief
Xyalazine	Veterinary tranquilizer; reported contaminant in street drugs (fentanyl)

4. **What are the most common side effects of alpha-2 agonists?**
The most commonly reported side effects are:
- Sedation
- Dry mouth
- Bradycardia
- Fatigue
- Constipation
- Orthostatic hypotension

Catecholamine reduction during treatment characteristically reduces both blood pressure and heart rate. Because an intact sympathetic response is essential to respond to a rapid change in posture, this may produce or worsen orthostatic hypotension. Patients with depression may not be a suitable candidate for treatment because mental alterations such as sedation and depression are also relatively common.

Considerations specific to individual medications include the following:
- Methyldopa can cause abnormal liver function tests, autoimmune reactions such as Coomb's positive hemolytic anemia and antinuclear antibody positivity.
- Clonidine can accumulate in advanced kidney disease due to reduced clearance, which can lead to hypotension and exacerbation of side effects.
- Guanfacine is a CYP3A4 substrate and can accumulate during administration of strong inhibitors.
- Tizanidine accumulates in liver failure and during coadministration with CYP1A2 inhibitors (e.g., fluoroquinolones or fluvoxamine) and is contraindicated in these settings.
- The transdermal clonidine patch may cause local skin irritation, which is typically an allergic reaction to the adhesive. It does not typically preclude the use of oral clonidine.
- Eye drops containing brimonidine can be absorbed after lacrimal drainage into the nasal mucosa or gastrointestinal tract and can rarely produce systemic side effects such as bradycardia and hypotension.

5. **What issues can arise when discontinuing alpha-2 agonists?**
Abrupt withdrawal of alpha-2 agonists in patients taking these medications long-term will produce rebound hypertension, which can sometimes be severe (see Chapter 13). Therefore alternative medications are preferred in patients who cannot reliably adhere to a regular medication schedule.[2]

6. **How does alpha-2 agonist rebound hypertension (drug withdrawal) present?**
- Hyperadrenergic symptoms (anxiety, palpitations, sweating) as a result of norepinephrine excess
- Hypertension with tachycardia

Rebound hypertension due to central alpha-2 agonist withdrawal is characterized by hypertension with tachycardia due to excess sympathetic activation. In contrast, hypertension due to vasoconstrictor sympathetic agents (e.g., phenylephrine) is usually accompanied by a reduction in heart rate due to baroreflex activation. Hyperadrenergic symptoms and hypertension can appear abruptly within the first 1 to 2 days after stopping an alpha-2 agonist, with maximal effect at 3 to 5 days if untreated, as a result of norepinephrine excess at peak withdrawal. Hypertension may be worsened by concurrent use of a β_1-selective beta-blocker, which can prevent tachycardia and relieve symptoms during norepinephrine excess but does not block the vascular alpha-1 receptor–mediated vasoconstriction and hypertension. Chronic beta-blocker use also increases receptor sensitivity, resulting in heightened response to norepinephrine if both agents are withdrawn simultaneously.

Patients are frequently unaware of the risk of rebound hypertension. In particular, patients and physicians using alpha-2 agonists for indications other than hypertension are often unaware of this risk. Patient education about withdrawal hypertension may improve medication adherence and reduce the risk of its occurrence. Patients presenting with withdrawal have often discontinued the drug due to conditions out of their control, such as hospital admission, incapacitation, or medication unavailability. A thorough comparison of home versus hospital medications should be performed, and physicians should have a high index of suspicion when an abrupt change in blood pressure occurs.

7. How can alpha-2 agonist rebound hypertension (drug withdrawal) be prevented or treated?
   - When a physician wants to discontinue clonidine or another alpha-2 agonist, the medication can be tapered slowly over a period of weeks during replacement with an alternative medication if needed. When tapering a clonidine patch, transition to a lower dose patch requires a new prescription for the lower dose patch because the patches should not be cut.
   - Use of a longer-acting agent such as guanfacine may reduce the risk of rebound hypertension due to missed doses or abrupt cessation.
   - Treatment of alpha-2 agonist withdrawal hypertension can be rapidly and specifically treated by restarting the drug or replacing with an alternative alpha-2 agonist. Guanfacine is longer acting and can be used to taper over a longer period.
   - Alternatively, combined beta- and alpha-blockade may be used if unable to tolerate alpha-2 agonists.

8. What conditions, other than hypertension, are treated by use of alpha-2 agonists?
   - Chronic pain syndromes
   - Muscle spasticity or musculoskeletal pain
   - Attention deficit/hyperactivity disorder
   - Withdrawal syndromes, which provoke significant hyperadrenergic syndromes, including alcohol and opioid withdrawal
   - Sedation and analgesia
   - Glaucoma
   - Clonidine suppression testing is used to determine if catecholamine secretion is autonomous in suspected pheochromocytoma
   - Clonidine and other alpha-2 agonists may produce an initial paradoxical vasoconstrictor response, which increases blood pressure, particularly at a high dose, and this effect can rarely be used therapeutically in patients with refractory autonomic failure

9. What commonly used muscle relaxer is primarily an alpha-2 agonist?
   - Tizanidine is an alpha-2 agonist approved for treatment of muscle spasticity in multiple sclerosis. It is commonly used as an alternative to opioids for treatment of chronic pain.
   - Tizanidine has major drug interactions with CYP1A2 inhibitors (e.g., fluoroquinolones, fluvoxamine), which can produce marked hypotension.
   - During long-term use, tizanidine can cause severe rebound hypertension or daily rebound hypertension if used once daily.
   - With the increased attention to avoid chronic opioid use, tizanidine use has increased as adjunctive therapy in postoperative pain management. Pain practitioners may not be aware of the risk of hypotension or rebound hypertension.

10. Should an alpha-2 agonist be the preferred agent in specific settings?
    - Methyldopa has traditionally been the preferred antihypertensive medication in pregnancy due to its demonstrated safety for the fetus. The primacy of methyldopa in pregnancy has recently been called into question with a recent open-label, randomized controlled study that suggests that nifedipine more effectively achieves blood pressure control in pregnancy, although it may have higher fetal risks of intensive care admission (see Chapter 23).[3]
    - Clonidine is available as a transdermal patch once weekly, which is beneficial for patients who are unable to take oral medications and thus may improve adherence.

11. Should these drugs be avoided in certain settings?
    - Moxonidine should be avoided in heart failure due to increased mortality and cardiovascular complications.[4]
    - Clonidine causes initial vasoconstriction when given intravenously and should not be administered via this route.
    - Tizanidine should be avoided in liver failure or during administration of strong CYP1A2 inhibitors.
    - Clonidine or other alpha-2 agonists can have a paradoxical pressor effect in autonomic failure, which may be an adverse or beneficial effect depending on the circumstance.

KEY POINTS

1. When tapering a clonidine patch, transition to lower dose patch requires a new prescription for the lower dose patch because the patches should not be cut.
2. Clonidine and other α2-agonists may produce an initial paradoxical vasoconstrictor response which increases blood pressure, particularly at a high dose.
3. Clonidine causes initial vasoconstriction when given intravenously, and should not be administered via this route.

REFERENCES

1. Sica DA. Centrally acting antihypertensive agents: An update. *J Clin Hypertens.* 2007;9:399–405.
2. Geyskes GG, Boer P, Dorhout Mees EJ. Clonidine withdrawal. Mechanism and frequency of rebound hypertension. *Br J Clin Pharmacol.* 1979;7:55–62.
3. Easterling T, Mundle S, Bracken H, et al. Oral antihypertensive regimens (nifedipine retard, labetalol, and methyldopa) for management of severe hypertension in pregnancy: an open-label, randomised controlled trial. *Lancet.* 2019;394:1011–1021.
4. Cohn JN, Pfeffer MA, Rouleau J, et al. Adverse mortality effect of central sympathetic inhibition with sustained-release moxonidine in patients with heart failure (moxcon). *Eur J Heart Fail.* 2003;5:659–667.

CHAPTER 39

DRUG-DRUG AND PHARMACOGENETIC INTERACTIONS

Jonathan D. Mosley, MD

QUESTIONS

1. What are the possible mechanisms by which medications or supplements affect antihypertensive medication effectiveness?

   The mechanisms by which medications or supplements may impact antihypertensive effectiveness include modulating the metabolism of the antihypertensive medication and activating molecular mechanisms which counteract the targeted blood pressure–lowering mechanisms. Drug metabolism is mediated, in part, by the cytochrome P450 proteins, which are monooxygenases which participate in activation, inactivation, and clearance of drugs.[1] Cytochrome P450 3A4 (CYP3A4), for instance, participates in the oxidation, inactivation, and removal from the circulation for a number of drugs including dihydropyridine calcium channel blockers such as nifedipine. Rifampin, an antibiotic often used in the treatment of tuberculosis, causes an induction of CYP3A4 which leads to decreased systemic concentrations of nifedipine and worsening hypertension.[2–6] Nonsteroidal antiinflammatory drugs (NSAIDs), by contrast, lead to increased blood pressure without altering drug metabolism. NSAIDS inhibit the cyclo-oxygenase pathway of arachidonic acid metabolism and decrease the formation of prostaglandins which modulate blood pressure though a number of mechanisms including altered tubular secretion of salt and water and modulation of the renin-angiotensin-aldosterone system. The overlap between these mechanisms and those modulated by thiazide diuretics[7,8] and angiotensin converting enzyme inhibitors/angiotensin receptor blockers (ACEi/ARBs)[9] results in attenuated activity of these classes of antihypertensives in the presence of NSAIDS. Additional mechanisms are presented in Table 39.1. Antihypertensive medications affected by cytochrome P450 are listed in Table 39.2.

Table 39.1 Notable Antihypertensive Medication Drug-Drug Interactions

DRUG	INTERACTING DRUGS	MECHANISM	EFFECT
ACE inhibitor	Angiotensin receptor blocker	↑RAS inhibition	↑Risk of renal dysfunction
	Neprilysin inhibitor	Likely due to altered vasoactive peptide degradation	↑Risk of angioedema
	DPP4 inhibitor	Likely due to altered vasoactive peptide degradation	↑Risk of angioedema ↑Blood pressure at high dose ACEi
Alpha blockers	PDE5 inhibitors Nitrates	Shared side effect profile	↑Risk of severe hypotension
Beta blockers	Verapamil Diltiazem Clonidine	Shared side effect profile	Bradycardia, AV nodal block
Calcium channel blockers (dihydropyridine)	Alpha blockers Hydralazine Minoxidil	Shared side effect profile	↑Risk of peripheral edema
K-sparing diuretics (Amiloride, Spironolactone, Eplerenone)	Trimethoprim Pentamidine ACEi/ARBs	Shared mechanism	↑Risk of hyperkalemia

Table 39.1 Notable Antihypertensive Medication Drug-Drug Interactions (*Cont.*)

DRUG	INTERACTING DRUGS	MECHANISM	EFFECT
NSAIDs	Thiazides/ACEi/ARB	↓Prostanoid biosynthesis	↓Antihypertensive efficacy
Renin inhibitors	ACE inhibitor or angiotensin receptor blocker	↑RAS inhibition	↑Risk of stroke, Hyperkalemia, renal failure in diabetics
Rifampin	CCBs, others	CYP3A4 induction	↓Drug, CCB concentration
Thiazides	Loop diuretics	Augmented mechanism	↑Risk of hypokalemia and hyponatremia, volume depletion
	Selective serotonin re-uptake inhibitors (SSRIs)	Additive mechanisms, ADH stimulation	↑Risk of hyponatremia
	Lithium	↑Renal reabsorption (↓ renal clearance)	Lithium toxicity
	Digoxin	Hypokalemia augments digoxin binding to receptor	Digitalis toxicity
Diltiazem Verapamil	CYP3A4-metabolized drugs	CYP3A4 inhibition	↑Concentration of CYP3A4-metabolized drugs

ACE, Angiotensin converting enzyme; *ADH,* antidiuretic hormone; *ARB,* angiotensin receptor blocker; *AV,* atrioventricular; *CCB,* calcium channel blocker, *DPP4,* dipeptidyl-peptidase 4; *NSAID,* nonsteroidal antiinflammatory drug; *PDE5,* phosphodiesterase type 5; *RAS,* renin angiotensin system.

Table 39.2 Antihypertensive Medication Cytochrome P450 Substrates and Inhibitors

P450 ISOFORM	1A2	2C8	2C9	2C19	2D6	3A4/5
Substrates	**Tizanidine** Triamterene Verapamil	Torsemide	Irbesartan Losartan Torsemide	Labetalol	Carvedilol Clonidine Lofexidine *Metoprolol* **Nebivolol** *Propranolol* Tamsulosin Timolol	Aliskiren Amlodipine Diltiazem **Eplerenone** **Felodipine** Guanfacine Lercanidipine Nifedipine **Nisoldipine** Nitrendipine Propranolol Verapamil
Inhibitors					Labetalol	**Diltiazem** *Verapamil*

No antihypertensive agents are known to commonly induce P450 activity.

Selected drugs are emphasized **in bold** (≥fivefold change in drug AUC exposure) or *in italics* (two- to fivefold change in drug AUC exposure) due to their predicted effects by the FDA. This list is limited only to antihypertensive drugs. A more complete list can be found at the Indiana University Clinical Pharmacology website, Cytochrome P450 Drug Interaction Table - Drug Interactions. https://drug-interactions.medicine.iu.edu/MainTable.aspx.

2. **What commonly used drugs are associated with drug interactions with antihypertensive medications?**

   Some drug-drug interactions among antihypertensives are due to either overlapping mechanisms of action or shared side effect profiles, which increase the risk of either exaggerated action or side effects. For instance, simultaneous use of combinations of nondihydropyridine calcium channel blockers, beta-blockers and central-acting alpha-blockers, all of which lower heart rate, increases the risk of bradycardia and heart block. Hyperkalemia can be a side effect of inhibitors of the components of the renin-angiotensin-aldosterone system and combinations of ACEis, ARBs, and direct renin inhibitor increases the risk of this side effect.[10,11] Thiazide diuretics can cause drug interactions due to either their direct effects or as a consequence of side effects. Thiazide-induced hypokalemia leads to digoxin toxicity by promoting increased affinity of digoxin to its receptor. Thiazides cause lithium toxicity by promoting increase reabsorption of this drug through the renal tubules.[12,13] Finally, thiazides, due to reasons directly related to their mechanism of action, lead to increased renal water reabsorption by way of increased antidiuretic hormone (ADH) levels and, when coupled with selective serotonin reuptake inhibitors (SS-RIs) which stimulate ADH, can cause hyponatremia.[14,15] Additional drug-drug interactions are listed in Table 39.1. The list of potential drug interactions is not exhaustive but a more complete list of drugs which inhibit or induce metabolizing enzymes can be found on the Food and Drugs Administration (FDA) website.[16]

3. How does rifampin interact with antihypertensive mediations, and how should you alter treatment?

Rifampin induces the expression of multiple hepatic and gastrointestinal drug-metabolizing cytochrome P450 enzymes and intestine P-glycoprotein, resulting in decreased drug concentration and half-life. Calcium channel blockers are notably affected, although effects on multiple drugs within other classes including propranolol, enalapril, and losartan have also been described.[17] When rifampin is started, you should anticipate worsening of hypertension if hepatically metabolized drugs are used. Alternative medications can be used, with selection of drugs which do not have any CYP450 drug interactions. Induction of these enzymes occurs within the first 2 to 7 days and may require 2 to 4 weeks to return to baseline after stopping rifampin. Other medications such as phenobarbital also induce multiple cytochrome P450 enzymes.

4. Are there any known genetic variants that affect antihypertensive medication effectiveness?

Although genetic variants that impact the actions of antihypertensive medications have been identified, testing for these variants is not standard in clinical practice. These variants typically modulate drug efficacy due to mechanisms that are similar to those leading to drug-drug interactions. These mechanisms include altered drug metabolism, altered receptor affinity and alteration of the basal levels of molecular pathways that are modulated by the antihypertensive (Table 39.3). There have been several loss of function variants within the cytochrome P450 gene *CYP2D5* that lead to increased plasma concentrations of metoprolol.[18–20] A missense variant in the beta-1 adrenergic receptor gene (*ADRB1*) decreases its affinity to beta blockers, thereby increasing dose requirements.[21,22] Multiple studies have addressed variants affecting thiazide response, and have identified several variants that have validated across studies. A variant in the gene *NEDD4L* decreases basal sodium reabsorption rates in the kidney and, in the presence of this variant, there is a relatively larger blood-pressure lowering response to thiazide diuretics.[23–25] Variants in *PRKCA*, *TET2*, and *CSMD1* have also been associated with altered thiazide response. A missense variant in the gene *NPHS1*, through mechanisms that are not well-defined, and common loss-of-function variants in CYP2C9 are associated with an attenuated blood-pressure lowering response to losartan.[26–28]

Table 39.3 Notable Antihypertensive Medication Drug-Gene Interactions

DRUG OR DRUG CLASS	GENE VARIANT	MECHANISM	CONSEQUENCE
Metoprolol	*CYP2D6* (multiple decreased function alleles)[a]	↑Plasma concentrations	↓Dose requirement
Beta blocker	*ADRB1* (R389G)	↓Receptor sensitivity	↓Medication response
	GRK4, multiple SNPs	Altered receptor response	↓Medication response
Losartan	*NPHS1* Glu117Lys (rs3814995)	Possibly altered nephrin function	↓SBP and DBP response to medication
	CYP2C9, multiple variants	reduced conversion to potent active metabolite	↓medication response
Thiazides	*NEDD4L* (rs4149601 G/A)	Decreased sodium reabsorption	↑Response to thiazide with A allele
	PRKCA (rs16960228A)	Increased PRKCA expression	↑Response to thiazide with A allele
	TET2 (rs12505746)	Unknown; aldosterone responsive gene	↑Response to thiazide
	CSMD1, multiple SNPs	Unknown	↑Response to thiazide
	SLCO2A1 (rs34550074)	Reduced prostaglandin E2 uptake	↑Risk of thiazide-induced hyponatremia

[a]BP response not consistent, compared to HR response.

DBP, Diastolic blood pressure; *SBP*, systolic blood pressure; *SNP*, single nucleotide polymorphism.

5. What genetic variants alter the risk of antihypertensive medication side effects?
   Genetic association studies have identified single nucleotide polymorphisms (SNPs) that associate with some adverse drug effects. For instance, a SNP located near the gene *KCNIP4* has been associated with cough due to ACEis.[29] A genetic variant in *SLCO2A1* which reduces the uptake of prostaglandin E2 is associated with increased risk of thiazide-induced hyponatremia.[30] As genetic testing and documentation of side effects improves, more associations are likely to emerge which provide insight into side effect mechanisms. However, to date, there have been no genetic variants of *clinical significance* that are associated with medications side effects, and routine genetic testing is not currently indicated.

6. Are there any genetic variants that should be tested for prior to starting an antihypertensive medication?
   In clinical practice, antihypertensive medications are titrated until blood pressure targets are realized. The magnitude of the blood pressure modulating effects of the genetic variants identified to date are too small either to enhance dose titration or to result in significant harm. Thus, genetic testing is not recommended prior to initiating antihypertensive therapy.

KEY POINTS

1. Drugs may counteract the effectiveness of antihypertensive medications by altering drug metabolism or counteracting the targeted blood pressure-lowering mechanisms.
2. Adverse drug interactions with antihypertensives can be due to overlapping mechanisms of action or exaggerated shared side effect profiles.
3. Common genetic variants which alter the effectiveness or increase the risk of adverse reactions to antihypertensives have been identified.
4. Testing for genetic variants is not recommended before initiating or altering the doses of antihypertensive medications.

REFERENCES

1. Wilkinson GR. Drug metabolism and variability among patients in drug response. *N Engl J Med.* 2005;352:2211–2221.
2. Cordeanu EM, Gaertner S, Faller A, et al. Rifampicin reverses nicardipine effect inducing uncontrolled essential hypertension. *Fundam Clin Pharmacol.* 2017;31:587–589.
3. Tada Y, Tsuda Y, Otsuka T, et al. Case report: nifedipine-rifampicin interaction attenuates the effect on blood pressure in a patient with essential hypertension. *Am J Med Sci.* 1992;303:25–27.
4. Niemi M, Backman JT, Fromm MF, Neuvonen PJ, Kivistö KT. Pharmacokinetic interactions with rifampicin, clinical relevance. *Clin Pharmacokinet.* 2003;42:819–850.
5. Xu Y, Zhou Y, Hayashi M, Shou M, Skiles GL. Simulation of clinical drug-drug interactions from hepatocyte CYP3A4 induction data and its potential utility in trial designs. *Drug Metab Dispos.* 2011;39:1139–1148.
6. Agrawal A, Agarwal SK, Kaleekal T, Gupta YK. Rifampicin and anti-hypertensive drugs in chronic kidney disease: pharmacokinetic interactions and their clinical impact. *Indian J Nephrol.* 2016;26:322–328.
7. Webster J. Interactions of NSAIDs with diuretics and beta-blockers mechanisms and clinical implications. *Drugs.* 1985;30:32–41.
8. Koopmans PP, Kateman WG, Tan Y, van Ginneken CA, Gribnau FW. Effects of indomethacin and sulindac on hydrochlorothiazide kinetics. *Clin Pharmacol Ther.* 1985;37:625–628.
9. Houston MC. Nonsteroidal anti-inflammatory drugs and antihypertensives. *Am J Med.* 1991;90:42S–47S.
10. Parving HH, et al. Cardiorenal end points in a trial of aliskiren for type 2 diabetes. *N Engl J Med.* 2012;367:2204–2213.
11. Zheng SL, Roddick AJ, Ayis S. Effects of aliskiren on mortality, cardiovascular outcomes and adverse events in patients with diabetes and cardiovascular disease or risk: a systematic review and meta-analysis of 13,395 patients. *Diab Vasc Dis Res.* 2017;14:400–406.
12. Petersen V, Hvidt S, Thomsen K, Schou M. Effect of prolonged thiazide treatment on renal lithium clearance. *Br Med J.* 1974;3:143–145.
13. Thomsen K, Schou M. The effect of prolonged administration of hydrochlorothiazide on the renal lithium clearance and the urine flow of ordinary rats and rats with diabetes insipidus. *Pharmakopsychiatr Neuropsychopharmakol.* 1973;6:264–269.
14. Rosner MH. Severe hyponatremia associated with the combined use of thiazide diuretics and selective serotonin reuptake inhibitors. *Am J Med. Sci.* 2004;327:109–111.
15. Jacob S, Spinler SA. Hyponatremia associated with selective serotonin-reuptake inhibitors in older adults. *Ann Pharmacother.* 2006;40:1618–1622.
16. Drug Development and Drug Interactions | Table of Substrates, Inhibitors and Inducers. *FDA* https://www.fda.gov/drugs/drug-interactions-labeling/drug-development-and-drug-interactions-table-substrates-inhibitors-and-inducers (2020).
17. Holtbecker N. Fromm MF, Kroemer HK, Ohnhaus EE, Heidemann H. The nifedipine-rifampin interaction. Evidence for induction of gut wall metabolism. *Drug Metab Dispos.* 1996;24:1121–1123.
18. Metoprolol therapy and CYP2D6 genotype. In: Dean L, Pratt V, eds. *Medical Genetics Summaries.* National Center for Biotechnology Information (US); 2012.
19. Hamadeh IS, et al. Impact of CYP2D6 polymorphisms on clinical efficacy and tolerability of metoprolol tartrate. *Clin Pharmacol Ther.* 2014;96:175–181.

20. Bijl MJ, et al. Genetic variation in the CYP2D6 gene is associated with a lower heart rate and blood pressure in beta-blocker users. *Clin Pharmacol Ther*. 2009;85:45–50.
21. Pacanowski MA, et al. beta-adrenergic receptor gene polymorphisms and beta-blocker treatment outcomes in hypertension. *Clin Pharmacol Ther*. 2008;84:715–721.
22. Sandilands A, Yeo G, Brown MJ, O'Shaughnessy KM. Functional responses of human beta1 adrenoceptors with defined haplotypes for the common 389R > G and 49S > G polymorphisms. *Pharmacogenetics*. 2004;14:343–349.
23. Luo F, et al. A functional variant of NEDD4L is associated with hypertension, antihypertensive response, and orthostatic hypotension. *Hypertension*. 2009;54:796–801.
24. Manunta P, et al. Physiological interaction between alpha-adducin and WNK1-NEDD4L pathways on sodium-related blood pressure regulation. *Hypertension*. 2008;52:366–372.
25. McDonough CW, et al. Association of variants in NEDD4L with blood pressure response and adverse cardiovascular outcomes in hypertensive patients treated with thiazide diuretics. *J Hypertens*. 2013;31:698–704.
26. Hiltunen TP, et al. Pharmacogenomics of hypertension: a genome-wide, placebo-controlled cross-over study, using four classes of antihypertensive drugs. *J Am Heart Assoc*. 2015;4:e001521.
27. Rimpelä JM, et al. Replicated evidence for aminoacylase 3 and nephrin gene variations to predict antihypertensive drug responses. *Pharmacogenomics*. 2017;18:445–458.
28. Eadon MT, Maddatu J, Moe SM, Sinha AD, Melo Ferreira R, Miller BW, Sher SJ, Su J, Pratt VM, Chapman AB, Skaar TS, Moorthi RN. Pharmacogenomics of hypertension in chronic kidney disease: the CKD-PGX study. Kidney360. 2021;doi: 10.34067/kid.0005362021:10.34067/KID.0005362021.
29. Mosley JD, et al. A genome-wide association study identifies variants in KCNIP4 associated with ACE inhibitor-induced cough. *Pharmacogenomics J*. 2016;16:231–237.
30. Ware JS, et al. Phenotypic and pharmacogenetic evaluation of patients with thiazide-induced hyponatremia. *J Clin Invest*. 2017;127:3367–3374.

CHAPTER 40

ROLE OF DEVICE THERAPY

Swapnil Hiremath, MD

QUESTIONS

1. **What do we mean by device therapies in hypertension?**
   Device therapies refers to interventions that are used to reduce blood pressure (BP). These interventions can be surgical, or with interventional angiographic procedures targeting the mechanism of hypertension. The device therapies that have undergone research in this area include
   - Renal denervation
   - Baroreceptor activation or modulation
   - Central arteriovenous fistula (AVF) creation
     A brief summary of the effect of these interventions and their current status is presented in Table 40.1.
     Renal Denervation:
   Catheter based radiofrequency (Simplicity and Spyral catheters, Medtronic Inc, Dublin, Ireland; EnligHTN system, St Jude Medical Inc, St Paul, MN)
   Catheter based ultrasound (Paradise system, ReCor Medical, Palo Alto, CA)
   Catheter based alcohol (Peregrin system, Ablative Solutions, Wakefield, MA)
     Baroreceptor:
   Baroreceptor activation: Bilateral multielectrode system (Rheos) and unilateral (CVRx Inc, Minneapolis, MN)
   Baroreceptor modulation: MobiusHD system (Vascular dynamics Inc, Mountain View, CA)
   Central Arteriovenous Fistula: ROX coupler (ROX Medical, San Clemente, CA)

2. **What is the history of interventions for hypertension?**
   In 1923, Bruning had suggested sympathectomy for control of hypertension as the role of the efferent sympathetic system in maintaining BP had already been discovered then. A few years later, following the observation that sympathectomy, performed for peripheral arterial disease, results in prolonged vasodilation, Adson and Brown performed the section of the nerve roots from D6 to L2 and noted a dramatic decrease in BP from 250/180 to 170/120.[1] Over the next few years, this procedure was used in severe cases of hypertension, but it was quickly noted that the impressive BP drop was accompanied by impressive adverse effects, such as loss of sensation,

Table 40.1 Summary of Device Therapies, Effect on BP, Adverse Effects, and Current Status

INTERVENTION	EFFECT ON BP	POSSIBLE ADVERSE EFFECTS	CURRENT STATUS
Lumbar sympathectomy	~ 70 mm Hg decrease	Paralytic ileus, impotence, loss of sweating, sensation, death	Abandoned
Renal denervation	Initial reports 20–30 mm Hg Sham controlled decrease in ABPM ~ 4/2 mm Hg	Low risk of procedural complications Potential risk of shock with hypovolemia or hemorrhage	Approved in Europe and some other countries Not approved in North America as of 2021
Baroreceptor	~ 16 mm Hg decrease in office BP compared to 9 mm Hg in control group in pivotal RCT	~ 4%–5 % developed facial nerve injury or damage with initial device Dysphagia, paresthesia	Approved in Europe Barostim Neo being pursued for heart failure MobiusHD in pilot trials
Central arteriovenous fistula	~ 13 mm Hg decrease in ABPM	30% risk of procedural complications and venous stenosis (early) Potential late complications include heart failure	Abandoned

ABPM, Ambulatory blood pressure monitoring; *BP*, blood pressure; *RCT*, randomized controlled trial.

paralytic ileus, problems with ejaculation, loss of sweating, and the occasional mortality. Once effective pharmacological therapy became available, this procedure fell into disfavor and was abandoned.

3. **How does renal denervation work?**
Renal denervation was rejuvenated by clinical research that demonstrated the role of afferent nerves from the kidney which increase the efferent sympathetic tone. Using catheter-based radiofrequency ablation, it was found that targeting the nerves in the renal artery resulted in a BP decrease. The BP decrease was initially reported to be in the initial case report, and in the first two clinical trials, which were performed in patients with severe, resistant hypertension.[2,3]

4. **What is the current evaluation of the effect of renal denervation?**
The initial bubbling enthusiasm in renal denervation defervesced after the reporting of the SYMPLICITY HTN-3 trial.[4] This was the first sham controlled randomized clinical trial (RCT), which also used 24-hour ambulatory blood pressure monitoring (ABPM) as the outcome. Though there was a decrease in BP from baseline with renal denervation, this was no different than the change in BP in the control group. Subsequent analysis suggested that the cause of this discrepancy may have been related to the expertise in denervation, and varying adherence. Subsequent trials were designed to overcome these potential flaws by using a multielectrode catheter, or an ultrasound-based denervation procedure. They also enrolled participants with mild hypertension (on no medications) or on less than three medications who underwent direct observed therapy before measurement of ABPM. These subsequent trials have demonstrated a reduction in ABPM of about 4/2 mm Hg compared to sham control.[4–8]

5. **What are the possible advantages of renal denervation over medications?**
The proponents of renal denervation point to a few potential advantages of renal denervation. Firstly, with the procedural effect of BP lowering, the variable effect of adherence, or lack thereof, is eliminated. Secondly, denervation may provide a smoother decrease in BP compared to the peaks and troughs seen with pharmacological BP lowering (Fig. 40.1).

6. **What about long-term efficacy and effect on clinical outcomes?**
The clinical trials reported do not extend beyond 6 months. There is concern that the ablated nerves could possibly regrow, and the BP lowering effect may be attenuated. The Global SYMPLICITY Registry does not report this; however, it is a registry and not a clinical trial. The existing RCTs have not been powered for clinical outcomes. Unfortunately, in the setting of resistant hypertension, the incidence of adverse cardiovascular outcomes is high, however, the variance is also high, so a properly powered RCT will be prohibitively infeasible.

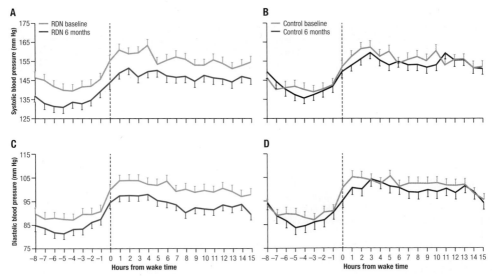

Fig. 40.1 24 Hourly ambulatory systolic blood pressure and diastolic blood pressure at baseline and 6 months, according to patient-recorded individual wake times. *RDN,* Renal denervation. (From Kandzari DE, Böhm M, Mahfoud F, et al. Effect of renal denervation on blood pressure in the presence of antihypertensive drugs: 6-month efficacy and safety results from the SPYRAL HTN-ON MED proof-of-concept randomised trial. *Lancet.* 2018;391(10137):2352)

7. What are the potential safety issues or disadvantages of renal denervation?

In the RCTs, there was a low risk of procedural complications, such as the risks associated with femoral puncture, and rare cases of arterial trauma. There is concern about the long-term effect of renal sympathetic denervation in the setting of hypovolemic shock, when the counterregulatory effect of an activated sympathetic system might be essential. In animal (sheep) studies, renal denervation and subsequent hemorrhage has been demonstrated to result in severe shock. A similar case report in a patient has also been reported in a patient with sepsis. However, these effects are still thought to be uncommon or rare. The risk of adverse outcomes in the global SYMPLICITY registry is low, providing a modicum of reassurance.

8. Why was there a discrepancy between early studies and later?

The initial studies with renal denervation suggested that the effect of this procedure might be as much as a decrease in systolic BP of 20 to 30 mm Hg. This hope was belied, and the final effect seems to be about 4/2 mm Hg. This effect is similar to the effect of a single BP lowering medication.

An elegant analysis explores the various causes for the difference.[9] The initial uncontrolled trial may reflect regression to mean, due to selection of patients with very high BP, which would be expected to be lower at the next measurement, irrespective of any action or intervention. In the controlled trials which were not blinded, observer bias during measurement of BP, and participant bias on change in adherence to BP lowering medications, may cause an inflation in the observed effect. Hence the subsequent trials were performed in a population not taking BP medications, or withholding medication for the trial period, or if on BP medications by confirming adherence the best way you can during the trial. One can see the effect of the major trials in Table 40.2. Note that in SYMPLICITY HTN-3, there was a significant lowering of BP in the sham arm (about 12/5 mm Hg) with no change in medications, which might reflect greater adherence in patients who believed they had the procedure.

9. Who should have renal denervation?

Renal denervation has, at the time of this writing, not yet been approved in North America, though it has been approved and has been in use in Europe and other jurisdictions. Paradoxically, though one might expect that the role of renal denervation would be in patients with resistant hypertension, or even refractory hypertension (i.e., after addition of a mineralocorticoid antagonist as the fourth agent), few trials have reported the efficacy of renal

Table 40.2 Major Sham Controlled Randomized Trials of Renal Denervation

	SYMPLIC-ITY 3	SPYRAL ON PILOT	RADIANCE TRIO	SPYRAL OFF PIVOTAL	RADIANCE SOLO
Denervation method	Simplicity (single electrode) Main renal artery	Simplicity G-3 or SPYRAL (multi-electrode) Main + branch, accessory >3 mm	Paradise system (ultrasound) Main renal artery, 2 spots 5 mm apart	Simplicity G-3 or SPYRAL (multi-electrode) Main + branch, accessory >3 mm	Paradise system (ultrasound) Main renal artery, 2 spots 5 mm apart
Other features	–	Direct observed therapy before ABPM pre/post	On medications; single pill combination of 3 drugs Drug levels measured	Off medications Drug levels measured	Off medications
Follow up measurement	6 months	6 months	2 months	3 months	2 months
Change in 24-hour ABPM in Denervation	−14.1/−6.75	−9.0/−6.0	−8.0/−4.9	−4.7/−3.7	−7.0/−4.4
Change in 24-hour ABPM in Sham	−11.7/−4.8	−1.6/−1.9	−3.0/−2.0	−0.6/−0.8	−3.1/−3.0
Difference in the arms	−2.4/−1.96	−7.4/−4.1	−4.5/−1.8	−3.9/−2.9	−4.1/−1.8

ABPM, Ambulatory blood pressure monitoring.

denervation in this setting. Nevertheless, the case might be made that an additional effect may be obtained in these patients, who are at an otherwise higher risk of adverse outcomes from the consequence of uncontrolled hypertension. In addition, a case has also been made for the use of renal denervation in patients who are not adherent or are intolerant of BP lowering medications.

10. **What is the evidence in baroreceptor stimulation or modulation?**
Baroreceptor activation therapy (BAT, Rheos system, CVRx Inc, Minneapolis, MN) relies on the activation of the myogenic stretch reflex in the carotid body, which would reduce central sympathetic activity and lower BP. The initial system consisted of multiple electrodes placed around both carotid sinuses, connected to a subcutaneous pulse generator, which could be switched on or off. After the initial promising pilot RCT data, the pivotal double blind Rheos RCT did not demonstrate a significant BP lowering with BAT compared to sham.[10] The proportion of responders in the group in whom the device was activated was 54% compared to 46% in the control arm ($P = .97$). The decrease in office systolic BP was 16 ± 29 mm Hg for the active group and 9 ± 29 mm Hg for the control ($P = .08$). More importantly, 25% of participants developed procedural adverse events. Subsequently, a second-generation device (Barostim Neo) has been developed which has a single disc electrode, is inserted unilaterally with a potentially safer safety profile, and is undergoing ongoing trials, though focused on heart failure. Another endovascularly delivered implant device, Mobius HD (Vascular dynamics Inc, Mountain View, CA), which increases wall strain in the carotid sinus, thus more of a baroreceptor modulator than activation, has similarly shown promise in a single arm pilot RCT (lowering of ABPM by ~21 mm Hg) and is undergoing a larger double blind RCT (CALM-2, NCT03179800).

11. **What is the role of a central arteriovenous fistula in controlling hypertension?**
Creation of an AVF adds a low-resistance, high-compliance venous segment to the central arterial tree to potentially exploit the natural mechanical effects and lower BP. A high output AVF in other settings (trauma, and dialysis) has been known to have hemodynamic effects. An RCT of a device (ROX coupler, ROX Medical, San Clemente, CA) which created an iliac AVF reported a decrease in office systolic BP of 27 mm Hg and ABPM of 13 mm Hg.[11] However, more than 50% of participants had procedural complications, and 30% developed venous stenosis requiring intervention during follow-up. In addition, high output heart failure is a known complication of AVF from other settings.[12] Unsurprisingly, further development of this intervention has been wisely abandoned.

12. **What are the other device therapy options that have been tried?**
A few other interventions have been attempted over the years, but robust definitive data are still awaited to show that these reliably decrease BP. These include median nerve stimulation, device guided breathing, and a microvascular decompression surgery for refractory hypertension of possible neurogenic etiology.

KEY POINTS

1. Device therapy in the modern era refers to denervation of renal sympathetic afferent nerves, activation or modulation of the baroreceptors, and central arteriovenous fistula creation. We have most data supporting a blood pressure lowering effect with renal denervation.
2. Despite initial reports of huge blood pressure decrease from uncontrolled and unblinded studies, properly conducted trials demonstrate a more modest 4 to 7 mm Hg decrease with renal denervation, approximately the effect seen with the addition of one blood pressure lowering drug.
3. Design issues such as blinding to avoid varying adherence and measurement bias, sham procedures to enforce blinding, monitoring adherence, and measurement of blood pressure with ambulatory monitoring are essential to provide robust results in device therapy trials.
4. Central arteriovenous fistula may lower blood pressure, but with high complication rates, and should not be pursued at this time.
5. Baroreceptor modulation/activation seems to have interesting physiologic effects, however, data from ongoing trials on safety and efficacy are needed before widespread use.

REFERENCES

1. Adson AW, Brown GE. Malignant hypertension: report of case treated by bilateral section of anterior spinal nerve roots from the sixth thoracic to the second lumbar, inclusive. *JAMA*. 1934;102(14):1115–1118.
2. Esler MD, Krum H, Sobotka PA, et al. Renal sympathetic denervation in patients with treatment-resistant hypertension (The SYMPLICITY HTN-2 Trial): a randomised controlled trial. *Lancet*. 2010;376(9756):1903–1909. https://doi.org/10.1016/S0140-6736(10)62039-9.
3. Schlaich MP, Sobotka PA, Krum H, et al. Renal sympathetic-nerve ablation for uncontrolled hypertension. *N Engl J Med*. 2009;361(9):932–934. https://doi.org/10.1056/NEJMc0904179.

4. Bhatt DL, Kandzari DE, O'Neill WW, et al. A controlled trial of renal denervation for resistant hypertension. *N Engl J Med.* 2014;370(15):1393–1401. https://doi.org/10.1056/NEJMoa1402670.
5. Kandzari DE, Böhm M, Mahfoud F, et al. Effect of renal denervation on blood pressure in the presence of antihypertensive drugs: 6-month efficacy and safety results from the SPYRAL HTN-ON MED proof-of-concept randomised trial. *Lancet.* 2018;391(10137):2346–2355. https://doi.org/10.1016/S0140-6736(18)30951-6.
6. Azizi M, Schmieder RE, Mahfoud F, et al. Endovascular ultrasound renal denervation to treat hypertension (RADIANCE-HTN SOLO): a multicentre, international, single-blind, randomised, sham-controlled trial. *Lancet.* 2018;391(10137):2335–2345. https://doi.org/10.1016/S0140-6736(18)31082-1.
7. Böhm M, Kario K, Kandzari DE, et al. Efficacy of catheter-based renal denervation in the absence of antihypertensive medications (SPYRAL HTN-OFF MED Pivotal): a multicentre, randomised, sham-controlled trial. *Lancet.* 2020;395(10234):1444–1451. https://doi.org/10.1016/S0140-6736(20)30554-7.
8. Azizi M, Sanghvi K, Saxena M, et al. Ultrasound renal denervation for hypertension resistant to a triple medication pill (RADIANCE-HTN TRIO): a randomised, multicentre, single-blind, sham-controlled trial [Published online May 16, 2021]. *Lancet.* 2021;397(10293):2476–2486. https://doi.org/10.1016/S0140-6736(21)00788-1.
9. Howard JP, Shun-Shin MJ, Hartley A, et al. Quantifying the 3 biases that lead to unintentional overestimation of the blood pressure-lowering effect of renal denervation. *Circ Cardiovasc Qual Outcomes.* 2016;9(1):14–22. https://doi.org/10.1161/CIRCOUTCOMES.115.002533.
10. Bisognano JD, Bakris G, Nadim MK, et al. Baroreflex activation therapy lowers blood pressure in patients with resistant hypertension: results from the double-blind, randomized, placebo-controlled Rheos pivotal trial. *J Am Coll Cardiol.* 2011;58(7):765–773. https://doi.org/10.1016/j.jacc.2011.06.008.
11. Lobo MD, Ott C, Sobotka PA, et al. Central iliac arteriovenous anastomosis for uncontrolled hypertension: one-year results from the ROX CONTROL HTN trial. *Hypertension.* 2017;70(6):1099–1105.
12. MacRae JM, Dipchand C, Oliver M, et al. Arteriovenous access: infection, neuropathy, and other complications. *Can J Kidney Health Dis.* January 2016;. https://doi.org/10.1177/2054358116669127.

CHAPTER 41

ORTHOSTATIC HYPOTENSION

Maureen C. Farrell, MS, and Cyndya A. Shibao, MD MSCI

QUESTIONS

1. **What physiologic responses prevent blood pressure from decreasing acutely when we stand?**
   After assuming the upright position, gravitational forces shift ~700 mL of blood volume to the lower part of the body, mostly in the splanchnic vascular circulation. This fluid shift is detected by the baroreceptors in the carotid sinus and aortic arch This information is transmitted through the glossopharyngeal and vagus nerves to the nucleus tractus solitarii (NTS) in the medulla oblongata. These neurochemical stimuli trigger changes within the hypothalamus that upregulate sympathetic activity and downregulate parasympathetic activity of the heart. Subsequently, the heart rate (HR) increases and the vasculature in the peripheral and splanchnic beds constrict to maintain the cardiac output and prevent a decrease in blood pressure. In addition to the autonomic response, the renin-angiotensin-aldosterone system (RAAS) becomes activated, generating angiotensin II as a potent vasoconstrictor. The RAAS response time is delayed compared to sympathetic nervous system activation.

2. **What is orthostatic hypotension?**
   Orthostatic hypotension (OH) describes a sustained reduction in systolic blood pressure of at least 20 mm Hg or diastolic blood pressure of 10 mm Hg within 3 minutes of standing or head-up tilt to at least 60 degrees on a tilt table.[1] Such drops in blood pressure often cause dizziness, blurry or tunnel vision, fatigue, dull neck and shoulder pain, and increased fall risk. Symptoms improve when seated or in recumbent position. Importantly, OH is associated with reduced functional capacity and mortality in elderly patients (Fig. 41.1).[2]

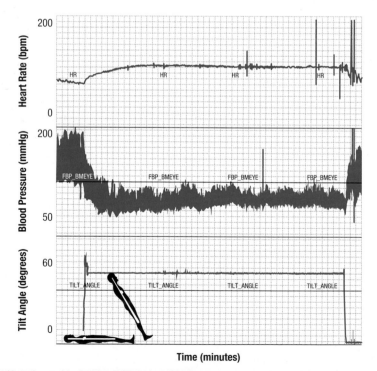

Fig. 41.1 Tilt table testing consists of continuous heart rate and blood pressure measurements during 60-degree tilt on an adjustable table. In patients with autonomic failure, blood pressure does not respond to increases in heart rate during tilt. Orthostatic symptoms result.

3. How should blood pressure be measured to diagnose OH?

The most sensitive and precise measurements should be obtained during fasting conditions, early in the morning. Blood pressure and HR measurements should be taken after the patient has been lying supine for at least 5 minutes and twice more after standing at 1 and 3 minutes. If time precludes the acquisition of orthostatic vital signs, blood pressure and HR can be measured in the seated position and after standing.[3] However, these measurements have low sensitivity to detect OH. Concomitant HR changes on standing provide additional information on the cardiovascular autonomic reflexes. Elevations in HR below 10 bpm during OH episodes should raise high suspicion for an autonomic neuropathy, and autonomic testing may be warranted.

4. Describe the most common causes of OH.

The most common cause of OH is polypharmacy. Medications, including alpha-1 blockers such as terazosin, prazosin, and tamsulosin, can predispose the patient to developing OH. In addition, tricyclic antidepressants, overuse of diuretics, and tizanidine (muscle relaxant) can also induce OH.[4] Transient conditions such as dehydration (poor oral intake, vomiting, diarrhea, or blood loss) may also cause OH and are often accompanied by significant orthostatic tachycardia. Less common causes of OH include primary autonomic neuropathies such as pure autonomic failure, multiple system atrophy (MSA), and Parkinson disease.[5] Secondary causes of autonomic neuropathies are diabetes mellitus, amyloidosis and autoimmune autonomic failure, and paraneoplastic syndromes.

5. How should a differential diagnosis be established for orthostatic hypotension in a hypertensive patient?

Although the definition of OH indicates a drop in systolic blood pressure of >20 mm Hg, for hypertensive patients, reduction of >30 mm Hg is required to be considered OH.[1] In hypertensive patients, the differential diagnosis includes the following etiologies:

- **Neurogenic orthostatic hypotension with supine hypertension (HTN):** patients with this condition have significant OH with a decrease in blood pressure of 60 to 70 mm Hg and evidence of autonomic neuropathy with abnormal autonomic function. About 50% of these patients develop supine HTN defined as a sustained nocturnal systolic blood pressure above 150 mm Hg.[6] Consider ambulatory blood pressure monitoring to detect supine HTN at night.
- **Baroreflex failure:** Suspect baroreflex failure in patients with a history of head or neck radiation, which may have occurred over 10 years prior to the development of OH.[7] You must also inquire about past surgical history, especially for neck surgery for carotid tumor excision or stenting for significant carotid artery atherosclerosis as they are iatrogenic causes of OH. Hypertensive episodes can be triggered by pain, stress, or other stimuli including exposure to light or cold. They resolve with sympatholytic agents such as oral clonidine at bedtime or as needed. Long-acting antihypertensive agents are not recommended in patients with baroreflex failure as they worsen OH.[8]
- **Pheochromocytoma:** these patients present with episodes of HTN and diaphoresis alternating with episodes of OH due to volume contraction caused by pressure natriuresis.[9] The suggested screening and initial evaluation in patients with suspected pheochromocytoma is detailed in Chapter 10 Pheochromocytoma, typically starting with fractionated metanephrines in either the plasma or the urine. The evaluation of patients with positive confirmatory testing should include an adrenal computed tomography scan with and without contrast to localize the adrenal pheochromocytoma. In certain cases, positron emission tomography (PET) imaging is required to localize extraadrenal tumors.
- **Other causes:** alpha-2 agonist medications such as tizanidine or clonidine can cause rebound HTN and OH when taking supratherapeutic doses Chapter 38.[4] Plasma catecholamines are markedly elevated during the withdrawal period, but suppressed if measured during drug administration.

6. Which patients are most likely to develop neurogenic OH?

Neurogenic OH is most common in adults over 75 years old and is responsible for 233 hospitalizations out of every 100,000 annually.[10] Several physiological changes occur with aging that predispose older patients to develop OH:

- the baroreceptors become less sensitive in detecting blood pressure fluctuations.
- alpha-1 mediated vasoconstriction response is diminished.
- the kidney has reduced capacity to concentrate urine.
- the aging heart becomes stiff and less compliant to accommodate large blood volumes and increased cardiac output.

In addition to advanced age, movement disorders like Parkinson disease are associated with the development of OH due to autonomic failure.

7. What are the best clinical assessments for accurately diagnosing neurogenic OH?

Orthostatic vital signs should be performed in all patient with suspicious of autonomic neuropathy. Autonomic function testing can be used to diagnose neurogenic OH (nOH); these tests are usually performed in specialized clinical centers. However, the ratio of increase in HR to decrease in systolic blood pressure ($\Delta HR/\Delta BP$) provides a validated clinical tool to identify patients with OH secondary to structural lesions within the baroreflex arch.[11] These values can be measured at the bedside either by measuring supine, seated, and upright vital signs or by continuous monitoring during a Valsalva maneuver. Baroreflex gain, the change in HR in response to changes in blood pressure, less than 0.49 bpm/mm Hg suggests autonomic neuropathy. Patients with diagnosed autonomic neuropathy should undergo clinical evaluation with blood testing for serum B12 levels, hemoglobin A1C, serum protein electrophoresis (SPEP), urine protein electrophoresis (UPEP), and a paraneoplastic antibody panel to rule out secondary causes of nOH. In cases that raise suspicion for pheochromocytoma, consider checking plasma and urine metanephrine levels as well as imaging studies to identify and localize the tumor.

8. **What are the characteristic clinical findings in patients with neurogenic OH?**
Patients with nOH commonly complain of fainting spells, dizziness, weakness, blurred vision, and pain in the shoulder blade. These symptoms worsen on standing and improve after sitting down or resting in the supine position. They are also worse in the mornings because these patients develop significant nocturia and lose volume overnight. This effect is most pronounced in nOH patients with supine HTN.[12,13] Furthermore, patients with nOH have concomitant postprandial hypotension, which causes significant lightheadedness and weakness immediately after eating. This effect is amplified after large, carbohydrate-rich meals.

9. **What are the physical examination findings commonly observed in patients with neurogenic OH?**
The prominent physical finding is the presence of OH associated with presyncopal symptoms on standing challenge. A subset of patients may experience localized hyperhidrosis in certain areas of the body to compensate for anhidrosis which could be secondary to sympathetic postganglionic denervation. Other physical findings depend on the underlying etiology. For example, in patients with nOH who present with a slow, shuffling gait, bradykinesia, cogwheel rigidity, and hypophonia, Parkinson disease or MSA should be considered in the differential diagnosis. In cases of nOH concomitant with dementia and visual hallucinations, Lewy body dementia should be considered.

10. **Describe the most commonly used therapeutic agents to treat OH.**
Treatment goals for nOH are aimed at symptomatic and functional improvement with reduction of syncopal symptoms and falls rather than aggressive blood pressure control. Clinical improvement can be achieved after careful review of medications and incorporation of nonpharmacological measures (Table 41.1). Pharmacological interventions are recommended when nonpharmacological measures fail. In reviewing medications, look for agents that may exacerbate nOH including diuretics, tricyclic antidepressants, tizanidine (a hidden sympatholytic), and alpha blockers, which are commonly used in the treatment of benign prostatic hyperplasia. Nonpharmacological measures include drinking 16 oz of water, which increases blood pressure by ~30 mm Hg in patients with nOH within 30 minutes. A mild pressor response of ~11 mm Hg is expected in elderly patients, but not detectable in young adults. Postural physiological countermeasures include gradual postural changes, squatting or contracting leg muscles, and crossing legs while standing to prevent venous pooling. Abdominal binders or biker shorts prevent pooling in the splanchnic circulation and may be a more comfortable option for some patients.

   If presyncopal symptoms persist despite use of nonpharmacological measures, then the addition of pharmacological interventions may be appropriate (see Table 41.1). In patients with mild nOH and severe HTN, the first line agent is pyridostigmine. The recommended starting dose is 30 mg three times a day (t.i.d.), which could be titrated up to 60 mg t.i.d. Pyridostigmine enhances neurotransmission at autonomic ganglia, increasing blood pressure while standing but not while lying supine. Though the blood pressure effects are mild, some patients report long-lasting benefits.[14] If a patient has supine HTN, one of the medications that must be stopped is fludrocortisone. Midodrine should be administered 30 minutes prior to standing activity as needed to improve orthostatic symptoms. It should not be administered prior to sleep due to the risk of worsening supine HTN.

   The most recent agent approved for the treatment of nOH is droxidopa, a norepinephrine precursor. This medication is effective in patients with severe nOH, particularly those with amyloidosis.[15] In patients with supine HTN, we recommend dosing twice a day (b.i.d.) instead of the recommended t.i.d. schedule. The initial recommended dose is 100 mg b.i.d., which can be titrated up to a therapeutic dose with the greatest effects occurring between 300 and 400 mg b.i.d. Importantly, the treatment plan must be individualized based on the patient's comorbid conditions.

11. **What additional factors must be considered for hospitalized patients?**
Hospitalized patients with OH represent a unique subset of OH patients because they are often bedbound lying supine. Bedrest limits the use of pressor agents as they can exacerbate supine HTN. If used, administration of pressor agents should be coordinated with the initiation of inpatient physical therapy to appropriately assess the effect of the drug on OH-related symptoms. Pressor agents given at fixed intervals should be avoided. It is recommended that patients remain seated or in a recliner during the day to avoid supine HTN that can occur while lying flat.

Table 41.1 Nonpharmacological Strategies and Pharmacological Agents Used in the Treatment of Neurogenic Orthostatic Hypotension and Postprandial Hypotension

NONPHARMACOLOGIC STRATEGIES		
NONPHARMACOLOGIC STRATEGY	EXAMPLE	EFFECT
Careful review of medications	1. Diuretics 2. Tricyclic antidepressants 3. Tizanidine (a hidden sympatholytic) 4. Alpha-1 blockers for benign prostatic hyperplasia	1. Diuresis reduces volume status 2. Anticholinergic and alpha-1 blockade 3. Alpha-2 agonist decreases sympathetic tone 4. Vasodilation leads to OH
Nonpharmacological measures	Drink 16 oz water	Volume expansion increases blood pressure within 30 minutes
Gradual postural physiological countermeasures include	Gradual postural changes, squatting or contracting leg muscles, and crossing legs while standing	Prevents venous pooling
Compression garments	Abdominal binders or biker shorts	Prevents venous pooling in splanchnic circulation
PHARMACOLOGIC AGENTS		
MEDICATION	MECHANISM OF ACTION	DOSING
Pyridostigmine	Peripheral acting acetylcholinesterase inhibitor, which enhances ganglionic transmission and SNS activity	30–60 mg t.i.d.
Midodrine[a]	Alpha-1 adrenergic agonist that acts as direct vasoconstrictor	2.5–10 mg t.i.d.
Droxidopa[b]	Norepinephrine precursor, which increases norepinephrine levels	100–600 mg t.i.d. *only b.i.d. in supine HTN*

[a]FDA-approved for the treatment of orthostatic hypotension (OH)
[b]FDA-approved for the treatment of neurogenic orthostatic hypotension
b.i.d., Twice daily; *FDA,* Food and Drug Administration; *HTN,* hypertension; SNS, sympathetic nervous system; *t.i.d.,* three times per day.

12. **How is OH managed in a patient with severe hypertension?**
    Patients with OH and supine HTN are counseled to avoid lying supine, elevate their beds by 6 to 9 inches during sleep, or to sleep in a recumbent chair. If necessary, short-acting antihypertensive agents can be prescribed to prevent HTN during sleep. The use of the antihypertensive therapy should be addressed based on the patient's co-morbid conditions and severity of the HTN. Uncontrolled HTN can lead to pressure diuresis, which can exacerbate OH. Furthermore, long-standing uncontrolled HTN has been associated with the development of left ventricular hypertrophy and increased creatinine levels.[16] Low dose angiotensin converting enzyme-inhibitors and angiotensin receptor blockers are recommended with careful titration and monitoring of orthostatic blood pressure. We prefer to initiate therapy with Losartan 25 to 50 mg at bedtime, based on a previous study that showed a blood pressure lowering effect in patients with supine HTN secondary to reduced pressure natriuresis.[17]

13. **What are the best pharmacological agents used to treat supine hypertension in the setting of autonomic failure?**
    Losartan, eplerenone, nitroglycerin transdermal patch, nifedipine, clonidine, and nebivolol can be used to treat supine HTN in patients with autonomic failure (Table 41.2).

KEY POINTS

1. Orthostatic hypotension increases the risk of falls, syncope, and hospitalizations especially in the elderly.
2. Treatment of orthostatic hypotension aims to provide symptomatic relief rather than strict blood pressure control and consists of nonpharmacological measures supplemented with pharmacological interventions in severe cases.
3. Supine hypertension may occur in patients with orthostatic hypotension and should be treated to prevent long-term complications (including left ventricular hypertrophy and renal failure) and reduce symptom burden.

Table 41.2 Pharmacological Agents Used in the Treatment of Supine Hypertension in Autonomic Failure

MEDICATION	MECHANISM OF ACTION	DOSING
Losartan	AT1 receptor blocker, which targets the elevated angiotensin II levels in autonomic failure	50 mg bedtime
Eplerenone	Selective mineralocorticoid antagonist, which targets inappropriate MR receptor activation in autonomic failure	50 mg bedtime
Nitroglycerin transdermal patch	Nitric oxide donor, vasodilator	0.1-0.2 mg/h applied at bedtime, remove in the morning
Nifedipine	Short-acting calcium channel blocker, which causes vasodilation. Recommended in patients with refractory supine HTN	10-30 mg bedtime
Clonidine	Central sympatholytic agent, which reduces residual sympathetic activity. Drug of choice in MSA patients with supine HTN	0.1 mg evening
Nebivolol	Third generation beta blocker with vasodilatory properties. Potentiates nitric oxide function	2.5-5 mg bedtime

HTN, Hypertension; *MR,* mineralocorticoid receptor; *MSA,* multiple system atrophy.

REFERENCES

1. Gibbons CH, Schmidt P, Biaggioni I, et al. The recommendations of a consensus panel for the screening, diagnosis, and treatment of neurogenic orthostatic hypotension and associated supine hypertension. *J Neurol.* 2017;264(8):1567–1582.
2. Luukinen H, Koski K, Laippala P, Kivela SL. Prognosis of diastolic and systolic orthostatic hypotension in older persons. *Arch Intern Med.* 1999;159(3):273–280.
3. Shaw BH, Garland EM, Black BK, et al. Optimal diagnostic thresholds for diagnosis of orthostatic hypotension with a 'sit-to-stand test'. *J Hypertens.* 2017;35(5):1019–1025.
4. Farrell MC, Biaggioni I, Shibao CA. Neurogenic orthostatic hypotension induced by tizanidine. *Clin Auton Res.* 2019;30(2):173–175.
5. McDonell KE, Shibao CA, Claassen DO. Clinical relevance of orthostatic hypotension in neurodegenerative disease. *Curr Neurol Neurosci Rep.* 2015;15(12):78.
6. Okamoto LE, Gamboa A, Shibao C, et al. Nocturnal blood pressure dipping in the hypertension of autonomic failure. *Hypertension.* 2009;53(2):363–369.
7. Sharabi Y, Dendi R, Holmes C, Goldstein DS. Baroreflex failure as a late sequela of neck irradiation. *Hypertension.* 2003;42(1):110–116.
8. Biaggioni I, Shibao CA, Diedrich A, Muldowney JAS, Laffer CL, Jordan J. Blood pressure management in afferent baroreflex failure: JACC review topic of the week. *J Am Coll Cardiol.* 2019;74(23):2939–2947.
9. Lenders JW, Eisenhofer G, Mannelli M, Pacak K. Phaeochromocytoma. *Lancet.* 2005;366(9486):665–675.
10. Shibao C, Grijalva CG, Raj SR, Biaggioni I, Griffin MR. Orthostatic hypotension-related hospitalizations in the United States. *Am J Med.* 2007;120(11):975–980.
11. Norcliffe-Kaufmann L, Palma JA, Kaufmann H. A validated test for neurogenic orthostatic hypotension at the bedside. *Ann Neurol.* 2018;84(6):959–960.
12. Goldstein DS, Pechnik S, Holmes C, Eldadah B, Sharabi Y. Association between supine hypertension and orthostatic hypotension in autonomic failure. *Hypertension.* 2003;42(2):136–142.
13. Gangavati A, Hajjar I, Quach L, et al. Hypertension, orthostatic hypotension, and the risk of falls in a community-dwelling elderly population: the maintenance of balance, independent living, intellect, and zest in the elderly of Boston study. *J Am Geriatr Soc.* 2011;59(3):383–389.
14. Singer W, Sandroni P, Opfer-Gehrking TL, et al. Pyridostigmine treatment trial in neurogenic orthostatic hypotension. *Arch Neurol.* 2006;63(4):513–518.
15. McDonell KE, Preheim BA, Diedrich A, et al. Initiation of droxidopa during hospital admission for management of refractory neurogenic orthostatic hypotension in severely ill patients. *J Clin Hypertens (Greenwich).* 2019;21(9):1308–1314.
16. Messerli FH, Williams B, Ritz E. Essential hypertension. *Lancet.* 2007;370(9587):591–603.
17. Arnold AC, Okamoto LE, Gamboa A, Angiotensin II. et al. independent of plasma renin activity, contributes to the hypertension of autonomic failure. *Hypertension.* 2013;61(3):701–706.

CHAPTER 42

BAROREFLEX DYSFUNCTION

Matthew Lloyd, PhD, and Satish R. Raj, MD MSCI

QUESTIONS

1. **What is the baroreflex?**
   The baroreflex is a critical mechanism in the homeostatic regulation of blood pressure. Blood pressure is monitored continually by receptors located in the carotid arteries, aorta, lungs, coronary arteries, and the splanchnic vasculature of the gut,[1,2] termed "baroreceptors." These receptors consist of mechanosensory neurons that form macroscopic "claws" that circumnavigate large arteries, and are activated when increased blood pressure causes the arterial lumen to expand, stretching the arterial wall. In response, baroreceptor neuron firing rate increases (Fig. 42.1).[3] The baroreceptors have classically been separated into "high-pressure" and "low-pressure" receptors based on their relative responses to varying levels of blood pressure. The carotid and aortic baroreceptors are considered "high-pressure" receptors, and are thought to be the primary controllers of heart rate and vascular resistance.[4] The "low-pressure" cardiopulmonary receptors sense changes in central blood volume and blood pressure.

2. **How does the baroreflex respond to increased blood pressure?**
   A rise in blood pressure stretches the arterial wall, resulting in an increase in baroreceptor action potentials. Baroreceptor afferent neurons travel via the glossopharyngeal and vagal nerves to synapse in the nucleus tractus solitarius in the medulla.[5,6] From here, excitatory interneurons activate preganglionic parasympathetic neurons in the dorsal motor nucleus of the vagus, and the nucleus ambiguous. Activation of these neurons results in acetylcholine release at the sinoatrial node in the heart, reducing heart rate.[5,6]
   The nucleus tractus solitarius also projects to inhibitory interneurons in the caudal ventrolateral medulla. These interneurons inhibit tonically active preganglionic sympathetic neurons in the rostral ventrolateral medulla, and reduce the firing rate of sympathetic neurons.[5,7] As both the heart and peripheral vasculature receive

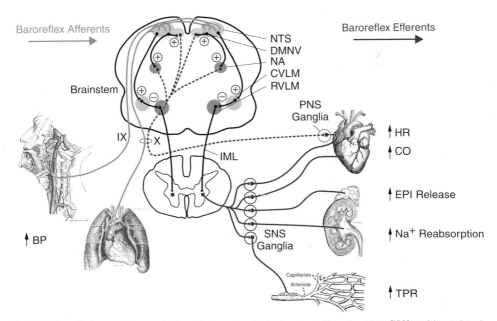

Fig. 42.1 Schematic diagram of the neurocircuitry of the baroreflex. *BP*, Blood pressure; *CO*, cardiac output; *CVLM*, caudal ventrolateral medulla; *DMNV*, dorsal motor nucleus of the vagus; *EPI*, epinephrine; *HR*, heart rate; *IML*, intermediolateral nucleus; *IX*, glossopharyngeal nerve; *NA*, nucleus ambiguus; *NTS*, nucleus tractus solitarius; *PNS*, parasympathetic nervous system; *RVLM*, rostral ventrolateral medulla; *SNS*, sympathetic nervous system; *TPR*, total peripheral resistance; *X*, vagus nerve.

sympathetic innervation, reduced sympathetic activity reduces the heart rate and contractility, as well as systemic vascular resistance.

In summary, a rise in blood pressure is modulated by the baroreflex via two mechanisms: (1) reduced heart rate and cardiac output, due to reduced sympathetic outflow, and increased parasympathetic outflow; and (2) reduced systemic vascular resistance due to reduced sympathetic outflow only.

3. How does the baroreflex respond to decreased blood pressure?

Baroreceptors are tonically active, and a *reduction* in blood pressure results in reduced baroreceptor firing rate.[5] This results in increased sympathetic outflow, resulting in increased systemic vascular resistance, heart rate, and contractility. Parasympathetic outflow through the vagus nerve is reduced, causing an increase in heart rate.

In summary, during a *decrease* in blood pressure (such as during an active stand), tonic baroreceptor firing rate decreases, and blood pressure is maintained via (1) increased total peripheral resistance, and (2) increased heart rate and cardiac output.

4. What role does the baroreflex play in the long-term control of blood pressure?

Although the baroreflex has traditionally been thought of as a short-term regulator of blood pressure, it plays a central role in the long-term regulation of blood pressure as well.[8] The baroreflex-mediated response during hypotensive periods acts to increase renal sympathetic nerve activity, resulting in increased sodium reabsorption by the kidney via the renin-angiotensin-aldosterone system.[9] This results in fluid retention, increased blood volume and blood pressure.[10] Conversely, the baroreflex acts to reduce blood volume during periods of hypertension, and therefore acts as a central reflex in the long-term regulation of blood pressure.

5. How is baroreflex function assessed?

There are a number of autonomic function tests that examine the cardiac and vascular responses to baroreflex stimulation. Baroreflex function is typically expressed as baroreflex sensitivity (BRS), and relates the baroreflex response to a given change in blood pressure. Cardiac baroreflex sensitivity is expressed as the change in cardiac R-R interval (in ms) per mm Hg change in blood pressure.

Vascular or sympathetic baroreflex sensitivity is commonly expressed as the percent change in sympathetic nerve firing per mm Hg blood pressure change, or the change in vascular resistance per mm Hg blood pressure change. Disorders that act to reduce baroreflex function result in reduced BRS.

The Oxford method was the first autonomic test to assess baroreflex function.[11] Developed in 1969, it involved the use of vasoactive drugs to alter blood pressure. Phenylephrine, an alpha agonist, is administered intravenously to raise blood pressure via increased total peripheral resistance. The modified Oxford method also uses sodium nitroprusside to induce vasodilation (via breakdown to nitric oxide) and a reduction in blood pressure.[12] The resulting baroreflex-mediated change in heart rate could then be assessed, and full cardiac baroreflex sigmoid curves could be constructed (Fig. 42.2). The slope of the steepest portion of the curve is used to calculate BRS. Due to the invasive and time-consuming nature of the test, plus the inability to assess the vascular arm of the baroreflex, the Oxford method is no longer used as a first-line autonomic test.

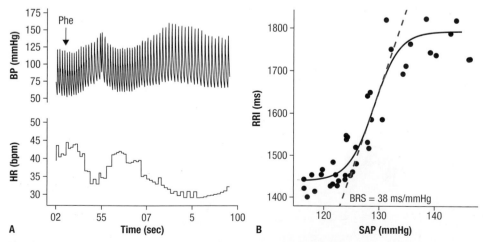

Fig. 42.2 Representative response from one healthy participant during assessment of baroreflex sensitivity with the Oxford Method. (A) Following infusion of phenylephrine (Phe), blood pressure rises rapidly. This elicits a baroreflex-mediated reduction in heart rate. (B) The maximum slope (indicated by the *dashed red line*) of the sigmoid baroreflex curve is used to calculate baroreflex sensitivity. *BP,* Blood pressure; *BRS,* baroreflex sensitivity; *HR,* heart rate; *Phe,* phenylephrine; *RRI,* R-R interval; *SAP,* systolic arterial pressure.

Other assessments of baroreflex function involve measuring the baroreflex response to altered blood pressure via orthostasis (head-up tilt,[13] lower body negative pressure,[14] active stand), direct stimulation of the carotid baroreceptors (via neck suction devices[15]), assessment of physiologic oscillations in blood pressure (cross-spectral analysis,[16] alpha index,[17] sequence analysis[18]), or forced exhalation into a tube (Valsalva maneuver). These autonomic tests require beat-to-beat blood pressure monitoring and specialized equipment (e.g., tilt table), and are therefore usually limited to autonomic clinics and laboratories.

6. What is the Valsalva maneuver?

Currently, the mainstay of autonomic function tests is the Valsalva maneuver, due to its short duration, limited required equipment, and the wealth of information it provides regarding baroreflex function (Fig. 42.3).[19] In short, the patient exhales forcefully into a tube to 40 mm Hg for 15 seconds, causing reductions in venous return, cardiac output, and blood pressure, due to occlusion of the vena cavae and pulmonary veins. The reduction in blood pressure should elicit a baroreflex-mediated increase in heart rate and systemic vascular resistance. The Valsalva maneuver therefore allows for assessment of both the cardiac and vascular arms of the baroreflex.[19] Baroreflex dysfunction can be observed when patients display reduced cardiac or vascular responses during (or immediately following) the maneuver.[20]

The Valsalva maneuver is divided into four distinct phases. Phase I of the maneuver involves an initial rise in intrathoracic pressure upon initiation of the forced expiration, which corresponds with a transient increase in blood pressure. As intrathoracic pressure rises, the pulmonary veins and venae cavae are occluded, and venous return drops, causing a fall in blood pressure during phase IIa. This reduction in blood pressure elicits a baroreflex-mediated increase in heart rate, as well as a burst of muscle sympathetic nerve activity (MSNA).[21] Due to the rise in heart rate and vasoconstriction, blood pressure rises during phase IIb. Upon release of the forced expiratory pressure, blood pressure falls transiently during phase III before venous return is rapidly restored as the vena cava are decompressed. In phase IV, a blood pressure overshoot is commonly seen due to the rapid recovery of venous return (see Fig. 42.3).[19]

Cardiac baroreflex function is commonly expressed as the Valsalva ratio, or the maximum heart rate observed in phase II (or just after) divided by the minimum heart rate in phase IV (see Fig. 42.3). Cardiac baroreflex sensitivity can also be derived from the blood pressure changes in phase IIa,[22] and phase IV,[23] and their corresponding baroreflex-mediated changes in heart rate.

Sympathetic vascular baroreflex function is commonly expressed using pressure recovery time (PRT),[20] which is the time it takes systolic blood pressure to recover following release of the Valsalva maneuver. Patients who are unable to vasoconstrict during phase IIb exhibit a longer PRT.[20] Two additional indices of vascular baroreflex function have also been developed. Alpha adrenergic baroreflex sensitivity (BRSa) is calculated as the reduction in systolic pressure during phase III (from baseline) divided by PRT.[20]

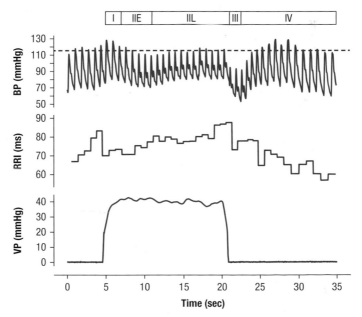

Fig. 42.3 Representative response from one healthy participant performing a Valsalva Maneuver. Note the systolic blood pressure in phase 4 overshoots baseline systolic pressure *(horizontal dashed line)*. *BP,* Blood pressure; *RRI,* R-R interval; *VP,* Valsalva pressure.

7. **What role does the baroreflex play in hypertension?**
The baroreflex has classically been considered as a short-term regulator of blood pressure, primarily because of baroreflex "resetting."[24] During acute elevations in blood pressure (e.g., exercise, nociception, emotional stimuli), the baroreflex regulates blood pressure at higher pressures, rather than counteracting the elevated blood pressure. This resetting was thought to also result in the baroreflex regulating blood pressure at a higher "set point" during hypertension, and would therefore not play a central role in the pathophysiology of hypertension.[8]

Several studies in the early 2000s demonstrated that baroreflex resetting is incomplete in some experimental models of hypertension, and the baroreflex is activated to reduce renal sympathetic nerve activity, resulting in reduced sodium reabsorption and reduced blood volume.[8] The baroreflex therefore appears to act chronically to reduce blood pressure in hypertension. Clearly, the ongoing presence of hypertension indicates that normal physiological baroreflex activation is insufficient to return blood pressure to normotensive levels. However, artificial baroreflex activation has been the focus of recently developed medical devices that stimulate carotid baroreflex afferents.[25]

Our understanding of the role of the baroreflex in hypertension is incomplete. Although the baroreflex is a central regulator of sympathetic outflow, there is still debate regarding the relative contribution of the sympathetic nervous system versus renal-centric mechanisms in essential hypertension.[26] Cardiac baroreflex sensitivity is reduced in chronic hypertension, although the underlying mechanisms are poorly understood.[27] Several mechanisms that contribute to the development of hypertension such as age, obesity, and sex, also impact baroreflex function.

8. **How does baroreflex function change with age?**
Cardiac BRS decreases with age.[15,28,29] Baroreflex-mediated heart rate responses are therefore larger in younger individuals versus older individuals.[30] The underlying mechanisms are poorly understood, but reduced sinoatrial node responsiveness to acetylcholine may contribute to declining cardiac BRS with age.[29] Age-related arterial stiffening has also been proposed to reduce baroreceptor stimulation during alterations in blood pressure.[31]

9. **How does baroreflex function change with obesity?**
Baroreflex sensitivity is reduced in patients with obesity.[32] The precise mechanism is not known, but may relate to high sympathetic activity and increased vascular stiffness that are observed in obese patients.[33] Given the well-established interaction between aging, obesity, and the risk of hypertension, both obesity- and age-related reductions in baroreflex sensitivity have important implications for the development and/or maintenance of hypertension.

10. **Is the role of the baroreflex in hypertension different between men and women?**
Resting sympathetic nerve activity, as measured with microneurography (direct nerve recordings), does not correlate with resting blood pressure in young men or women.[34] This absent relationship, particularly considering the high interindividual variability in resting sympathetic activity, had previously suggested that the sympathetic nervous system is less important in the long-term regulation of blood pressure. However, in the last 10 years our understanding of the physiology underlying the poor relationship between sympathetic nerve activity and blood pressure has improved.

In men, a reciprocal relationship between sympathetic outflow and cardiac output counteracts the increased vascular tone that results from higher levels of sympathetic outflow. Resting mean arterial pressure is therefore not different between young men with different resting sympathetic nervous activity.

Young women display no significant relationship between resting sympathetic tone and vascular resistance, likely due to estrogen-mediated increases in beta-2-adrenergic vasodilatory activity.[35] Resting sympathetic tone also does not appear to affect cardiac output. Sympathetic tone therefore does not correlate with mean arterial pressure in women.

It is well established that sympathetic nervous system activity increases in both men and women with age.[36,37] This increased sympathetic activity, with concomitant reductions in parasympathetic activity, has been termed "autonomic dysfunction," but is distinct from baroreflex dysfunction and autonomic failure that is discussed later.

In men, the reciprocal relationship between cardiac output and sympathetic outflow degrades with age, and resting sympathetic tone correlates robustly with blood pressure later in life. In women, the postmenopausal reduction in estrogen removes the beta-adrenergic vasodilatory response to sympathetic nerve activation, and blood pressure becomes more tightly coupled with sympathetic nerve activity. Therefore, sympathetic nerve activity increases with aging, becomes a greater contributing factor for the development of hypertension in later life.

11. **What is baroreflex dysfunction?**
Baroreflex dysfunction occurs with injury to any part of the baroreflex neural pathway: baroreceptors, afferent nerves, their brainstem connections, preganglionic efferent nerves, or postganglionic efferent nerves.[38] The clinical manifestation of the dysfunction depends on which aspect of the neural arc is affected. Disorders affecting the afferent limb of the baroreflex present differently from those affecting the efferent arm (Table 42.1). The lesion can be localized with clinical autonomic testing, and a detailed medical history.

Table 42.1 Afferent vs. Efferent Baroreflex Failure

	AFFERENT BAROREFLEX FAILURE	EFFERENT BAROREFLEX FAILURE
Common Term	Baroreflex failure	Autonomic failure
Defining Clinical Feature	Extremely labile blood pressure	Orthostatic hypotension
Supine Hypertension	Somewhat common	Extremely common
Most Common Causes	Radiation therapy or surgery to the head and neck	Diabetic neuropathy, Parkinson disease
Postprandial Hypotension	Somewhat common	Extremely common
Episodic Tachycardia	Extremely common	Rare
Hypertension with Tachycardia	Extremely common	Rare
Blood Pressure Fluctuations Initiated by Visual/Auditory Stimuli	Extremely common	Rare

12. What is efferent baroreflex dysfunction (a.k.a. autonomic failure)?
Disorders affecting baroreflex efferent nerves primarily reduce a patient's ability to vasoconstrict. The defining clinical manifestation of this is orthostatic hypotension, which is defined as a sustained reduction in blood pressure of 20/10 mm Hg within 3 minutes of assuming an upright posture.[39] This is often accompanied by symptoms of presyncope (e.g., lightheadedness, dimming vision, nausea) and syncope. The magnitude of orthostatic hypotension is similar in patients with preganglionic (e.g., multiple system atrophy) and postganglionic (e.g., pure autonomic failure, diabetes, amyloidosis) lesions. Efferent baroreflex dysfunction is most commonly caused by diabetic peripheral neuropathy. Neurodegenerative disorders such as Parkinson disease, dementia with Lewy bodies, and multiple system atrophy may also result in orthostatic hypotension via reduced vasoconstriction.[40] Efferent baroreflex dysfunction is covered in more detail in Chapter 41, Orthostatic Hypotension.

13. What is afferent baroreflex dysfunction?
Etiology
Afferent baroreflex failure is caused by damage to the baroreceptors, glossopharyngeal, and/or vagal nerves. Baroreceptor information is therefore not conducted to the nucleus tractus solitarius, and results in unrestrained sympathetic outflow, volatile blood pressure fluctuations, severe hypertensive crises, intermittent severe hypotension, and orthostatic hypotension.[41]

Afferent baroreflex failure is most commonly a late sequela of carotid sinus nerve damage during radiation therapy,[41,42] and may occur years after treatment. Neck surgery, as with carotid endarterectomy, carotid angioplasty, or bilateral resection of neck tumors (e.g., carotid paragangliomas), may cause acute afferent baroreflex failure. In carotid endarterectomy, baroreflex impairment is transient.[43] Patients with Guillain-Barre syndrome, an autoimmune disorder precipitated by an infectious disease, may also develop baroreflex afferent lesions that cause blood pressure instability.[44,45]

Congenital afferent baroreflex failure occurs in patients with Riley-Day syndrome (also known as familial dysautonomia or hereditary sensory and autonomic neuropathy III [HSAN III]), an autosomal recessive neuropathy caused by a point mutation in the IKBKAP gene on chromosome 9.[46] This mutation disrupts peripheral nervous system development, but the precise mechanism is unknown.

Presentation
The baroreflex acts as a buffer to changes in blood pressure; the loss of baroreflex function results in large, unopposed swings in blood pressure (up and down). This extreme lability of blood pressure is the hallmark of afferent baroreflex failure, with hypertensive episodes occurring in nearly all patients. The severity of fluctuations in blood pressure is related to the extent of damage to the afferent nerves, which can vary greatly. These fluctuations can be initiated by environmental stimuli such as bright lights or loud noises (hypertension), or physical relaxation and eating (hypotension).[47] The severity of the fluctuation is also influenced by the intensity of the stimulus.

Hypertensive episodes can be caused by mental stress, environmental stimuli, or physical exertion.[48] Without baroreflex modulation, activation of the sympathetic nervous system is unchecked, causing hypertension with tachycardia.[38,48] These hypertensive crises are extreme, and can cause pressures to rise above 240/110 mm Hg.[48] The administration of a cold pressor test (submerging the hand into ice water for 60–90 seconds) can provoke an exaggerated pressor response that is unique to afferent, but not efferent, baroreflex dysfunction.[41]

Management

Afferent baroreflex failure is one of the most challenging hypertensive or autonomic disorders to manage. To appropriately manage their expectations, patients should be informed that complete normalization of blood pressure is likely impossible, but blood pressure may be regulated well enough to improve their quality of life. Patients should be coached to reduce stimulations that may incite a hypertensive episode, for example by using earplugs or sunglasses.

Long-acting central sympatholytic drugs (e.g., methyldopa, guanfacine, clonidine patch) are the mainstay of treatment for afferent baroreflex failure in order to control labile hypertension and paroxysmal hypertensive crises. Oral clonidine can be used acutely during a hypertensive episode. Hypotensive episodes can be managed first with oral water bolus, abdominal binders, physical stimulation, and midodrine if needed.[41]

KEY POINTS

1. The baroreflex buffers changes in arterial blood pressure by altering total peripheral resistance (purely sympathetically mediated) and cardiac output (sympathetically and parasympathetically mediated).
2. The Valsalva maneuver is the mainstay of autonomic tests, and allows for evaluation of both the cardiac and vascular baroreflex responses to a change in blood pressure.
3. The baroreflex plays a central role in the long-term regulation of blood pressure.
4. The relationship between baroreflex function and hypertension is unknown, but recent evidence, as well as current baroreflex-modulation therapies, indicate a significant role for the baroreflex in the development of hypertension.
5. Baroreflex dysfunction occurs with injury to any part of the baroreflex neural pathway: baroreceptors, afferent nerves, their brainstem connections, preganglionic efferent nerves, or postganglionic efferent nerves.
6. Afferent baroreflex dysfunction results in extremely labile blood pressure, with periods of extreme hypertension *and* hypotension.
7. Afferent baroreflex failure is one of the most challenging hypertensive or autonomic disorders to manage, and treatment should focus on management of patients' expectations, reduction of stimuli (auditory, visual) that induce hypertensive crises, and pharmacological management of hypertension with long-acting sympatholytics.

REFERENCES

1. Doe CP, Drinkhill MJ, Myers DS, Self DA, Hainsworth R. Reflex vascular responses to abdominal venous distension in the anesthetized dog. *Am J Physiol.* 1996;271(3 Pt 2):H1049–H1056.
2. Cui J, Gao Z, Blaha C, Herr MD, Mast J, Sinoway LI. Distension of central great vein decreases sympathetic outflow in humans. *Am J Physiol - Hear Circ Physiol.* 2013;305(3):378–385. doi: 10.1152/ajpheart.00019.2013.
3. Armstrong M, Moore RA. *Physiology, Baroreceptors.* StatPearls Publishing; 2020. http://www.ncbi.nlm.nih.gov/pubmed/30844199.
4. Wieling W, de Lange FJ, Jardine DL. The heart cannot pump blood that it does not receive. *Front Physiol.* 2014;5:360. doi: 10.3389/fphys.2014.00360.
5. Zanutto BS, Valentinuzzi ME, Segura ET. Neural set point for the control of arterial pressure: role of the nucleus tractus solitarius. *Biomed Eng Online.* 2010;9:4. doi: 10.1186/1475-925X-9-4.
6. Kimmerly DS. A review of human neuroimaging investigations involved with central autonomic regulation of baroreflex-mediated cardiovascular control. *Auton Neurosci Basic Clin.* 2017;207(March):10–21. doi: 10.1016/j.autneu.2017.05.008.
7. Guyenet PG, Stornetta RL, Holloway BB, Souza GMPR, Abbott SBG. Rostral ventrolateral medulla and hypertension. *Hypertension.* 2018;72(3):559–566. doi: 10.1161/HYPERTENSIONAHA.118.10921.
8. Lohmeier TE, Iliescu R. The baroreflex as a long-term controller of arterial pressure. *Physiology.* 2015;30(2)doi: 10.1152/physiol.00035.2014.
9. Miller AJ, Arnold AC. The renin–angiotensin system in cardiovascular autonomic control: recent developments and clinical implications. *Clin Auton Res.* 2019;29(2):231–243. doi: 10.1007/s10286-018-0572-5.
10. Thames MD, Ballon BJ. Occlusive summation of carotid and aortic baroreflexes in control of renal nerve activity. *Am J Physiol - Hear Circ Physiol.* 1984;15(6):851–857. doi: 10.1152/ajpheart.1984.246.6.h851.
11. Smyth HS, Sleight P, Pickering GW. Reflex regulation of arterial pressure during sleep in man. A quantitative method of assessing baroreflex sensitivity. *Circ Res.* 1969;24(1):109–121.
12. Rudas L, Crossman AA, Morillo CA, et al. Human sympathetic and vagal baroreflex responses to sequential nitroprusside and phenylephrine. *Am J Physiol.* 1999;276(5 Pt 2):H1691–H1698.
13. Protheroe CL, Ravensbergen HRJC, Inskip JA, Claydon V. Tilt testing with combined lower body negative pressure: a "gold standard" for measuring orthostatic tolerance. *J Vis Exp.* 2013;(73):e4315. doi: 10.3791/4315.
14. Goswami N, Blaber AP, Hinghofer-Szalkay H, Convertino VA. Lower body negative pressure: physiological effects, applications, and implementation. *Physiol Rev.* 2019;99(1):807–851. doi: 10.1152/physrev.00006.2018.
15. Cooper V, Hainsworth R. Carotid baroreflex testing using the neck collar device. *Clin Auton Res Off J Clin Auton Res Soc.* 2009;19(2):102–112. doi: 10.1007/s10286-009-0518-z.
16. Robbe HW, Mulder LJ, Ruddel H, Langewitz WA, Veldman JB, Mulder G. Assessment of baroreceptor reflex sensitivity by means of spectral analysis techniques. 1987;10(5):538-543.
17. Pagani M, Somers V, Furlan R, et al. Changes in autonomic regulation induced by physical training in mild hypertension. *Hypertension.* 1988;12(6):600–610.

18. Blaber AP, Yamamoto Y, Hughson RL. Methodology of spontaneous baroreflex relationship assessed by surrogate data analysis. *Am J Physiol*. 1995;268(18):H1682–H1687.
19. Goldstein DS, Cheshire WP. Beat-to-beat blood pressure and heart rate responses to the Valsalva maneuver. *Clin Auton Res*. 2017;27(6):361–367. doi: 10.1007/s10286-017-0474-y.
20. Vogel ER, Sandroni P, Low PA. Blood pressure recovery from Valsalva maneuver in patients with autonomic failure. *Neurology*. 2005;65(10):1533–1537. doi: 10.1212/01.wnl.0000184504.13173.ef.
21. Schrezenmaier C, Singer W, Swift NM, Sletten D, Tanabe J, Low PA. Adrenergic and vagal baroreflex sensitivity in autonomic failure. *Arch Neurol*. 2007;64(3):381–386. doi: 10.1001/archneur.64.3.381.
22. Goldstein D, Horwitz D, Keiser H. Comparison of techniques for measuring baroreflex sensitivity in man. *Circulation*. 1982;66(2): 432–439.
23. Palmero HA, Caeiro TF, Iosa DJ, Bas J. Baroreceptor reflex sensitivity index derived from phase 4 of the Valsalva maneuver. *Hypertension*. 1981;3(6 Pt 2):134–137. doi: 10.1161/01.HYP.3.6.
24. Fadel PJ, Raven PB. Human investigations into the arterial and cardiopulmonary baroreflexes during exercise. *Exp Physiol*. 2012;97(1):39–50. doi: 10.1113/expphysiol.2011.057554.
25. Bolignano D, Coppolino G. Baroreflex stimulation for treating resistant hypertension: ready for the prime-time?. *Rev Cardiovasc Med*. 2018;19(3):89–95. doi: 10.31083/j.rcm.2018.03.3185.
26. Navar LG. Counterpoint: activation of the intrarenal renin-angiotensin system is the dominant contributor to systemic hypertension. *J Appl Physiol*. 2010;109(6):1998–2000. doi: 10.1152/japplphysiol.00182.2010a. discussion 2015.
27. Mussalo H, Vanninen E, Ikäheimo R, et al. Baroreflex sensitivity in essential and secondary hypertension. *Clin Auton Res*. 2002;12(6):465–471. doi: 10.1007/s10286-002-0069-z.
28. Huang CC, Sletten DM, Weigand SD, Low PA. Effect of age on adrenergic and vagal baroreflex sensitivity in normal subjects. *Muscle and Nerve*. 2007;36(5):637–642. doi: 10.1002/mus.20853.
29. Monahan KD. Effect of aging on baroreflex function in humans. *Am J Physiol*. 2007;293:3–12. doi: 10.1152/ajpregu.00031.2007.
30. Frey MA, Tomaselli CM, Hoffler WG. Cardiovascular responses to postural changes: differences with age for women and men. *J Clin Pharmacol*. 1994;34(5):394–402. doi: 10.1002/j.1552-4604.1994.tb04979.x.
31. Monahan KD, Dinenno FA, Seals DR, Clevenger CM, Desouza CA, Tanaka H. Age-associated changes in cardiovagal baroreflex sensitivity are related to central arterial compliance. *Am J Physiol Heart Circ Physiol*. 2001;281:H284–H289. doi: 10.1161/01.hyp.26.1.48.
32. Skrapari I, Tentolouris N, Katsilambros N. Baroreflex function: determinants in healthy subjects and disturbances in diabetes, obesity and metabolic syndrome. *Curr Diabetes Rev*. 2006;2(3):329–338.
33. Peterson HR, Rothschild M, Weinberg CR, Fell RD, McLeish KR, Pfiefer MA. Body fat and the activity of the autonomic nervous system. *N Engl J Med*. 1988;318(17):1077–1083. doi: 10.1056/NEJM198603273141302.
34. Joyner MJ, Limberg JK. Blood pressure: return of the sympathetics?. *Curr Hypertens Rep*. 2016;18(1):1–6. doi: 10.1007/s11906-015-0616-3.
35. Briant LJB, Charkoudian N, Hart EC. Sympathetic regulation of blood pressure in normotension and hypertension: when sex matters. *Exp Physiol*. 2016;101(2):219–229. doi: 10.1113/EP085368.
36. Sundlöf G, Wallin BG. Human muscle nerve sympathetic activity at rest. Relationship to blood pressure and age. *J Physiol*. 1978;274:621–637. doi: 10.1113/jphysiol.1978.sp012170.
37. Narkiewicz K, Phillips BG, Kato M, Hering D, Bieniaszewski L, Somers VK. Gender-selective interaction between aging, blood pressure, and sympathetic nerve activity. *Hypertension*. 2005;45(4):522–525. doi: 10.1161/01.HYP.0000160318.46725.46.
38. Ketch T, Biaggioni I, Robertson RM, Robertson D. Four faces of baroreflex failure: hypertensive crisis, volatile hypertension, orthostatic tachycardia, and malignant vagotonia. *Circulation*. 2002;105(21):2518–2523. doi: 10.1161/01.CIR.0000017186.52382.F4.
39. Freeman R, Wieling W, Axelrod FB, et al. Consensus statement on the definition of orthostatic hypotension, neurally mediated syncope and the postural tachycardia syndrome. *Clin Auton Res*. 2011;21(2):69–72. doi: 10.1007/s10286-011-0119-5.
40. Freeman R, Abuzinadah AR, Gibbons C, Jones P, Miglis MG, Sinn DI. Orthostatic hypotension: JACC state-of-the-art review. *J Am Coll Cardiol*. 2018;72(11):1294–1309. doi: 10.1016/j.jacc.2018.05.079.
41. Biaggioni I, Shibao CA, Diedrich A, Muldowney JAS, Laffer CL, Jordan J. Blood pressure management in afferent baroreflex failure: JACC review topic of the week. *J Am Coll Cardiol*. 2019;74(23):2939–2947. doi: 10.1016/j.jacc.2019.10.027.
42. Sharabi Y, Dendi R, Holmes C, Goldstein DS. Baroreflex failure as a late sequela of neck irradiation. *Hypertension*. 2003;42(1):110–116. doi: 10.1161/01.HYP.0000077441.45309.08.
43. Hirschl M, Kundi M, Blazek G. Five-year follow-up of patients after thromboendarterectomy of the internal carotid artery. *Stroke*. 1996;27(7):1167–1172. doi: 10.1161/01.STR.27.7.1167.
44. Willison HJ, Jacobs BC, van Doorn PA. Guillain-Barré syndrome. *Lancet*. 2016;388(10045):717–727. doi: 10.1016/S0140-6736(16)00339-1.
45. Van Den Berg B, Walgaard C, Drenthen J, Fokke C, Jacobs BC, Van Doorn PA. Guillain-Barré syndrome: pathogenesis, diagnosis, treatment and prognosis. *Nat Rev Neurol*. 2014;10(8):469–482. doi: 10.1038/nrneurol.2014.121.
46. Norcliffe-Kaufmann L, Slaugenhaupt SA, Kaufmann H. Familial dysautonomia: history, genotype, phenotype and translational research. *Prog Neurobiol*. 2017;152:131–148. doi: 10.1016/j.pneurobio.2016.06.003.
47. Kaufmann H, Kaufmann LN, Palma JA. Baroreflex dysfunction. *N Engl J Med*. 2020;:163–178. doi: 10.1056/NEJMra1509723.
48. Norcliffe-Kaufmann L, Palma JA, Kaufmann H. Mother-induced hypertension in familial dysautonomia. *Clin Auton Res*. 2016;26(1):79–81. doi: 10.1007/s10286-015-0323-9.

CHAPTER 43

HYPERTENSION – ORIGINS

Garabed Eknoyan, MD

QUESTIONS

1. **When did hypertension enter medical nosography as a disease?**

   It all started in antiquity with the recognition of the pulse as a sign of life, death, and disease. The Mesopotamian epic of Gilgamesh (c. 2600 BCE) records the lament of its protagonist, Gilgamesh, at the death of his best friend, Enkidu, "I touch his heart but it does not beat at all." How he touched the heart is not stated. That the pulse was synchronous wherever felt on the body and coincided with the heartbeat is recorded in ancient Egyptian medical texts of about 1500 BCE. Variations in the frequency and force of the pulse in the course of diseases was studied and refined in ancient Chinese medicine, where the diagnosis and site of disease was made by palpation of the pulse. Whereas examination of the pulse (*sphygmós*) was used and recorded in Greek medicine, its physiologic study was hampered by the concept of the circulation promulgated by Galen (130–210) that blood is made in the liver, from whence it flows to and fro in the vasculature, and that "vital spirits" are added to it in its course through the heart, an erroneous view that prevailed for fifteen centuries until the discovery of the circulation in 1628 by William Harvey (1578–1657). Harvey showed that blood circulates and that ventricular systole provides the force that drives it through the arteries and causes their pulsation. It is from these foundations that the force of the blood pressure which had been assessed from the pulse came to be identified as a clinical condition that deserved better scrutiny in the 18th century.

   That an arterial pulse that is hard to compress is an omen of poor health has been recognized since antiquity. Its association with shortened life and lesions of the brain, heart, and the kidneys began to be studied in the 19th century, after the report that a hard pulse was associated with ventricular hypertrophy in patients with kidney disease by Richard Bright (1789–1858) in 1836. However, it was only with measurement of the blood pressure by sphygmography (writing of the pulse, from the Greek for pulse, *sphygmós* and from Latin for writing, *graphia*) that quantification rather than mere qualitative description of the arterial pulse began to be studied in the 20th century. The epidemiologic data that accrued thereafter documented the clinical relevance of elevated blood pressure and identified hypertension as a disease rather than a mere sign of disease.

2. **How did the measurement of blood pressure evolve?**

   The actual measurement of arterial blood pressure can be traced to an English clergyman, the Reverend Stephen Hales (1677–1761) who, in 1733, reported on the "force of the blood" from the height of a blood column connected to the femoral artery of horses and dogs. It would be another century before the French physicist Jean Poiseuille (1797–1869) introduced a mercury manometer for the measurement of the force of the blood in 1828, thereby reducing the awkwardness of the height of the column (9 feet) used to measure the arterial pressure directly. Shortly thereafter, in 1847, the German physiologist Carl Ludwig (1816–95) added a float to the mercury manometer connected to an arm which inscribed the pressure on a rotating drum (*kymograph*), thereby providing a permanent record of studies on pulse pressure, rate, and rhythm.

   The clinical determination of blood pressure had to wait for the development of noninvasive methods of measurement. Several attempts at doing that with a mercury manometer applied to the radial artery were tried. The turning point came in 1896 when the Italian pediatrician Scipione Riva-Rocci (1863–1937) developed a clinically useful sphygmomanometer (*sphygmós* from Greek for pulse; *manométre* from French for measuring instrument) which connected a mercury manometer to a wrap-around inflatable cuff applied around the upper arm and inflated to occlude the pulse palpated in the radial artery. That allowed for the estimation of systolic pressure. The accuracy of the procedure was increased in 1901 when the width of the inflatable cuff was increased from 5 to 13 centimeters by the German physician Heinrich von Recklinghausen (1867–1942).

   The next breakthrough in the clinical assessment of blood pressure was introduced in 1905 by a Russian surgeon from St. Petersburg, Nikolai Korotkov (1874–1920) who described the sounds heard through a stethoscope over the brachial artery below the inflatable cuff during its deflation. He reported the auscultated sounds from their initial tapping to their disappearance in a one-page article. For all the fame that Korotkov achieved, he had no interest in hypertension. His quest was that of a surgeon in evaluating the blood supply to the extremities of patients with vascular disease before surgery. Another surgeon who actually popularized the clinical measurement of blood pressure using the stethoscope was the American neurosurgeon Harvey Cushing (1869–1939), who visited Riva-Rocci in Turin in 1901 and on his return introduced the procedure in the United States. The clinical utility of the procedure was then promoted by the physiologist Walter Cannon (1871–1945) who went on to use it in his studies of shock. By 1912, the regular measurement of the blood pressure of patients admitted to the Massachusetts General Hospital was required and soon became an established routine in clinical practice.

It was this marriage of the stethoscope to the sphygmomanometer adopted in clinical practice early in the 20th century that generated the data base that would lead to the identification of hypertension as a disease. The 1925 report of the Actuarial Society of America was the first landmark report on the detrimental effects of elevated blood pressure on survival based on data derived from office blood pressure recordings. It made a transformative statement which convinced the medical profession of the ill effects of hypertension that had been long suggested from its tactile description as hard pulse pressure.

3. **How were the effects of hypertension on organs recognized?**
A hard-wiry radial pulse had long been associated with concerns of poor health. But it was the association of albuminuria, dropsy, and kidney disease in 1827 by Richard Bright that would open the door to its investigation. Actually, it was Bright's subsequent report in 1836 of the association of ventricular hypertrophy with the fullness of a hard pulse in patients with kidney disease which launched the studies that would eventuate in identifying the systemic effects of hypertension as a disease rather than merely a sign of disease.

Most of the studies that followed were based on pathological observations of the vasculature in general, and that of the kidney in particular. A contemporary of Bright, the London physician George Johnson (1818–96) was the first to argue that it was the increased resistance of the narrowed vasculature which necessitated an increase in blood pressure to overcome their resistance. Stated otherwise, a rise in blood pressure was essential to maintain blood supply to organs. This concept was strengthened by the studies of two other London physicians, William Gull (1816–90) and his junior colleague Henry Sutton (1837–91), who, in 1872, described "arterio-capillary fibrosis" and "hyaline-fibrinoid" changes in arterioles throughout the body of patients with ventricular hypertrophy, with and without kidney disease. They proposed that these generalized vascular changes accounted for the renal disease and cardiac hypertrophy.

A primary role of high arterial pressure causing vascular sclerosis and ventricular hypertrophy had been proposed in 1856 by a founder of experimental pathology in Germany, Ludwig Taube (1818–76). Actually, a fibrous hardening and medial muscular hypertrophy of the arteries had been reported earlier by the French pathologist Jean Lobstein (1777–1835) as "arteriosclerosis" in 1833, but they were not linked to blood pressure or kidney disease until then.

The first clinical evidence of these pathological observations was presented by Frederick Mahomed (1849–84) working at Guy's Hospital in London who, in 1874, started using a modified Poiseuille manometer to measure the blood pressure of his patients. In 1879, Mahomed reported what he termed the "pre-albuminuric stage of Bright's disease," wherein the blood pressure was elevated in the absence of evident kidney disease. He went on to propose that high blood pressure itself, in the absence of Bright's disease, could give rise to the vascular lesions described by Gull and Sutton.

The clinical findings of Mahomed were supported by the Cambridge professor of medicine T. Clifford Allbutt (1836–1925) who, in a series of reports, argued that renal disease was not necessary for the presence of elevated blood pressure, which in 1896 he termed "*hyperpiesis*" as a manifestation of the primary malady he dubbed "*hyperpiesia*," rather than one merely secondary to kidney disease. Based on detailed studies of cases of severe hypertension (up to 250/140 mm Hg) the first professor of medicine at Johns Hopkins, Theodor Janeway (1872–1917), proposed in 1904 naming the disease "hypertensive cardiovascular disease," specifically to differentiate it from that associated with Bright's disease. Actually, the term hypertension had been introduced in 1889 by the French cardiologist Henri Huchard (1814–1910) in his report that elevated blood pressure can occur independent of nephritis. It was revived in 1911 as essential hypertension ("*essentielle Hypertonie*") by the German physician from Wiesbaden Emil Frank, and came to prevail over those proposed by Allbutt and Janeway. Although characterizing hypertension as "essential" gained clinical acceptance, it has been and continues to be questioned by basic scientists who prefer its definition as "primary" or "idiopathic."

Subsequently, the German clinician Fanz Volhard (1872–1950), in cooperation with his pathology associate Theodor Fahr (1877–1945), went on to differentiate essential hypertension into the so-called red or benign (*guttartig*) hypertension from that of white or malignant (*bösartig*) hypertension. The classification of hypertension with particular emphasis on the retinal changes in differentiating benign from malignant hypertension was reported from the Mayo Clinic by Norman Keith (1885–1976) in 1927. The following meticulous clinical studies of hypertensive subjects by George Pickering (1904–80) from Oxford University ultimately established hypertension as a quantitative disease of graded severity that appeared to be related to the level of blood pressure.

4. **How did the treatment of hypertension evolve?**
The data available early in the 20th century on the detrimental effects of hypertension was derived from cases of severe or malignant hypertension (> 180/110 mm Hg). As a result, the treatment of hypertension continued to be debated and even recommended not to be lowered. As late as 1937, the eminent cardiologist Paul Dudley White (1886–1973) declared that "hypertension may be an important compensatory mechanism which should not be tampered with, even if we were certain that we could control it." The effectiveness and wisdom of treating hypertension would continue to be questioned well into the 1950s. The classic example of this conundrum is

that of President Franklin Roosevelt (1882–1945) who succumbed to a massive intracranial hemorrhage due to malignant hypertension that had been treated with rest, massage, and sedatives.

In the absence of effective antihypertensive drugs, surgical procedures such as bilateral thoraco-lumbar sympathectomy and nephrectomy of unilateral atrophic kidneys came into vogue in the 1940s. Both approaches proved to be only temporally effective, definitely ineffective in the long run, and were abandoned by the 1960s as new antihypertensives became available.

The antihypertensive properties of most drugs introduced then were discovered accidentally. Sulfanilamide, introduced as an antimicrobial, was found to have diuretic properties that led to the synthesis of chlorothiazide (*Diuril*) in 1958. Methyldopa, developed for the treatment of carcinoid syndrome, was introduced as an antihypertensive (*Aldomet*) in 1960. Clonidine, developed for the treatment of allergic rhinitis, caused drowsiness due to hypotension and was approved as an antihypertensive (*Catapres*) in 1966. The beta-blocker propranolol (*Inderal*), introduced for the treatment of angina, was found to lower blood pressure and was approved as an antihypertensive in 1964. Similarly, the calcium channel blocker nifedipine (*Adalat*), introduced for the treatment of angina, was approved for the treatment of hypertension in 1969.

The availability of potentially effective antihypertensives corresponded to that of the entry of randomized clinical trials in medicine in 1952, and the study of antihypertensives proved to be one of the first beneficiaries of these early ventures into evidence-based medicine in the 1960s. The first multicenter double-blind randomized trial designed for the treatment of hypertension was the Veterans Administration Cooperative Study on Antihypertensive Agents begun in 1964 at the initiative of Edward Fries (1912–2005). This placebo-controlled study used the three antihypertensive drugs available then, the vasodilator hydralazine, the adrenergic suppressor reserpine, and the diuretic chlorothiazide. The results showed a major salutary effect on severe hypertension and a favorable outcome of those with milder hypertension.

The series of landmark studies that followed clearly established the efficacy of antihypertensive drug therapy. The increasing recognition of hypertension as a common and serious public health problem that is potentially preventable led to the establishment of the National High Blood Pressure Education Program in 1972, a forerunner of programs that followed under the auspices of the National Heart Lung and Blood Institute (NHLBI). Notable amongst those was the establishment of the Joint National Committee (JNC) on Detection and Treatment of High Blood Pressure which published the first set of guidelines for the treatment of hypertension in 1977. Since then, the definition of hypertension and the target level for its treatment have been a downward moving target, with lower targets recommended for diabetics and those with kidney disease.

KEY POINTS

1. Blood pressure was assessed from the hardness of the pulse until 1896 when the sphygmomanometer was introduced.
2. Hypertension as a disease, rather than a sign of disease, was established in the late 1920s from epidemiologic data collected by insurance companies.
3. The treatment of hypertension was questioned until the 1950s. The first randomized clinical trial to establish the effectiveness of hypertension treatment was published in 1967.
4. The antihypertensive effects of drugs introduced initially were accidentally discovered. The first drugs specifically developed for treatment of hypertension were the angiotensin-converting enzyme inhibitors introduced in the 1980s.

BIBLIOGRAPHY

Bedford DE. The ancient art of feeling the pulse. *Br Heart J.* 1951;13:423–436.
Cameron JS. Villain and victim: the kidney and high blood pressure in the 19th century. *J R Coll Physicians London.* 1999;33:382–394.
Eknoyan G. On the contribution of studies on kidney in the recognition, conceptual evolution, and understanding of hypertension. *Adv Chronic Kid Dis.* 2004;11:192–196.
Folkow B. Physiological aspects of primary hypertension. *Physiol Rev.* 1982;62:347–504.
Ruskin A. *Classics in Arterial Hypertension.* Springfield IL: Charles C. Thomas; 1956.
Wakerlin GE. From Bright toward light: the story of hypertension research. *Circulation.* 1962;26:1–6.

INDEX

Note: Page numbers followed by '*f*' indicate figures those followed by '*t*' indicate tables and '*b*' indicate boxes.